AOSpine Masters Series

Primary Spinal Tumors

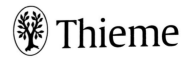

AOSpine Masters Series

Primary Spinal Tumors

Series Editor:
Luiz Roberto Vialle, MD, PhD
Professor of Orthopedics, School of Medicine
Catholic University of Parana State
Spine Unit
Curitiba, Brazil

Guest Editors:
Ziya L. Gokaslan, MD, FACS
Donlin M. Long Professor
Professor of Neurosurgery, Oncology, and Orthopaedic Surgery
Director, Neurosurgical Spine Program
Vice Chair, Department of Neurosurgery
Johns Hopkins University School of Medicine
Baltimore, Maryland

Charles G. Fisher, MD, MHSc, FRCSC
Professor and Head
Division of Spine Surgery
Department of Orthopaedic Surgery
University of British Columbia
Vancouver, British Columbia

Stefano Boriani, MD
Unit of Oncologic and Degenerative Spine Surgery
Rizzoli Orthopedic Institute
Bologna, Italy

With 86 figures

Thieme
New York • Stuttgart • Delhi • Rio

Thieme Medical Publishers, Inc.
333 Seventh Ave.
New York, NY 10001

Executive Editor: Kay Conerly
Managing Editor: Judith Tomat
Editorial Assistant: Haley Paskalides
Senior Vice President, Editorial and Electronic Product Development: Cornelia Schulze
Production Editor: Barbara A. Chernow
International Production Director: Andreas Schabert
International Marketing Director: Fiona Henderson
Director of Sales, North America: Mike Roseman
International Sales Director: Louisa Turrell
Vice President, Finance and Accounts: Sarah Vanderbilt
President: Brian D. Scanlan
Compositor: Carol Pierson, Chernow Editorial Services, Inc.

Library of Congress data is available from the publisher.

Important note: Medicine is an ever-changing science undergoing continual development. Research and clinical experience are continually expanding our knowledge, in particular our knowledge of proper treatment and drug therapy. Insofar as this book mentions any dosage or application, readers may rest assured that the authors, editors, and publishers have made every effort to ensure that such references are in accordance with **the state of knowledge at the time of production of the book.**

Nevertheless, this does not involve, imply, or express any guarantee or responsibility on the part of the publishers in respect to any dosage instructions and forms of applications stated in the book. **Every user is requested to examine carefully** the manufacturers' leaflets accompanying each drug and to check, if necessary in consultation with a physician or specialist, whether the dosage schedules mentioned therein or the contraindications stated by the manufacturers differ from the statements made in the present book. Such examination is particularly important with drugs that are eitherrarely used or have been newly released on the market. Every dosage schedule or every form of application used is entirely at the user's own risk and responsibility. The authors and publishers request every user to report to the publishers any discrepancies or inaccuracies noticed. If errors in thiswork are found after publication, errata will be posted at www.thieme.com on the product description page.

Some of the product names, patents, and registered designs referred to in this book are in fact registered trademarks or proprietary names even though specific reference to this fact is not always made in the text. Therefore, the appearance of a name without designation as proprietary is not to be construed as a representation by the publisher that it is in the public domain.

Printed in China by Everbest Printing Ltd.
5 4 3 2 1
ISBN 978-1-62623-047-7

Also available as an e-book:
eISBN 978-1-62623-049-1

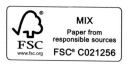

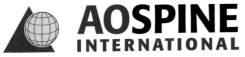

AOSpine Masters Series

Luiz Roberto Vialle, MD, PhD
Series Editor

Contents

Series Preface

Spine care is advancing at a rapid pace. The challenge for today's spine care professional is to quickly synthesize the best available evidence and expert opinion in the management of spine pathologies. The AOSpine Masters Series provides just that—each volume in the series delivers pathology-focused expert opinion on procedures, diagnosis, clinical wisdom, and pitfalls, and highlights today's top research papers.

To bring the value of its masters level educational courses and academic congresses to a wider audience, AOSpine has assembled internationally recognized spine pathology leaders to develop volumes in this Masters Series as a vehicle for sharing their experiences and expertise and providing links to the literature. Each volume focuses on a current compelling and sometimes controversial topic in spine care.

The unique and efficient format of the Masters Series volumes quickly focuses the attention of the reader on the core information critical to understanding the topic, while encouraging the reader to look further into the recommended literature.

Through this approach, AOSpine is advancing spine care worldwide.

Luiz Roberto Vialle, MD, PhD

Guest Editors' Preface

To practice evidence-based spine surgery a spine surgeon must combine a rigorous and critical approach to the evaluation of scientific literature with clinical expertise, and a strong commitment to patient centeredness and humanistic values. In no other domain of spine surgery are these principles more critical and relied upon then in the management of primary tumors of the spine, where a poor management decision can render a potentially curable patient, incurable. The goal of this guide is to balance critical appraisal of current evidence in spine oncology with opinion from experienced experts, to create a distinctive and meaningful clinical reference for the practicing spine oncology surgeon.

The chapters have been researched and written by key opinion leaders in spine oncology and range from general evaluation, staging and decision making principles to histology specific oncologic patient management. The 3 senior editors have reviewed each chapter to try and ensure consistency and the necessary synthesis of best available literature and expert opinion. Furthermore a conscious and very necessary effort to ensure multidisciplinary appraisal and input has been taken. In fact the input of the medical and radiation oncologist, radiology interventionalist, and pathologist, along with the spine surgeon is emphasized throughout this book, just as it should be in the day-to-day care of spine tumor patients. Multiple authors were encouraged for each chapter to ensure the most balanced, transparent, and comprehensive representation possible.

The oncologically appropriate management of primary tumors of the spine has been plagued by a lack of standardization; this begins with the basic terminology, and encompasses the staging and complex management of these rare, often lethal tumors. The basis of the problem is the fact that these elements used in managing spine tumors have all historically relied on the use of accepted general orthopedic and neurosurgical principles in the spine. The spinal community, however, has been generally reluctant to fully adopt the principles of appendicular musculoskeletal oncology developed by Enneking. This is because *en bloc* tumor resection in the spine entails complexities not always encountered in the extremities, such as restoring stability, and avoiding severe neurologic injury. Consequently, the adaptation of these relatively aggressive oncologic principles to the spine has been left open to the personal interpretation of the treating surgeon, as opposed to a universal evidence-based agreement on appropriate care. Fortunately through collaborative efforts of the world's spine oncology surgeons, many of whom are authors in this book, and education and research organizations such as AO, there is greater standardization and improved outcomes in the management of these patients.

We are hopeful that this guide will contribute to the evolving realization that evidence-based cancer treatment can be applied to primary spine tumor management as well. The shear immensity, morbidity, and resource consumption of many of these procedures, in a setting of patient quality of life, must be a take home message from this book. Furthermore the readers must recognize the absolute necessity for standardized staging and language, along with early multidisciplinary input in management, if we are going to provide these unique and challenging patients with the highest level of care possible.

Charles G. Fisher, MD, MHSc, FRCSC
Stefano Boriani, MD
Ziya L. Gokaslan, MD, FACS

Contributors

Luca Amendola, MD
Unit of Spine Surgery
Ospedale Maggiore
Bologna, Italy

Christopher P. Ames, MD
Professor
Clinical Neurological Surgery
Director
Spine Tumor and Spinal Deformity
  Surgery
Codirector
Spinal Surgery and University of California–
  San Francisco Spine Center
Director
Spinal Biomechanics Laboratory
San Francisco, California

Stefano Bandiera, MD
Unit of Oncologic and Degenerative Spine
  Surgery
Rizzoli Institute
Bologna, Italy

Stefano Boriani, MD
Unit of Oncologic and Degenerative Spine
  Surgery
Rizzoli Orthopedic Institute
Bologna, Italy

Justin M. Broyles, MD
Plastic Surgeon in Residence
Department of Plastic and Reconstructive
  Surgery
Johns Hopkins School of Medicine
Baltimore, Maryland

Simone Colangeli, MD
Unit of Oncologic and Degenerative Spine
  Surgery
Rizzoli Institute
Bologna, Italy

Nicolas Dea, MD, FRCSC
Neurosurgeon
Combined Neurosurgical and Orthopedic
  Spine Program
Vancouver General Hospital
University of British Columbia
Blusson Spinal Cord Center
Vancouver, British Columbia

Vedat Deviren, MD
Associate Professor
Clinical Orthopaedics
Orthopaedic Surgery
University of California–San Francisco Spine
  Center
San Francisco, California

Christian P. DiPaola, MD
Department of Orthopedics, Spine
   Surgery
University of Massachusetts Memorial
   Medical Center
Worcester, Massachusetts

Charles G. Fisher, MD, MHSc, FRCSC
Professor and Head
Division of Spine Surgery
Department of Orthopaedic Surgery
University of British Columbia
Vancouver, British Columbia

Daryl R. Fourney, MD, FRCSC, FACS
Assistant Professor
Division of Neurosurgery
Royal University Hospital
University of Saskatchewan
Saskatoon, Saskatchewan

Alessandro Gasbarrini MD
Unit of Oncologic and Degenerative Spine
   Surgery
Rizzoli Institute
Bologna, Italy

Riccardo Ghermandi, MD
Unit of Oncologic and Degenerative Spine
   Surgery
Rizzoli Institute
Bologna, Italy

Ziya L. Gokaslan, MD, FACS
Donlin M. Long Professor
Professor of Neurosurgery, Oncology,
   and Orthopaedic Surgery
Director, Neurosurgical Spine Program
Vice Chair, Department of Neurosurgery
Johns Hopkins University School
   of Medicine
Baltimore, Maryland

Mari L. Groves, MD
Assistant Resident
Department of Neurosurgery
Johns Hopkins Hospital University School
   of Medicine
Johns Hopkins Hospital
Baltimore, Maryland

Derek G. Ju, MD
Medical Student, MD Candidate
Department of Neurosurgery
Johns Hopkins University
Baltimore, Maryland

Sudhir Kathuria, MD
Assistant Professor
Radiology
Neurological Surgery and Neurology
Director
Spine Interventions, Interventional
   Neuroradiology
Baltimore, Maryland

Brent Y. Kimball, MD
Department of Neurosurgery
University of Tennessee Health Science Center
Memphis, Tennessee

Ilya Laufer, MD
Department of Neurosurgery
Memorial Sloan-Kettering Cancer Center
Department of Neurological Surgery
Weill Cornell Medical College
New York, New York

Mélissa Nadeau, MD, FRCSC
Adult Spine Fellow
Department of Orthopaedic Surgery
Vancouver General Hospital
University of British Columbia
Vancouver, British Columbia

Michael C. Oh, MD, PhD
Methodist Brain and Spine Institute
Dallas, Texas

Scott H. Okuno, MD
Professor
Department of Oncology
Mayo Clinic
Rochester, Minnesota

Shreyaskumar Patel, MD
Professor and Deputy Department Chair
Department of Sarcoma Medical Oncology
Division of Cancer Medicine
University of Texas M.D. Anderson Cancer Center
Houston, Texas

Y. Raja Rampersaud, MD, FRCS (C)
Orthopaedic Surgeon
Division of Orthopaedic Surgery
Arthritis Program
Toronto Western Hospital
University Health Network
Toronto, Ontario

Steven I. Robinson, MBBS
Instructor
Medicine and Oncology
Department of Oncology
Mayo Clinic
Rochester, Minnesota

Justin M. Sacks, MD FACS
Assistant Professor
Department of Plastic/Reconstructive Surgery
Johns Hopkins School of Medicine
Baltimore, Maryland

Rowan Schouten, FRACS, MBChB, BSc
Orthopaedic Surgeon
Forté Health Building
Christchurch, New Zealand

Daniel Michael Sciubba, MD
Associate Professor of Neurosurgery,
    Oncology & Orthopaedic Surgery
Johns Hopkins University
Baltimore, Maryland

Jackson Sui
Hospital and Health Care Professional
Birmingham, Michigan

Peter Paul Varga, MD
Director
National Center for Spinal Disorders
Budapest, Hungary

Jean-Paul Wolinsky
Associate Professor
Neurosurgery and Oncology
Department of Neurosurgery
Johns Hopkins University School of Medicine
Baltimore, Maryland

Yoshiya (Josh) Yamada, MD FRCPC
Department of Radiation Oncology
Memorial Sloan-Kettering Cancer Center
New York, New York

Patricia L. Zadnik, BA
Spinal Oncology Research Fellow
Sciubba Lab
Johns Hopkins Medicine
Baltimore, Maryland

1

Evaluation and Decision Making

Stefano Boriani and Charles G. Fisher

▨ Introduction

Primary bone tumors of the spine are very rare,[1,2] comprising only 10% or less of all bone tumors. In the United States about 7,500 new cases are estimated per year. The overall world occurrence can be expected to be 2.5 to 8.5 cases per million inhabitants per year. Compared with primary spinal tumors, metastatic tumors are much more common; the spine is the most common skeletal region for secondary tumors. The occurrence of spinal metastases in the clinical course of common solid tumors is reported to be 20 to 70%; therefore, a 30 to 50 times more frequent incidence is reported compared with that of primary bone tumors of the spine.

Of 43,735 primary bone tumors reviewed in the literature on bone tumors, 1,851 (4.2%) were located in the spine above the sacrum. These figures explain why they are often unsuspected, misdiagnosed, and, in many cases, unfortunately, incorrectly treated.

As the occurrence of lumbar stenosis, cervical radiculopathy, and acute spinal cord injury is estimated at 300 cases, 83 cases, and 5 cases per 100,000 persons per year, respectively,[2] an expertise in diagnosis and treatment strategy is required for early recognition of a spine tumor and for differentiating a primary tumor from a metastatic tumor.

▨ Clinical Findings and Imaging

Back and neck pain related to activity are very frequent symptoms, particularly in adults, and mostly related to disk prolapse, degenerative changes, and myofascial strains. Conversely a spine tumor should be first suspected when a patient with a history of cancer (current, recent, or in the past) complains of back or neck pain, particularly if it is progressive, unrelenting, not closely related to activity, and increasing during the night. Tumor growth may cause expansion of the bony cortex of the vertebral body, which results in pathological fracture and invasion of paravertebral soft tissues. Pain in these cases can be associated with acute or chronic compression of neurologic structures that can result in radiculopathy and or myelopathy. Some lesions do not cause pain. Latent lesions (hemangiomas, fibrous dysplasia, exostosis) are asymptomatic by definition, and diagnosis is achieved incidentally on imaging performed for other reasons. Cases of incidental detection of chordoma are also reported. This malignant tumor is characterized by very slow growth and, in anatomically voluminous regions such as the sacrum, can grow to very large sizes before detected.

Painful scoliosis in an adolescent is strongly suggestive of osteoid osteoma or osteoblastoma.

Usually not visible on standard radiograms, the fixed curve without a compensatory curve and rotation is strongly suggestive. Technetium isotope bone scan helps to localize the lesion. A computed tomography (CT) scan, performed at the level of intense uptake, displays the pathognomonic image of osteoid osteoma: a small island of pathological ossification surrounded by a lytic halo and frequently by a wide rim of reactive bone formation.

Technetium isotope bone scan is also able to localize multiple lesions. The role of positron emission tomography (PET) scan is becoming more relevant, particularly in its ability to differentiate tumors from infectious diseases.

Imaging studies (CT scan and magnetic resonance imaging [MRI]) can generate a working diagnosis, as some patterns are quite characteristic. Giant cell tumor and Ewing's sarcoma are lytic conditions, and most osteosarcomas are characterized by extensile aggressive pathological bone formation with ill-defined borders. A multicameral balloon-like pattern with double-density content is typical of aneurysmal bone cysts. Infiltrating erosions inside the cancellous bone of a vertebral body arising from the posterior wall is suggestive of chordoma. Soft tissue masses arising from the posterior elements with rounded calcifications are typical of peripheral chondrosarcomas.

Angiography shows pathological vascularity, and selective arterial embolization has become an indispensable tool to reduce intraoperative bleeding.

Histological diagnosis should always be achieved by biopsy, but clinical, laboratory, and imaging studies are important to orientate diagnosis and to select the biopsy technique.

▥ Biopsy

The goal of a biopsy is to obtain a specimen of the tumor, which is representative of the lesion and large enough to allow histological and ultrastructural analysis as well as immunologic stains. The surgeon must recognize the vital part of the tumor and discard the necrotic or reactive part. Cultures should be taken to rule out infection. There are three traditional biopsy techniques: incisional, needle or trocar, and excisional.

A number of basic principles should be observed when performing incisional and excisional biopsies in order to prevent tumor contamination of the surrounding tissue, which is the major risk of biopsy. Transverse incisions and flaps should be avoided; the tumor should be approached in the most direct manner possible, avoiding the anatomic interspaces (so-called extracompartmental spaces) commonly followed in orthopedic surgery. The approach should cross muscular structures. Tissues should be handled carefully, hemostasis should be meticulous, and suturing performed in all the anatomic layers. Bleeding from exposed bone or from uncauterized vessels and injured muscle will form a postoperative hematoma that may carry tumor cells beyond the margins of the intended excision and contaminate tissues proximal or distal to the primary lesion. The margin of the soft tissue component of the mass is often the most helpful to biopsy, as central portions are frequently necrotic. The surgeon should take care not to crush or distort the specimen, so as to maintain its architecture. Finally, if the definitive excision follows the biopsy during the same session, it is essential that all instruments used during the biopsy be discarded. The field should be re-draped, and the surgeons should change gowns and gloves before the definitive excision. If fusion is planned, bone graft should be taken through a separate surgical setup. If the planned definitive procedure is an en-bloc resection, the biopsy incision from the skin to the tumor mass should be placed so that it may be excised in a single block with the tumor and its margins. This is rarely possible in the treatment of tumors of the spine, if the epidural space has been violated.

Frozen section biopsy can be obtained during the excisional procedure when the diagnosis is highly probable and just requires confirmation. In rare situations, a patient may have two separate primaries; if there is any doubt, the results of the frozen section should be received before proceeding with the resection, such as in a situation of an assumed spine metastasis. Excisional biopsy can be considered only for conditions whose radiographic pattern is pathognomonic, for example osteoid osteoma.

The correct way to obtain a tumor sample from a vertebral body without violating the epidural space is with a transpedicular biopsy. The pedicle must be perforated by a drill or trocar. The surgeon must be careful not to perforate the pedicle wall, causing epidural space contamination. A small straight curette is then introduced to remove the specimen. The perforated pedicle must be filled with acrylic cement to prevent tumor backflow. The soft tissue track can be removed together with the surrounding muscle.

Small trocar biopsies are subject to sampling errors and provide small specimens for evaluation. The authors' preferred technique is to biopsy with a 12-gauge trocar performed under CT guidance. This technique produces tissue cores that allow for histological architecture and immunohistochemical studies. CT guidance allows the interventional radiologist to reach even the smallest lesions inside the vertebral body.

Diagnosis should always be confirmed on histological diagnosis; biopsy is mandatory. Conversely, some latent, asymptomatic lesions such as hemangioma, fibrous dysplasia, and exostosis are characterized by such a pathognomonic imaging that a biopsy is not always necessary. When this is the case it is recommended to follow the evolution of the disease by sequential imaging, initially every 4 to 6 months, to fully assess the latency of the condition.

In rare situations a patient may present with neurologic deterioration in a setting of a possible primary tumor. The surgeon is faced with the decision to stage the tumor and obtain a diagnosis or proceed with neurologic decompression, potentially rendering the patient incurable due to the tumor being violated. Each case is different, and conditional probabilities must be considered and integrated in a shared decision-making process with the patient. Often some delay in the treatment can be achieved with the use of steroids.

▧ Oncological Staging

Enneking et al[3] proposed in 1980 a system to stage the biological behavior of tumors of bone and soft tissue. This system was later applied also to the spine in several reviews. This system divides benign tumors into three stages (S1, S2, and S3) and localized malignant tumors into four stages (IA, IB, IIA, and IIB). Two further stages include metastatic high-grade intra- and extracompartmental malignant tumors (IIIA and IIIB). This classification is based on clinical, imaging, and histological findings. Each stage is related to overall prognosis and, by necessity, directly linked to categories of surgical procedures based on the concept of "margin."[3,4]

Benign Tumors

The first stage of benign tumors (S1, latent, inactive; **Fig. 1.1**) includes asymptomatic lesions, bordered by a true capsule, which is usually seen as a sclerotic rim on plain radiograms. These tumors do not grow, or grow very slowly. No treatment is required, unless surgery is needed for decompression or stabilization. Benign stage 2 tumors (S2, active; **Fig. 1.2**) grow slowly, causing mild symptoms. The tumor is bordered by a thin capsule and by a layer of reactive tissue, sometimes found on plain radiograms as an enlargement of the tumor outline. The bone scan is positive. An intralesional

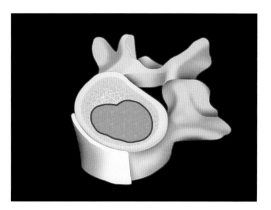

Fig. 1.1 Stage 1 benign tumor. The tumor is latent and inactive, and a capsule surrounds the lesion.

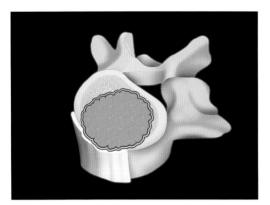

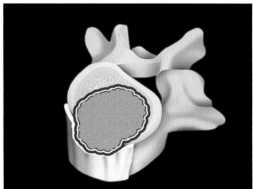

Fig. 1.2 Stage 2 benign tumor. The tumor grows slowly. The capsule is thinner. The tumor is surrounded by reactive tissue, as expression of local reaction to tumor growth.

Fig. 1.3 Stage 3 benign tumor. The tumor grows faster and invades early the epidural space or the perivertebral region. The capsule is very thin, and the reactive zone is wider.

excision can usually be performed with a low rate of recurrence. Based on very low quality evidence, the incidence of recurrences can be lowered further by local adjuvants (cryotherapy, embolization, radiation therapy). Benign stage 3 tumors (S3, aggressive; **Fig. 1.3**) are rapidly growing, with a capsule that is very thin, discontinued, or absent. The tumor invades neighboring compartments, and a wide reactive hypervascularized tissue (pseudocapsule) is often found, sometimes permeated by neoplastic digitations. The bone scan is highly positive. Indistinct margins are seen on plain X-rays, CT scan shows extracompartmental extension, and MRI clearly defines a pseudo-

capsule with significant edema and reaction. Intralesional excision (curettage), even if augmented by radiation, can be associated with a significant rate of local recurrence. En-bloc excision with marginal or wide margins is the treatment of choice.

Malignant Tumors

Low-grade malignant tumors are assigned stage I, subdivided into IA (the tumor remains inside the vertebra; **Fig. 1.4**) and IB (tumor invades paravertebral compartments; **Fig. 1.5**). No true capsule is associated with these lesions, but a thick pseudocapsule of reactive

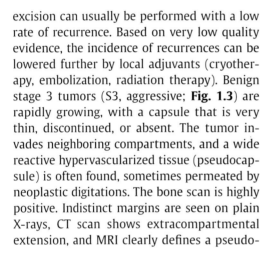

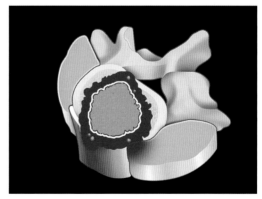

Fig. 1.4 Stage IA malignant tumor: low grade, intracompartmental. The pseudocapsule may include a small island of tumor.

Fig. 1.5 Stage IB malignant tumor: low grade, extracompartmental. The pseudocapsule may include a small island of tumor.

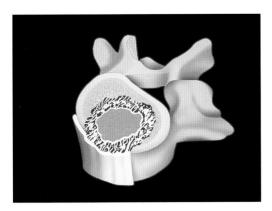

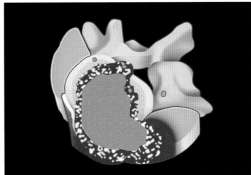

Fig. 1.6 Stage IIA malignant tumor: high grade, intracompartmental. The pseudocapsule is fully invaded by the tumor.

Fig. 1.7 Stage IIB malignant tumor: high grade, extracompartmental. The pseudocapsule is fully invaded by the tumor. A small island of tumor can be found outside the main tumor mass.

tissue permeated by small microscopic islands of tumor is seen. A resection performed along the pseudocapsule (marginal) can leave residual foci of active tumor; stereotactic radiation or proton-beam therapy can be added to reduce the risk of recurrence. The treatment of choice, if feasible, is a wide en-bloc resection, and careful marginal dissection if neurologic tissues are involved. High-grade malignancies are defined as IIA (**Fig. 1.6**) and IIB (**Fig. 1.7**). The neoplastic growth is so rapid that the host has no time to form a continuous reactive tissue. There is continuous seeding with neoplastic nodules (satellites). Moreover, these tumors can have neoplastic nodules at some distance from the main tumor mass (skip metastases). These malignancies are generally seen on plain radiograms as radiolucent and destructive and in many cases are associated with a pathological fracture. Invasion of the epidural space is rapid in stage B, particularly in small cell tumors (Ewing's sarcoma, lymphomas) characterized by semifluid tissue, which are able to occupy the epidural space after infiltrating the cortical border of the vertebra.

The margin of the resection must be wide (it is not possible to achieve a "radical" margin, in the spine), and courses of radiation and chemotherapy (according to the tumor type) must be considered for the local control and for the avoidance of distant spread. Often in areas of anatomic constraints, marginal margins (discussed below) or planned intralesional trans-

gressions must be accepted, or consideration given to the sacrifice of neurologic structures.

Stages IIIA and IIIB describe the same lesions as IIA and IIB, but are associated with distant metastasis, and in the majority of situations would be considered incurable.

■ Margins and Surgical Planning

As staging must be based on the natural history, surgical planning must be based on what the procedure achieves in relation to the margin of the lesion. The final pathological margin achieved through surgical technique is directly related to prognosis. Stener and Johnsen[5] were the first (to our knowledge) to apply extremity oncological principles to the spine; these concepts were published in exhaustive reports of en-bloc resections in the spine. Roy-Camille and Tomita later popularized the techniques of en-bloc resection. Many papers reviewed series of patients and provided tips and details for various techniques.[1,6–9] Since the late 1980s Weinstein and Boriani[10] tried to focus on a unified classification that proposed envelopes of resection as Enneking et al[3] had done for the extremities. By retrospectively reviewing his large case series, Boriani was able to establish significant relationships between margin and outcome specific to the spine.

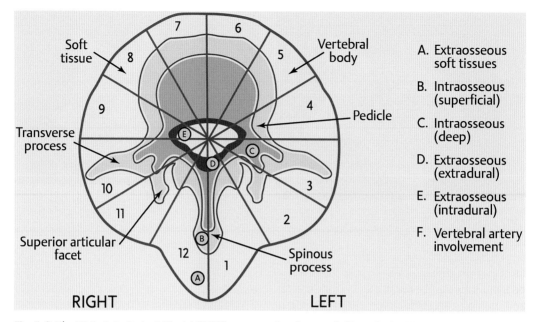

Fig. 1.8 The Weinstein-Boriani-Biagini (WBB) surgical staging system. On the transverse plane, the vertebra is divided into 12 radiating zones (numbered 1 to 12 in a clockwise order) and into vie layers (A to E from the prevertebral to the dural involvement). (From Boriani S, Biagini R, De Iure F, et al. En bloc resections of bone tumors of the thoracolumbar spine. A preliminary report on 29 patients. Spine 1996;21:1927–1931. Reproduced with permission.)

The Weinstein-Boriani-Biagini (WBB) staging system (**Fig. 1.8**) has been subjected to several clinical evaluations and recently submitted to a study of its reliability and validity by an international multidisciplinary group of spine tumor experts,[10] which found moderate interobserver reliability and substantial intraobserver reliability.

The WBB staging system focuses on the extent and location of the tumor. In the transverse plane, the vertebra is divided into 12 radiating zones (numbered 1 to 12 in a clockwise order) and into five layers from the prevertebral to the dural involvement (A through E). The longitudinal extent of the tumor is recorded by identifying the specific vertebrae involved. This system allowed for a more rational approach to surgical planning, provided that all efforts are made to perform surgery along the required margins.

Terminology

The application of a common terminology is mandatory for exchanging information and for doing multicenter studies, which are so important in this chronically underpowered population. A common terminology is required because if an en-bloc resection and a gross total excision are erroneously described with the same terms, it is difficult, if not impossible, to compare results. Surprisingly, many authors neglect or simply ignore the issue of true margins. Without a clear description of surgical and histopathological margins, it is impossible to evaluate the outcome of any surgical treatment. To stress the importance of a common language, the terms proposed by Enneking et al[3] and later applied to the spine[9] serve as examples.

Radical Resection

This term should be applied to the en-bloc removal of the tumor together with the whole compartment of origin. An example would be a thigh amputation for a tumor arising in the tibia, or a scapulectomy for a tumor arising and still contained in the scapula. Consequently, a radical resection in the spine defines an en-bloc resection of a full vertebra, provided that the tumor is fully confined inside the vertebra, including the spinal cord above and below. Even in this dramatic case, if the tumor has grown into the epidural space, the term *radical resection* will not be appropriate, as the epidural space is to be considered an extracompartmental area extending from the skull to the sacrum.

Intralesional Excision

Intralesional excision means a piecemeal removal of the tumor (also called curettage, gross total resection, and debulking). It is an intralesional procedure; the tumor is violated and any chance of obtaining tumor-free margins is lost. This procedure is appropriate for stage 2 benign tumors and for metastases. Microscopic and possible macroscopic tumor is always left after these procedures, and local progression can be expected according to the growing potential of the disease.

En-Bloc Resection

En-bloc resection entails the removal of the tumor as a single intact whole, fully encased by a cuff of healthy tissue (a circumferential margin of tumor-free normal tissue). For the en-bloc resection to have achieved its surgical goal, the pathologist must confirm that the resected tissue around the tumor mass (the so-called margin) is tumor free. En-bloc resections can be carried out with marginal margins or even planned transgressions, with the final margin outcome again determined by the pathologist.

The effectiveness of the margin as a barrier depends on its quality and also on the aggressiveness of the tumor. The margin is defined as "wide" when the plane of dissection has been peripheral to the reactive zone through normal tissue. The quality of the margin and thickness are relevant but not well quantified. A fascial barrier represents a wide margin, whereas 1 cm of muscle or cancellous bone may be inadequate to represent an appropriate barrier. The major issue in the decision-making process of planning en-bloc resection in the spine is the functional implications (for example, nerve roots) related to structures being resected with

the tumor in order to achieve a wide margin. *Marginal margin* means that the plane of dissection has been performed along the reactive zone. This is very close to the tumor and the possibility that satellites of tumor may be transgressed or left behind is real. *Intralesional margin* means that the tumor has been violated, and the tumor specimen is not covered by healthy tissue. Tumor cells will be left behind.

Palliative Procedure

This term describes all the surgical procedures generally directed toward a functional purpose, for example to decompress neurologic structures or stabilize the spine. This type of procedure is generally performed for metastatic disease.

▦ Surgical Techniques: En-Bloc Resections

The techniques of en-bloc resection for tumors of the vertebral body are well known.[6] The WBB staging system[9] can be helpful in standardizing the surgical planning of en-bloc resection according to the region of the spine and the tumor extent and location within that region. The great variability of these two parameters dictates that the same surgical procedure cannot be performed in all cases and that surgical planning is usually different for each case. Under the guidance of WBB staging system, six different approaches can be standardized: only anterior; only posterior; anterior first, posterior second; posterior first, double anterior second and third; posterior first, combined anterior and posterior second; anterior first, posterior second, combined anterior (contralateral) and posterior. These six approaches can be combined to create 10 different types of surgery. Detailed description of how to apply the WBB system is beyond the scope of this chapter, but it becomes clear as one plans to do an en-bloc resection and considers all the anatomic and functional issues related to safely and effectively removing a tumor en bloc.

Unique to bone tumors in the spine is the proximity of functionally relevant vital structures (e.g., spinal cord, nerve roots, large arteries and veins) that represent the margin. In such cases sacrifice of these structures must be proposed for performing oncologically appropriate surgery. Specific techniques of en-bloc resection have been reported, with the sacrifice of the following structures: dura,[11] cauda equina,[12] cervical nerve roots,[7] spinal cord,[13] and visceral organs.[14] Planning of the appropriate en-bloc resection must therefore consider the margins to be achieved. The approach or the approaches required and the timing can be decided according to the WBB surgical staging system.

The single anterior approach enables en-bloc resection of small tumors of the thoracic and lumbar vertebral bodies. They must be enclosed inside sectors 8 to 5, arising in layer A

and B, but not extending to layer C. In this case a posterior approach is required to provide an appropriate margin under direct visual control by entering the canal and releasing the dura.

The single posterior approach can be appropriate, as described by Roy-Camille and Tomita to remove as a whole a tumor arising in the vertebral body of a thoracic vertebra. Criteria to achieve appropriate margins include sector 9 or 4 free from tumor. If the tumor grows in layer D, the margin will be intralesional during the release from the dura. If the tumor grows in layer A, the margin will be intralesional during the release from the anterior structures (**Fig. 1.9**).

The single posterior approach with sagittal osteotomy enables en-bloc resection of a tumor eccentrically growing in the thoracic and lum-

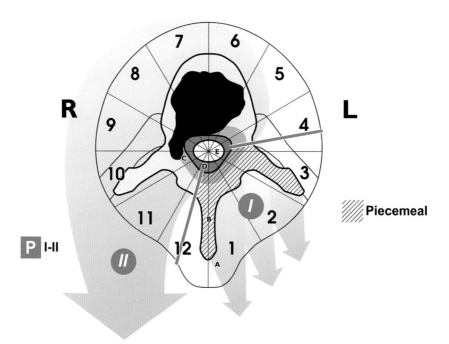

Fig. 1.9 Single posterior approach. It enables the removal by en-bloc resection of a tumor arising in the vertebral body of a thoracic vertebra. Criteria to achieve appropriate margins include sector 9 or 4 free from tumor. If the tumor grows in layer D, the margin will be intralesional during the release from the dura. If the tumor grows in layer A, the margin will be intralesional during the release from the anterior structures. This is a two-step procedure, as shown by roman numerals on the figure: (I) Piece-meal excision of the posterior arch not involved by the tumor. At least four sectors are required, starting from sector 4 or from sector 9. Release from the dura and section of the nerve root(s) involved by the tumor. (II) Blunt dissection of the anterior part of the vertebral body from the mediastinum, osteotomy, or diskectomy above and below the tumor, with full release from the dura and finalizing the resection.

bar spine (**Fig. 1.10**), provided the body is not involved over sector 5 at left and over sector 8 at right. At least three sectors posteriorly must not be involved by the tumor (4 to 1–2 or 12–11 to 9).

A combination of anterior approach first and posterior approach second enables en-bloc resection of a tumor located in the thoracic and lumbar spine (**Fig. 1.11**) and in the cervical spine growing anteriorly (layer A). When the tumor is growing anteriorly (layer A) an anterior approach must be performed as the first step to provide a wide/marginal margin under visual control. If the tumor extension is mostly eccentric (i.e., involving sectors 5 to 11), a sag-

ittal osteotomy from posterior to anterior can be performed to complete the resection (**Fig. 1.12**).

Huge lumbar tumors can also be removed by en-bloc resection via two surgical stages: the first stage posterior, and the second an anterior approach followed by a final posterior approach (**Fig. 1.13**). This technique was described by Roy-Camille for lumbar tumors and is associated with the highest rate of morbidity and complications.[15] The combination of anterior and posterior approaches is preferred when it is assumed that complex maneuvers will be necessary to remove the specimen. To resect a tumor of L5, three stages are suggested: first, anterior approach to the contralateral side of

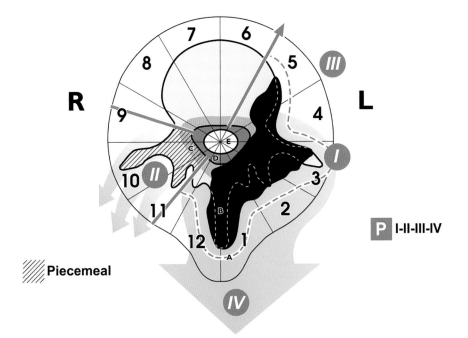

Fig. 1.10 Single posterior approach with sagittal osteotomy. A tumor excentrically growing in the lumbar spine can be removed en bloc by a single posterior approach provided that the body is not involved over sector 5 at left and over sector 8 at right. At least three sectors posteriorly must not be involved by the tumor (4 to 1–2 or 12–11 to 9). This is a four-step procedure, as shown by roman numerals on the figure: (I) Provide the appropriate margin over the tumor posteriorly growing by resecting inside the posterior muscles covering the tumor mass if it is expanding in layer A. The release will proceed laterally until the lateral side of the vertebral body. In the thoracic spine the pleura can be left on the tumor, and in the lumbar spine the posterior part of the psoas must be dissected, but the segmental vessels must be found and ligated. (II) Piecemeal excision of the posterior arch not involved by the tumor. This step includes the approach to the canal, release of the dura from the tumor (if the tumor grows in layer D, the margin will result intralesional), and section of the nerve root(s) involved by the tumor. (III) Displace carefully the dura and perform the osteotomy from posterior to anterior in sector 8 or 5. (IV) The specimen is removed.

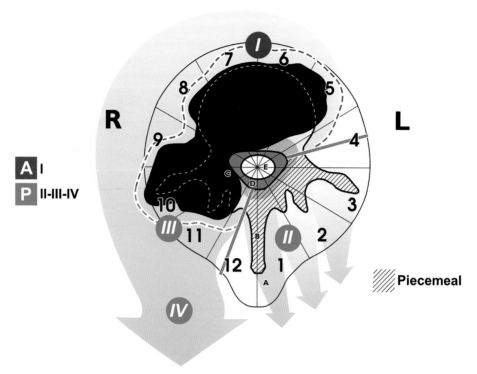

Fig. 1.11 Two approaches: anterior first, posterior second in the thoracic and in the lumbar spine. When the tumor is growing anteriorly (layer A), an anterior approach must be performed as the first step to provide a wide/marginal margin under visual control. This is a four-step procedure, as shown by roman numerals on the figure: (I) In case of tumors mostly occupying the vertebral body, the anterior approach can be the first step to release from mediastinum or retroperitoneal, eventually leaving involved structures as the margin. A sheet of Silastic or similar material can be left as protection. (II) Posterior approach: piecemeal excision of the posterior arch not involved by the tumor. At least three or four sectors are required, starting from sector 4 or from sector 9. (III) Release of the dura from the tumor, section of the nerve root(s) involved by the tumor, and then provide the appropriate margin over the tumor posteriorly growing by resecting inside the posterior muscles covering the tumor mass if it is expanding in layer A. (IV) The specimen is removed by rotating around the dural sac.

the tumor to release the aorta/cava bifurcation; second, posterior; third, anterior and posterior approach.

In planning the surgical procedure the cord vascularity must be considered. During these procedures, particularly when the resection is multilevel or the tumor particularly huge, the functional integrity of the spinal cord is at risk mostly due to the manipulation of the cord during maneuvers to deliver the tumor. For example, an anatomic feature unique to the higher thoracic spine (T1 to T4) is easier release of the vertebrae from the aorta, as no segmental arteries are closely connected to the verte-bral body.[16] Below T5 the intercostal arteries run around the vertebral body and keep the aorta closely related to bone; therefore, careful retraction is needed when en-bloc resection of the vertebral body is performed by the posterior approach. At the thoracolumbar junction the diaphragm pillar can extend to T12, making the dissection posteriorly more difficult. Sometimes this is best approached anteriorly for a safer release.

The role of the artery of Adamkiewicz as a single, exclusive feeding for the anterior spinal artery is controversial. It seems reasonable that cord vascularity is not dependent on one artery.

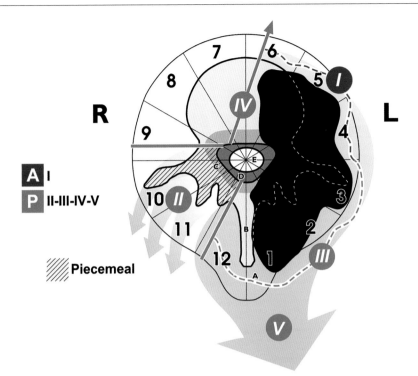

Fig. 1.12 This procedure can be planned in case the tumor is eccentrically growing. Anterior first, posterior second in the thoracic and lumbar spine, and sagittal osteotomy posterior to anterior. This is a five-step procedure, as shown by roman numerals on the figure: (I) In the first stage the anterior approach provides a wide/marginal margin under visual control, releasing from mediastinum or from peritoneal, eventually leaving involved structures as the margin. Diskectomies or transversal grooves in vertebral bodies are performed to define the upper and lower margins. A sheet of Silastic or any other tissue can be left as protection. In the second stage, the posterior approach, piecemeal excision of the posterior arch not involved by the tumor is performed. (II) At least three sectors are required, starting from sector 4 or from sector 9. (III) Provide the appropriate margin over the tumor posteriorly growing by resecting inside the posterior muscles covering the tumor mass if it is expanding in layer A. (IV) Release of the dura from the tumor, section of the nerve roots crossing the tumor, and osteotomy posterior to anterior at some distance from the tumor in order to leave uninvolved bone as margin. (V) The resected specimen can be removed once the upper and lower diskectomies or osteotomies are finalized.

Previously, we performed angiographic studies before surgery to identify the radiculomedullary artery feeding the artery of Adamkiewicz. In four cases the nerve root was sacrificed without any damage to cord vascularity. Since then, the role of such a study was felt to be less critical and did not affect the planning. Tomita and his group[16–18] had the same experience, and demonstrated that the risk of cord ischemia is mostly related to the number of contiguous radicular arteries sacrificed rather that to a single artery. Furthermore, there is some evidence in the literature of multiple feeders to the anterior spinal artery. We now recommend taking no more than three nerve roots bilaterally in the thoracic spine, and avoiding acute shortening or distraction during the resection.[19]

▨ Complications

The morbidity associated with en-bloc resections is high, often combining the risks and complications of anterior spine surgery with those of major posterior surgery.

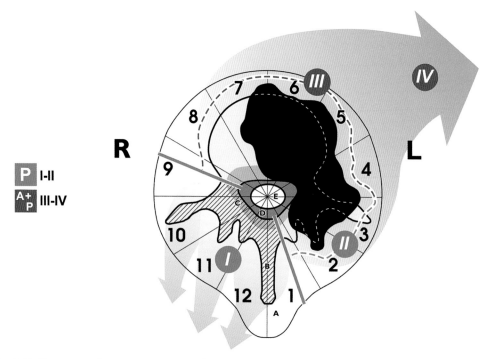

Fig. 1.13 Two stages: first posterior approach, second contemporary anterior and posterior approaches. This technique is typical and more appropriate for lumbar tumors and is associated with the highest rate of morbidity and complications. In thoracic spine it is less advisable. The first steps are performed with the patient in the prone position: piecemeal excision of the posterior arch not involved by the tumor. This is a four-step procedure, as shown by roman numerals on the figure: (I) At least three sectors are required, starting from sector 4 or from sector 9. (II) In cases of a tumor posteriorly growing and invading layer A, an appropriate margin must be provided by resecting inside the posterior muscles covering the tumor mass. Then release the dura from the tumor (if the tumor grows in layer D, the margin will result intralesional) and section the nerve root(s) crossing the tumor. Diskectomies or transversal grooves in vertebral bodies are performed to define the upper and lower margins. The second stage is performed with the patient in the lateral position. Anterolateral approach (thoracotomy, thoracoabdominal, retroperitoneal) and reopening of the posterior approach. (III) To provide an appropriate margin over the tumor, it must remain covered by pleura or by psoas. Spiral wires are used to embolize the segmental arteries to facilitate the release of the aorta on the contralateral side. (IV) Once the upper and lower diskectomies or osteotomies are finalized, the specimen is removed by combined maneuvers.

Previous surgery, radiation, and prolonged combined approaches increase the risk of complications, with infection being particularly threatening, due to the wide prolonged exposure and the compromised immune status of many of these patients.[15] Two cases of late aortic dissection occurred after radiation therapy (doses of 42 and 44 Gy). In both cases an anterior vertebrectomy was performed following release of the aorta from the tumor[15]. Nonunion is a common late complication due to the hostile environment in which to achieve a solid bony fusion. Mortality is not negligible, with a rate of 2.2%.[15]

▪ Chapter Summary

Obtaining a diagnosis is the first critical step in the management of primary tumors of the spine. This is achieved through staging that culminates in a carefully planned CT-guided biopsy. To determine management, the clinical, imaging, and histological information is reviewed by a multidisciplinary team. Expertise in the biological behavior of the different tumor types is mandatory in deciding the most appropriate surgical margin and the surgical technique to obtain it. To facilitate this process, the Enneking staging system is used. A surgical staging system (such as the WBB) is also required for planning the surgical procedure in order to achieve such margins. Decision making should include in-depth discussions with the patient to ensure that all issues, including probability of local recurrence, survival, and risk, are clearly understood. The intrinsic morbidity of en-bloc resections and the anatomic sacrifices required to achieve appropriate margins must be weighed against the increasing risk of local recurrence associated with less than optimal intralesional margins, but this may be the only option in some cases.

The combination of Enneking and WBB staging systems should

- prevent high morbidity surgery when not necessary (for example, in stage 2 benign or in metastatic tumors);
- achieve the appropriate margin by correctly performing en-bloc resections in selected cases; and
- advance the knowledge of these tumors by comparing uniform reports on outcomes of homogeneously treated tumors.

It is important to consider the complications in the treatment of primary tumors of the spine, as sometimes management of complications is more difficult than management of the tumor itself. To this end, the first chance is not only the most important, but may be the only chance to cure the patient. Second chances are often too late. The ability to integrate the best surgical and nonsurgical treatments can affect not only the immediate care of the patient, but also, and more importantly, the long-term survival.

Tumors of the spine are unique and require highly skilled teams to deal with the difficult decisions invoked by every case. These cases are not for the routine spine surgeon or traditional oncological surgeon.

Acknowledgment
The authors acknowledge the outstanding contribution of Carlo Piovani for data collection and original drawings.

Pearls

◆ The decision-making process for the treatment of primary bone tumors of the spine is based on a thorough understanding of the biology and the behavior of each tumor. This is achieved by diagnosis and oncological staging (Enneking), which dictates the oncologically appropriate treatment (including surgery, radiation therapy, chemotherapy, and other medical treatments).
◆ The decision-making process of primary bone tumors is performed by a multidisciplinary team and includes the following steps:
  ◦ Clinical findings and imaging provide the working diagnosis.
  ◦ Histology and oncological staging indicate biological behavior and direct the treatment.
  ◦ Surgery of primary tumors has a curative intent.
◆ Computer tomography–guided trocar biopsy is the method of choice to provide an appropriate specimen and the least possible contamination of the surrounding tissues. The biopsy should be done by the same center that will administer the treatment.
◆ Surgery of primary tumors has a curative purpose. Oncologically appropriate surgical treatment can substantially improve the prognosis and can be considered a lifesaving procedure.
◆ Shared decision making with the patient is imperative in all cases of primary tumor resection. The patient's acceptance of functional loss to achieve better local control and prognosis, versus a preference for saving function despite the increased risk of local recurrence and decreased survival, must be discussed.
◆ Intentional violation of oncological principles such as planned intralesional transgression to preserve vital structures or reduce morbidity[1] can be considered and should be discussed with the patient and a multidisciplinary team. In this setting the role of further adjuvant therapy becomes critically important.

Pitfalls

◆ Treating a patient without a diagnosis and appropriate staging could lead to rendering a potentially curable patient incurable.
◆ Do not perform an ill-conceived open biopsy. Tumors submitted to open biopsy had a five to

seven times higher rate of local recurrence, independent of diagnosis.

◆ Do not create unnecessarily compromising margins, especially in low-grade malignancies (chordoma, chondrosarcoma), and assume that adjuvant treatments will compensate for violation of oncological principles.

◆ In attempting a "cure," assuming this is possible and the patient understands the risks and benefits of such a treatment, an appropriate margin must be achieved even if it requires major vascular and neurologic sacrifices. In the decision-making process, this should never be offered in cases with metastases or benign stage 1 and the majority of stage 2.

◆ The assumption that an en-bloc resection done with an intralesional or marginal margin along the dura is associated with the same rate of local control (recurrence) as intralesional piecemeal excision (gross total resection) is wrong. A piecemeal approach is always intralesional and always associated with local recurrence unless the specific tumor is sensitive to adjuvant therapies such as radiation therapy.

References
Five Must-Read References

1. Fisher CG, Keynan O, Boyd MC, Dvorak MF. The surgical management of primary tumors of the spine: initial results of an ongoing prospective cohort study. Spine 2005;30:1899–1908
2. Chi JH, Bydon A, Hsieh P, Witham T, Wolinsky JP, Gokaslan ZL. Epidemiology and demographics for primary vertebral tumors. Neurosurg Clin N Am 2008;19:1–4
3. Enneking WF, Spanier SS, Goodman MA. A system for the surgical staging of musculoskeletal sarcoma. Clin Orthop Relat Res 1980;153:106–120
4. Simon MA. Surgical margins. In: Simon MA, Springfield D, eds. Surgery for Bone and Soft Tissue Tumors. Philadelphia: Lippincott-Raven, 1998:77–92
5. Stener B, Johnsen OE. Complete removal of three vertebrae for giant-cell tumour. J Bone Joint Surg Br 1971;53:278–287
6. Yao KC, Boriani S, Gokaslan ZL, Sundaresan N. En bloc spondylectomy for spinal metastases: a review of techniques. Neurosurg Focus 2003;15:E6–E12
7. Rhines LD, Fourney DR, Siadati A, Suk I, Gokaslan ZL. En bloc resection of multilevel cervical chordoma with C-2 involvement. Case report and description of operative technique. J Neurosurg Spine 2005;2:199–205
8. Bailey CS, Fisher CG, Boyd MC, Dvorak MF. En bloc marginal excision of a multilevel cervical chordoma. Case report. J Neurosurg Spine 2006;4:409–414
9. Currier BL, Papagelopoulos PJ, Krauss WE, Unni KK, Yaszemski MJ. Total en bloc spondylectomy of C5 vertebra for chordoma. Spine 2007;32:E294–E299
10. Boriani S, Weinstein JN, Biagini R. Spine Update. A surgical staging system for therapeutic planning of primary bone tumors of the spine. A contribution to a common terminology. Spine 1997;22:1036–1044
11. Chan P, Boriani S, Fourney DR, et al. An assessment of the reliability of the Enneking and Weinstein-Boriani-Biagini classifications for staging of primary spinal tumors by the Spine Oncology Study Group. Spine 2009;34:384–391
12. Biagini R, Casadei R, Boriani S, et al. En bloc vertebrectomy and dural resection for chordoma: a case report. Spine 2003;28:E368–E372
13. Keynan O, Fisher CG, Boyd MC, O'Connell JX, Dvorak MF. Ligation and partial excision of the cauda equina as part of a wide resection of vertebral osteosarcoma: a case report and description of surgical technique. Spine 2005;30:E97–E102
14. Murakami H, Tomita K, Kawahara N, Oda M, Yahata T, Yamaguchi T. Complete segmental resection of the spine, including the spinal cord, for telangiectatic osteosarcoma: a report of 2 cases. Spine (Phila Pa 1976) 2006;31:E117–122
15. Druschel C, Disch AC, Melcher I, et al. Surgical management of recurrent thoracolumbar spinal sarcoma with 4-level total en bloc spondylectomy: description of technique and report of two cases. Eur Spine J 2012;21:1–9
16. Boriani S, Bandiera S, Donthineni R, et al. Morbidity of en bloc resections in the spine. Eur Spine J 2010;19:231–241
17. Kawahara N, Tomita K, Baba H, et al. Cadaveric vascular anatomy for total en bloc spondylectomy in malignant vertebral tumors. Spine 1996;21:1401–1407
18. Kato S, Kawahara N, Tomita K, Murakami H, Demura S, Fujimaki Y. Effects on spinal cord blood flow and neurologic function secondary to interruption of bilateral segmental arteries which supply the artery of Adamkiewicz: an experimental study using a dog model. Spine 2008;33:1533–1541
19. Kawahara N, Tomita K, Kobayashi T, Abdel-Wanis ME, Murakami H, Akamaru T. Influence of acute shortening on the spinal cord: an experimental study. Spine 2005;30:613–620

Safety and Efficacy of Surgery for Primary Tumors of the Spine

Daryl R. Fourney, Charles G. Fisher, and Stefano Boriani

▣ Introduction

The rarity of primary spine tumors and the slow growth rate of many types (e.g., chordoma, low-grade chondrosarcoma, giant cell tumor) make them difficult to study, especially with regard to the results of surgery and other treatments. The overwhelming majority of studies are retrospective, and the few prospective studies are limited by a short follow-up time.[1] It is difficult to compare older studies because of loose interpretation of the terminology and a lack of standardization in staging and management. Even in individual case series, patient management often varies over time due to advances in diagnosis, surgical technique, and adjuvant therapies. All of these factors have combined to yield a heterogeneous group of published reports,[2-9] but has not obscured the principal fact that an oncologically valid approach to these diseases leads to improved disease control and survival.[10]

The work of Weinstein, Boriani, and Biagini[2,3,11,12] and others[5,6] has shown that the principles of musculoskeletal oncology originally developed by Enneking[13,14] can be applied to the spine. The principles of primary tumor management are outlined in **Table 2.1**, and these principles are revisited throughout this book, with variations in how they are addressed based on the pathology, the location and extent of disease, and patient factors (e.g., medical fitness, exposure to previous therapies, and treatment preference). It is important to emphasize the extensive nature of en-bloc resection surgery, its inherent morbidity, and its cost. In fact, the high rate of intraoperative and early postoperative complications are often weighed against the probability of survival and local control, begging the question of whether en-bloc surgery is justified in the spine.[1,5,7]

Efficacy is a broad concept that evaluates the overall value or usefulness of an intervention. It includes an analysis of clinical outcomes and resource utilization. For primary spine tumors, the main clinical outcome of interest is disease control and, ideally, cure. This chapter assesses the efficacy of en-bloc or oncologically appropriate surgery for primary spine tumors to achieve disease control, and discusses the potential for morbidity and strategies to promote safety.

▣ Long-Term Results of Surgery

Recently, the first population-based study on malignant primary osseous tumors of the spine that had sufficient power to evaluate the role of surgical resection on survival was reported by Mukherjee et al.[15] The Surveillance, Epidemiology, and End Results (SEER) registry was analyzed for cases of histologically confirmed primary (nonmetastatic) tumor of the mobile spine or pelvis over a 30-year period (1973–2003). A major limitation of this study was that

Table 2.1 Principles and Pitfalls that Affect the Efficacy of Surgery for Primary Tumors

Principle	Pitfall
High index of suspicion	• Diagnosis after intralesional resection with contaminated tumor margins
Biopsy before treatment (percutaneous CT-guided core biopsy)	• Biopsy tract not incorporated in later excision • Fine-needle aspiration limits ability to assess tissue architecture
Consistent terminology	• Lack of precision describing surgical approach or margins
Staging with Enneking and WBB classification	• Enneking inappropriate surgery associated with higher rates of local recurrence and mortality
Multidisciplinary management/ experienced centers	• All aspects of care not fully appreciated (e.g., pathology, local and systemic staging, surgical feasibility, technical points to reduce surgical morbidity, need for adjuvant and neoadjuvant therapy, soft tissue coverage, patient preferences, etc.)
Long term follow-up	• Delayed diagnosis of recurrence many years after excision of slow-growing tumor types (e.g., chordoma, low-grade chondrosarcoma)

Abbreviations: CT, computed tomography; WBB, Weinstein–Boriani–Biagini.

the surgical margins and the functional outcome of surgery were not reported. The authors performed a multivariate analysis, and after adjusting for age, radiation therapy, and extent of local tumor invasion, surgical resection was independently associated with significantly improved survival for chordoma (hazard ratio [HR], 0.617; 95% confidence interval [CI], 0.25–0.98), chondrosarcoma (HR, 0.153; 95% CI, 0.07–0.36], osteosarcoma (HR, 0.382; 95% CI, 0.21–0.69), and Ewing's sarcoma (HR, 0.494; 95% CI, 0.26–0.96). Radiation therapy was associated with prolonged survival for patients with osteosarcoma and chordomas, but not for patients with Ewing's sarcoma and chondrosarcoma.

into two groups based on surgical margins: Enneking appropriate (EA) and Enneking inappropriate (EI). There were 147 patients with a median follow-up of 4 years (range, 2–7 years). There was a significantly higher risk of local recurrence after EI surgery, and there was a strong correlation between the first local recurrence and mortality with an odds ratio of 4.69 ($p < 0.0001$). EI surgery was associated with a higher risk of mortality (HR, 3.10; $p = 0.0485$) compared with an EA approach. The most significant limitation of this study was that the EI cohort had more high-grade tumors; however, the EI group also had a significantly higher rate of adjuvant therapy, which should bias toward the null hypothesis, thus strengthening the conclusions.

▓ Applying Enneking's Principles to the Spine

A predominantly prospective cohort study by Fisher et al[6] of patients with primary spine tumors from four spine centers in Canada treated between 1982 and 2008 was analyzed to determine whether applying Enneking's principles to the surgical management of primary bone tumors of the spine significantly decreases local recurrence or mortality. Cases were divided

▓ Feasibility of Obtaining Acceptable Margins

In a systematic review published in 2009, Yamazaki et al[1] assessed the early efficacy of en-bloc resection techniques by determining the number of wide/marginal resections versus the number of intralesional resections. The results varied significantly among studies. All of the studies included in the systematic review reported the postoperative margins, but not the *expected* margins based on the preoperative surgical staging. The one exception was a prospective study by Fisher et al.[5] Among the 26 patients with primary spine tumors reported by Fisher et al., post operative margins were wide in 15, marginal in four (all planned wide), and intralesional in seven (two planned wide, one planned marginal). Thus, Weinstein–Boriani–Biagini (WBB) staging accurately predicted the margins in 19 of 26 cases (73%). However, if the general goal of surgery was attainment of a wide or marginal en-bloc resection (i.e., excluding the four cases that were expected to be intralesional), the WBB staging accurately predicted the attainment of wide or marginal en-bloc resection in 23 of 26 cases (88%). In experienced hands, en-bloc resection with acceptable margins is achievable if WBB staging determines that it is feasible.

Long-Term Results of En-Bloc Resection for Chordoma and Chondrosarcoma

Boriani et al[2] reviewed 52 consecutive chordomas of the mobile spine over a 50-year period. The series included a retrospective review of 15 cases treated prior to 1991 and a prospective group of 37 cases treated from 1991 to 2002. All patients were staged and subjected to one of five protocols: (1) radiation therapy with or without palliative surgery (n = 10); (2) intralesional extracapsular excision (n = 8); (3) intralesional excision plus radiation therapy (n = 16); (4) attempted en-bloc resection, intralesional or contaminated, combined with radiation therapy (n = 8); and (5) en-bloc resection (n = 10). Every patient treated with radiation therapy alone or intralesional excision had recurrence within 2 years of surgery. Intralesional extracapsular excision plus radiation therapy also had a very high recurrence rate (12 of 16, mean 30 months) but three patients were continuously disease-free (mean, 52 months) and five patients were alive with stable disease (mean, 69 months) at last fol-

low-up. Twelve of 18 patients who received en-bloc resection were continuously disease-free for an average of 8 years (range, 48–155 months). For the six patients who recurred, it is notable that all of them had previously undergone surgery or had documented contaminated tumor margins. The only treatment protocol that resulted in greater than 5 years of continuously disease-free survival was en-bloc resection with marginal or wide margins.

Boriani et al[3] also retrospectively reviewed 32 cases of chondrosarcoma within the mobile spine. The average follow-up period was 81 months (range, 2–236 months). Recurrences occurred in 3 of 14 patients treated with en-bloc resection, compared with 100% of 18 patients treated with intralesional curettage.

A systematic review published in 2009 by Boriani et al[4] compared the effects of wide/marginal (en-bloc) resection with the effects of intralesional resection on local recurrence and survival for chordomas and chondrosarcomas of the spine. They also evaluated the effects of radiation therapy. The authors reported significantly decreased local recurrence and death for both tumor types after en-bloc resection, as compared with intralesional resection ($p < 0.0001$). The odds ratio for local recurrence with intralesional resection was 10.25. For chordoma, the odds ratio for death if local recurrence occurred was 15.03.

Radiation therapy is generally recommended in the event of intralesional or incomplete resection of chordoma or chondrosarcoma, but fairly high doses (60 to 65 Gy equivalents) are required.[4] Superior dose distribution may be achieved with proton beam therapy or stereotactic body radiosurgery (SBRT).[16–18] The published series using these treatments are mainly limited to skull base and cervical spine lesions, but we expect more studies utilizing SBRT for mobile spine chordomas and chondrosarcomas in the coming years.

Morbidity Rate of En-Bloc Resection

In a systematic evaluation of complications after surgery for primary spine tumors, Yamazaki et al[1] found tremendous variability in the reported rate of complications. Most studies were retrospective series and they reported lower rates of complications compared to the one prospective study.[5] However, the retrospective studies had greater long-term follow-up, and thus late complications, such as instrumentation failure and tumor recurrence, were more frequently described.[2,5,7,19] Only two studies used previously published criteria[20] to classify complications.[7,19]

Boriani et al[21] retrospectively assessed morbidity in 134 patients who underwent en-bloc resection for spine tumors between 1990 and 2007, including 90 with primary tumors and 44 with metastatic tumors. The rate of complications was 35.1%. The risk of major complications was more than twice as high in patients with contaminated tumor margins (odds ratio [OR], 2.52; 95% CI, 1.01–6.30; $p = 0.048$). A separately published analysis of the same data showed a higher rate of complications in patients referred from another center after an open biopsy or surgery who subsequently developed recurrence (72%) compared with previously untreated patients (20%).[19] On multivariate analysis, the independent predictors of major complications were multisegmental tumor (OR, 1.95; 95% CI, 1.07–3.56; $p = 0.03$) and use of a simultaneous combined anterior-posterior approach (OR, 3.79; 95% CI, 1.09–13.17; $p = 0.036$).[21]

For sacral tumors, Fourney et al[7] found a correlation between higher level of sacrectomy and nerve root sacrifice, with an increased complication rate and longer inpatient stay. The incidence of wound complications has been reduced by the use of specialized flap closure techniques, and this is perhaps best exemplified after sacrectomy, where soft tissue defects may be particularly large.

Mortality Rate of En-Bloc Resection

In the systematic review by Yamazaki et al,[1] mortality rates varied from 0 to 7.7%. The most common cause of death related to surgery was respiratory failure. The mortality rate after en-

bloc resection in the large series reported by Boriani et al[21] was 2.2%, occurring in three patients: one intraoperative death due to injury of the vena cava, one postoperative pulmonary embolism, and one late dissection of the wall of the aorta 8 months after surgery.

Safety Promotion Strategies

The morbidity of surgical resection for spine tumors derives from several factors, but there are many effective prevention strategies (**Table 2.2**).

Preoperative angiographic embolization is a worthwhile consideration, especially for highly vascularized lesions such as giant cell tumor. Sufficient vascular access, including the placement of large-bore intravenous catheters, is necessary in order to administer large volumes of fluids and blood. Central venous pressure monitoring is recommended for most cases of en-bloc resection. We have generally avoided use of the cell saver in primary tumors because of the potential for tumor dissemination. Tranexamic acid appears to be a safe, effective, low-cost method to reduce blood loss during and after surgery. After induction of anesthesia, the loading dose is 2 g in 100 mL for adults and 30 mg/kg for children administered over 20 minutes, followed immediately by a maintenance dose of 1 g in 100 mL infused at a rate of 100 mg/h for adults and 1 mg/kg/h for children.[22]

The length of these procedures, the degree of tissue resection, and the postoperative period of convalescence required are all risk factors for deep venous thrombosis and pulmonary embolism. We routinely utilize sequential pneumocompression stockings in the perioperative period and prophylactic low molecular weight heparin postoperatively.

Intraoperative complications are related to the manipulation of vital structures. The risk of injury increases in the case of reoperation or previously irradiation tissues, due to fibrous scar and tissue fragility. If a dural tear is encountered, immediate suturing with a muscu-

Table 2.2 Factors that Affect Morbidity After En-Bloc Resection for Primary Spine Tumors

Factor	Safety Promotion Strategy
Complex anatomy due to large tumor growth/extension	• Familiarity with anatomy • Experience with en-bloc resection of the spine/paraspinal structures
Excessive hemorrhage from the tumor or epidural vein	• Preoperative embolization • Tranexamic acid • Careful surgical technique
Manipulation or sacrifice of vascular or nervous structures	• Careful tissue handling with microsurgical techniques • Multimodality intraoperative neurophysiological monitoring
Epidural fibrosis due to previous surgery	• Prevent recurrence through careful staging and planning of the first resection
Wound dehiscence or infection	• Plan appropriate soft tissue coverage (flap if necessary) • Avoid operating through previously irradiated fields
Long-term hardware failure	• Circumferential reconstruction to enable a stable fusion

lar coverage is recommended. If a watertight closure cannot be obtained, cerebrospinal fluid (CSF) drainage is an option but carries its own risks (e.g., overdrainage, pneumocephalus, meningitis).

Manipulation of the spinal cord, especially in the thoracic spine, should be avoided. Careful microsurgical technique is required when handling nervous tissue. We recommend the use of multimodality intraoperative neurophysiological monitoring (somatosensory evoked potentials, motor evoked potentials, electromyography).

Late instrumentation failure has been reported in about 7% of cases.[19] En-bloc resection entails significant instability, and given the goal of long-term disease-free survival, circumferential reconstruction and long-segment stabilization is recommended. Most importantly, meticulous planning and thought must go into biological fixation. With long-term survival anticipated, fusion must be achieved, and this can be difficult in a biologically hostile environment. Vascularized strut grafts and augmented soft tissue coverage are often necessary in large resections.

Finally, the benefit of experience cannot be understated. The surgical anatomy is often complex due to tumor growth adjacent to the spinal cord and critical paraspinal structures. The entire treatment, from biopsy to resection to long-term follow-up, should ideally be performed at the same center, under the guidance of a multidisciplinary team led by an experienced spine oncology surgeon.

▪ Avoiding Problems

Open Biopsy

Poorly planned biopsies increase the risk of local recurrence by tumor dissemination along fascial planes and the biopsy tract.[8] In a series of patients with chordoma of the mobile spine and pelvis, Bergh et al[9] found that performance of an invasive diagnostic procedure outside the index center and inadequate surgical margins were associated with tumor recurrence and tumor-related death. In patients with primary tumors of the sacrum, Fourney et al[7] noted a 78% continuously disease-free survival for patients undergoing both biopsy and surgery at the index institution, compared with 55% for those patients who underwent a prior procedure at another institution.

Incisional biopsy or intralesional resection significantly increases the risk of local recurrence; therefore, transcutaneous computed tomography–guided trocar biopsy is recommended.[1] When there is a suspicion of a primary tumor, the surgeon who performs the definitive surgery should ideally be the one to perform or direct the biopsy procedure.

Permanent marking of the biopsy site is recommended so that it can be identified and included in the excision. Although fine-needle aspiration provides cytomorphological features that may yield a diagnosis, a trocar needle may improve accuracy by analysis of all histological features of the tissue.[1,23,24]

Inconsistent Terminology and Staging

Historically, the assessment and management of primary spine tumors have followed general principles of neurosurgery and orthopedics; however, the reluctance of spine surgeons to adopt Enneking's principles of musculoskeletal oncology has largely been overcome in recent years. Nevertheless, it is still common to receive consultations regarding contaminated margins after a poorly conceived excisional biopsy or intralesional resection. It is important to emphasize the correct use of terminology and staging methods inherent to the planning and execution of oncologically sound procedures.[11,14]

Underestimating the Technical Challenges and Functional Sacrifices of Surgery

The management of primary tumors of the spine is challenging. Many are slow growing and may be extensive by the time of presentation (e.g., chordoma, chondrosarcoma), involve complex anatomy, and only partially respond to adjuvant therapies.[2,3,5–8,19,21] Local recurrence of chordoma in particular is difficult to palliate as it often leads to multiple aggressive recurrences, debilitation, and eventual death.[2,8,10,19]

When staging determines that en-bloc excision is the procedure of choice, surgical planning needs to take into account not only the functional sacrifices necessary to achieve the oncological goals, but also the inherent morbidity of surgery and eventual health-related quality of life (HRQOL). Only one study has addressed this issue and found that at a mean follow-up of 3½ years after en-bloc resection for primary bone tumors the Short Form (SF)- 36 mental component score was 51 (essentially normal) and the physical component summary 38.[5]

Chapter Summary

The risk of complications and recurrence is highest after revision surgery. Therefore, the first treatment is a major determinant of outcome.[21] When there is a suspicion of primary spine tumor, referral to an experienced center is recommended, because the surgeon who performs the definitive excision should ideally perform (or at least direct) the biopsy.[1] This ensures that unrelated functional tissue is not contaminated with tumor. Contamination would necessitate the tissue's inclusion in subsequent en-bloc resection—something that would not occur with properly planned biopsy.

Local and systemic staging using Enneking's approach identifies patients who may be cured, or at least have a better chance at long-term disease control and reduced mortality with en-bloc resection. Oncologically sound margins are likely to be achieved when WBB staging determines that it is feasible.[1] However, the adverse-event profile of these surgeries is very high, even at experienced centers. Therefore, we recommend that only experienced, multidisciplinary teams perform them. The need for careful patient selection including detailed preoperative counseling cannot be overstated.

Pearls

- Enneking's principles of oncological staging are valid with respect to primary spine tumors.
- Adequate margins are feasible depending on the surgical staging (WBB system).
- En-bloc resection has a high rate of complications and therefore should only be performed at experienced centers.
- Multidisciplinary tumor boards are necessary to plan and carry out appropriate treatment.
- Biopsy is ideally planned or performed by the surgical oncologist who will ultimately perform the en-bloc resection so that the biopsy tract can be incorporated in the resected specimen.

Pitfalls

♦ A high index of suspicion for primary tumors is necessary to prevent incisional biopsy or intra-lesional resection that could make oncologically sound margins impossible to achieve.
♦ Inconsistent terminology (e.g., "gross total re-section," "radical resection")

♦ Inadequate staging
♦ Inadequate surgical planning (e.g., need for soft tissue coverage)
♦ Underestimating the technical challenges and functional consequences of surgery

References

Five Must-Read References

1. Yamazaki T, McLoughlin GS, Patel S, Rhines LD, Fourney DR. Feasibility and safety of en bloc resection for primary spine tumors: a systematic review by the Spine Oncology Study Group. Spine 2009;34(22, Suppl):S31–S38
2. Boriani S, Bandiera S, Biagini R, et al. Chordoma of the mobile spine: fifty years of experience. Spine 2006; 31:493–503
3. Boriani S, De Iure F, Bandiera S, et al. Chondrosarcoma of the mobile spine: report on 22 cases. Spine 2000;25:804–812
4. Boriani S, Saravanja D, Yamada Y, Varga PP, Biagini R, Fisher CG. Challenges of local recurrence and cure in low grade malignant tumors of the spine. Spine 2009;34(22, Suppl):S48–S57
5. Fisher CG, Keynan O, Boyd MC, Dvorak MF. The surgical management of primary tumors of the spine: initial results of an ongoing prospective cohort study. Spine 2005;30:1899–1908
6. Fisher CG, Saravanja DD, Dvorak MF, et al. Surgical management of primary bone tumors of the spine: validation of an approach to enhance cure and reduce local recurrence. Spine 2011;36:830–836
7. Fourney DR, Rhines LD, Hentschel SJ, et al. En bloc resection of primary sacral tumors: classification of surgical approaches and outcome. J Neurosurg Spine 2005;3:111–122
8. Sundaresan N, Rosen G, Boriani S. Primary malignant tumors of the spine. Orthop Clin North Am 2009; 40:21–36, v v.
9. Bergh P, Kindblom LG, Gunterberg B, Remotti F, Ryd W, Meis-Kindblom JM. Prognostic factors in chordoma of the sacrum and mobile spine: a study of 39 patients. Cancer 2000;88:2122–2134
10. Fourney DR, Gokaslan ZL. Current management of sacral chordoma. Neurosurg Focus 2003;15:E9
11. Boriani S, Weinstein JN, Biagini R. Primary bone tumors of the spine. Terminology and surgical staging. Spine 1997;22:1036–1044
12. Chan P, Boriani S, Fourney DR, et al. An assessment of the reliability of the Enneking and Weinstein-Boriani-Biagini classifications for staging of primary spinal tumors by the Spine Oncology Study Group. Spine 2009;34:384–391
13. Enneking WF, Spanier SS, Goodman MA. A system for the surgical staging of musculoskeletal sarcoma. Clin Orthop Relat Res 1980;153:106–120
14. Enneking WF. A system of staging musculoskeletal neoplasms. Clin Orthop Relat Res 1986;204:9–24
15. Mukherjee D, Chaichana KL, Parker SL, Gokaslan ZL, McGirt MJ. Association of surgical resection and survival in patients with malignant primary osseous spinal neoplasms from the Surveillance, Epidemiology, and End Results (SEER) database. Eur Spine J 2013;22:1375–1382
16. Gwak HS, Yoo HJ, Youn SM, et al. Hypofractionated stereotactic radiation therapy for skull base and upper cervical chordoma and chondrosarcoma: preliminary results. Stereotact Funct Neurosurg 2005; 83:233–243
17. Henderson FC, McCool K, Seigle J, Jean W, Harter W, Gagnon GJ. Treatment of chordomas with Cyber-Knife: Georgetown University experience and treatment recommendations. Neurosurgery 2009;64(2, Suppl):A44–A53
18. Park L, Delaney TF, Liebsch NJ, et al. Sacral chordomas: impact of high-dose proton/photon-beam radiation therapy combined with or without surgery for primary versus recurrent tumor. Int J Radiat Oncol Biol Phys 2006;65:1514–1521
19. Bandiera S, Boriani S, Donthineni R, Amendola L, Cappuccio M, Gasbarrini A. Complications of en bloc resections in the spine. Orthop Clin North Am 2009;40:125–131, vii vii.
20. McDonnell MF, Glassman SD, Dimar JR II, Puno RM, Johnson JR. Perioperative complications of anterior procedures on the spine. J Bone Joint Surg Am 1996; 78:839–847
21. Boriani S, Bandiera S, Donthineni R, et al. Morbidity of en bloc resections in the spine. Eur Spine J 2010; 19:231–241
22. Elwatidy S, Jamjoom Z, Elgamal E, Zakaria A, Turkistani A, El-Dawlatly A. Efficacy and safety of prophylactic large dose of tranexamic acid in spine surgery:

a prospective, randomized, double-blind, placebo-controlled study. Spine 2008;33:2577–2580

23. Lis E, Bilsky MH, Pisinski L, et al. Percutaneous CT-guided biopsy of osseous lesion of the spine in patients with known or suspected malignancy. AJNR Am J Neuroradiol 2004;25:1583–1588

24. Pierot L, Boulin A. Percutaneous biopsy of the thoracic and lumbar spine: transpedicular approach under fluoroscopic guidance. AJNR Am J Neuroradiol 1999;20:23–25

Interventional Options for Primary Tumors of the Spine

Sudhir Kathuria

Introduction

Minimally invasive image-guided interventions have undergone a rapid evolution in the last two decades. Most of this evolution has been technologically driven and has included advances in real-time use of high-resolution imaging during interventions; new and improved embolic agents, bone cements, and catheters; and guidewire technology. Percutaneous techniques are being increasingly utilized in both diagnostic and therapeutic interventions of primary spine tumors. This chapter discusses the interventional techniques of spine biopsy, vertebral augmentation, and preoperative embolization, with an emphasis on how they apply to primary tumors of the spine.

Image-Guided Spine Biopsy

The biopsy represents the final phase of the local workup for a spinal lesion. If primary spinal tumor is in the differential diagnosis, then the physician doing the biopsy should discuss the plan with the spine surgeon coordinating the patient care to ensure that the biopsy tract will not compromise definitive management. Ideally, the biopsy should be performed in the same center that will provide the definitive treatment, and should involve consultation with the musculoskeletal pathologist to consider any special precautions. Percutaneous image-guided spine biopsy is now commonly performed to diagnose a suspected neoplastic process. Compared with open surgical biopsy, it is less invasive and more cost-effective, with an overall lower risk of complications.[1] Determining whether a lesion is benign or malignant and its specific histological type and grade is vital for subsequent management and treatment planning.

The decision to perform a spine biopsy should be made after a thorough analysis of risks and benefits. The general risks of percutaneous spine biopsy include bleeding, injury to vascular or neural structures, and infection. In certain tumors, such as chordoma, disease can spread along the needle tract due to tumor implantation. Increasing use of image guidance and coaxial needle technique has decreased the incidence of these complications. Certain complications are specific to the anatomic structures that are in proximity or along the path of needle placement during the biopsy procedure. Pneumothorax can occur during biopsy of thoracic spine or lesions adjacent to the lung or pleura. Stroke due to injury to the carotid or vertebral artery is a concern when performing cervical spine biopsy.[2]

▦ Patient Preparation

Most spine biopsies can be performed on an outpatient basis using local anesthesia and moderate sedation. General anesthesia may be necessary in certain situations, such as cervical spine biopsy where patient motion is risky, transoral C2 lesion biopsy where intubation is required to avoid aspiration, and some underlying medical conditions.

The patient is generally positioned prone for thoracic or lumbosacral spine biopsy and supine for cervical spine biopsy, except for certain lesions located within the posterior elements for which the prone position may be more appropriate. In certain instances, for example, when a patient has a colostomy or gastrostomy tube and is unable to lie completely prone, biopsy can be performed in the lateral decubitus or semi-prone position. Strict aseptic technique should be used during this procedure to minimize any iatrogenic infections.

▦ Image Guidance

The imaging modalities available for guidance include X-ray fluoroscopy, computed tomography (CT) fluoroscopy, magnetic resonance imaging (MRI); they can be used singly or in combination. The choice of modality is determined by its availability, the size and location of the suspected lesion, and operator preference.

X-ray fluoroscopy has the advantage of being able to visualize and navigate the needle in real time using a two-dimensional projection format. Many simple biopsy procedures can be safely performed using this system. However, it lacks the spatial and soft tissue contrast resolution.

I prefer CT fluoroscopy in most cases as it provides excellent spatial and contrast resolution for precise lesion localization and identification of important intervening structures. This enables the operator to select a safe biopsy needle trajectory to access the target lesion. CT fluoroscopy provides a prompt display of continuously updated images that show the exact needle location in relation to the target lesion and important normal structures in the vicinity. This reduces the risk and significantly shortens the procedure time. CT fluoroscopy is extremely helpful in approaching lesions in anatomically difficult areas.[3]

Magnetic resonance (MR)-guided biopsy procedures can be safely performed in clinical practice. Although CT fluoroscopy currently is the modality of choice, MR guidance provides distinct advantages in certain situations. Most cystic lesions and certain bony lesions such as hemangiomas are better detected on MRI. A major advantage of an MR-guided procedure is the lack of radiation exposure to both patients and physicians, which is especially important in children and pregnant women. Current major limitations of this modality are longer procedure time, higher cost, and limited availability of machine and instruments. However, development of new MRI guidance methods and devices is rapidly evolving.

▦ Biopsy Needle Systems and Technique

There are several commercial biopsy needle systems available. The selection depends on lesion location and whether the lesion is soft tissue, cystic, or osseous in nature. Aspiration biopsy of a cystic or soft tissue lesion can be performed with 25-, 22-, or 20-gauge needles specially designed to aspirate cellular material. Core biopsies are performed using soft tissue cutting needles (16- or 18-gauge) or trephine and beveled tip bone biopsy needles.

We recommend using a coaxial needle technique where only a single guiding needle/cannula pass is made from the skin to the lesion. This technique requires only a single biopsy tract within the soft tissue, thus reducing procedure time and risk of soft tissue injury associated with additional passes. The guiding needle provides access for several biopsy needle passes inside the lesion. This technique also reduces the risk of infiltration of normal tissues with potential tumor cells from the biopsy needle.[2]

Biopsy Approaches for Spine Tumors

The appropriate biopsy approach depends on lesion size, location, and intervening anatomic structures. Thorough knowledge of the anatomy is essential for planning a safe route of access for needle placement. In the cervical spine, the critical anatomic structures include the vertebral and carotid artery, jugular vein, esophagus, trachea, pharynx and hypopharynx, thyroid gland, segmental nerves, and spinal cord. In the thoracic spine anatomic knowledge of the pleura, lung, aorta, radicular arteries, and neurologic structures is critical. In the lumbar spine, the conus and exiting roots, kidneys, bowel, and major blood vessels must all be considered.[4]

Posterior Approach

A posterior approach is generally used for sacral, lumbar, thoracic, and posterior cervical lesions. The patient is placed prone or in the lateral decubitus position. The biopsy needle can enter the vertebral body via a transpedicular (**Fig. 3.1**) or parapedicular approach. Generally the treating surgeon would prefer the biopsy tract to be as close to the midline as possible and to be marked with a suture or dye.

Anterior Approach

Due to smaller pedicle size, an anterior approach is often used for most cervical spine lesions. The needle is inserted adjacent to the medial border of the sternocleidomastoid muscle and advanced between the carotid sheath and neck airways (**Fig. 3.2**). Special attention should be paid to avoid the esophagus and hypopharynx. This procedure should be done with CT fluoroscopy guidance, and intermittent CT images should be obtained to check the needle trajectory.

Transoral Approach

The transoral approach can be very useful for accessing C2 vertebral body lesions. It can also be used to access lesions at adjacent levels including C1 and C3. This approach requires general anesthesia, as intubation is necessary to avoid any aspiration (**Fig. 3.3**). Prophylactic antibiotics should be used with this approach, as it is difficult to create a sterile field along the posterior pharyngeal wall though which the biopsy needle is inserted. This is a relatively

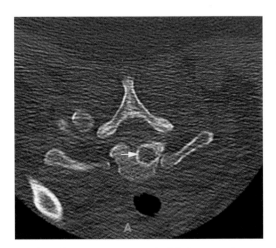

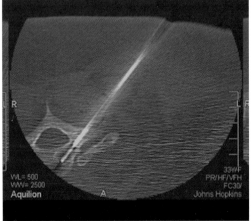

a

b

Fig. 3.1a,b Posterior approach. **(a)** Computed tomography (CT) scan of a patient in the prone position shows a well-defined lytic lesion (*arrow*) in the T1 vertebral body. **(b)** CT-fluoroscopy–guided transpedicular biopsy needle placement from the posterior approach inside the lesion.

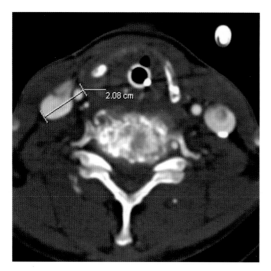
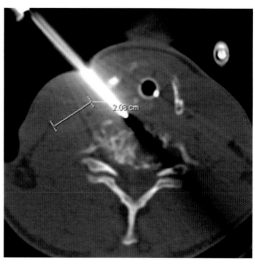

a   b

Fig. 3.2a,b Anterolateral approach. **(a)** Initial planning CT scan of a patient with an abnormal C5 lesion with a prevertebral component. The measurement bar shows the width of vascular compartment at the level of the planned needle path. **(b)** CT-fluoroscopy image shows a biopsy

needle inserted through the medial part of the sternocleidomastoid muscle and advanced between the airway and the carotid sheath inside the lesion. Note the use of the measurement bar to avoid needle injury to the carotid artery.

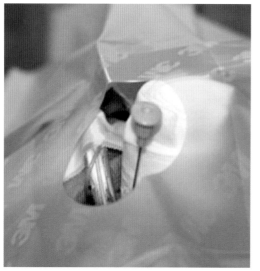
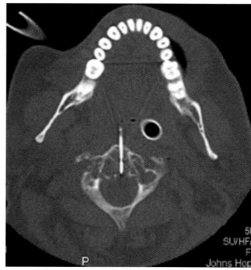

a   b

Fig. 3.3a,b Transoral approach. **(a)** Close-up view of the intubation tube and transoral biopsy needle inserted through an open mouth. Note the gauze roll

used to keep the mouth open. **(b)** CT-fluoroscopy image shows the biopsy needle tip inside the lesion.

safe approach, as no important structures lie between the posterior pharyngeal wall and the bone.[5]

Postprocedure Care

Direct compression is applied at the puncture site for about 5 to 10 minutes to achieve hemostasis. This is followed by placement of sterile dressing on the puncture site and adjacent skin. The patient should be kept in the recovery area for 1 to 2 hours to watch for any bleeding; to assess pain, weakness, and dizziness; and to monitor the general vital signs. The patient is discharged with a medication prescription and a contact number to reach a physician if any complications arise.

▨ Vertebral Augmentation for Spine Tumors and Pathological Fractures

Vertebral augmentation is a minimally invasive procedure primarily utilized for treating back pain associated with a vertebral compression fractures. This procedure was first introduced as a technique for the treatment of symptomatic vertebral hemangioma in 1987.[6] Since that time, it has become a valuable and frequently used therapeutic option in the management of back pain caused by osteoporotic and pathological fractures.

The fundamental goal of a vertebral augmentation procedure is to stabilize and improve the compressive strength of the vertebral body through the safe injection of stabilizing material. This can be achieved by both vertebroplasty and kyphoplasty. Vertebroplasty involves the injection of special bone cement inside the fractured vertebra using a needle under image guidance, generally X-ray or CT-fluoroscopy. There are several bone cements available, but the most commonly used is acrylic polymer polymethylmethacrylate (PMMA). Kyphoplasty, in comparison with vertebroplasty, involves an additional step of creating a cavity inside the diseased vertebral body by inflating a balloon

followed by injection of the bone cement in the cavity.

Patient Selection

Malignant lesions can spread to the spinal column by hematogenous, lymphatic, perineural, or direct extension.[7] Pain arises from cortical erosion, fracture, or impingement on the nerve roots or spinal cord. There are various treatment options that depend on the underlying nature of the disease and include surgery, medical therapy, radiation therapy, or a combination of them. Vertebral augmentation is now playing an increasing role in this patient population.

The decision regarding therapy should be made by a multidisciplinary team taking into consideration the nature and extent of the disease, the medical condition of the patient, the response to prior therapy, and the patient's life expectancy. The goal of vertebral augmentation in pathological fractures is to improve pain and structural stability of the bone. Radiation therapy is effective in many cases, but if there is spinal instability present, pain relief will not occur with radiation alone as there is no immediate bone strengthening.[8] Vertebral augmentation can be a good therapeutic option by itself or can be combined with radiation and surgical therapy.

Absolute contraindications for vertebral augmentation include ongoing local or systemic infection, compressive myelopathy secondary to retropulsed bone fragment or tumor, and any uncorrectable coagulopathy. Relative contraindications unique to pathological fractures depend on the operator expertise and the tools available.

Severely compressed vertebral bodies with epidural tumor extension are technically difficult to treat and may be made worse with injection of PMMA. Some of these cases can be treated by an experienced operator using a plasma-mediated tumor ablation system to first create a cavity within the tumor, followed by judicious PMMA cement injection.[9] The use of CT-fluoroscopy with excellent spatial and contrast resolution can be very useful in such cases, as they require precise needle placement and close monitoring of PMMA cement injection.

Preprocedural Imaging

Cross-sectional imaging, including MRI and CT, is extremely useful for identifying the location and extent of the disease. It also provides useful information about any canal or neural compromise. CT in particular is very helpful in demonstrating osseous destruction that can be a potential route of cement extravasation and for assessing transpedicular access.

Tools, Technique, and Special Considerations

A variety of disposable vertebroplasty and kyphoplasty needles are available. Needles range in sizes from 8 to 13 gauge. Smaller size 15-gauge needles are also available and more suitable for cervical spine. Several PMMA-based stabilizing agents with different characteristics are commercially available that can be used for vertebral augmentation.

The basic principles and techniques of safe needle placement described earlier in the spine biopsy section also apply to vertebral augmentation. A posterolateral approach is generally preferred for lumbar and thoracic spine lesions. Special attention should be paid to avoid breaking medial and inferior borders of the pedicles. Breach of these cortical walls can result in needle entry into the spinal canal or neural foramen, with potential injury to the spinal cord or to nerves. For cervical spine lesions, anterolateral approach is generally more suitable. For lesions within the C2 vertebral body, a transoral route may be more favorable.

The needle is advanced using continuous or intermittent fluoroscopy until the tip is placed in desired location, generally in the anterior part of the tumor. Most injection devices that are available are self-contained systems, with a reservoir into which the PMMA cement is filled. This device is then connected with the needle and the PMMA can be injected in a controlled fashion by rotation or trigger mechanism (**Fig. 3.4**). PMMA should be injected in small boluses with close attention to any leakage beyond the confines of the vertebral body, especially into pulmonary veins, epidural veins,

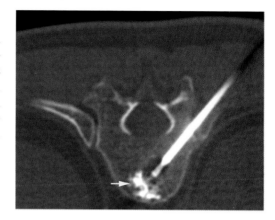

Fig. 3.4 CT fluoroscopy image obtained during vertebroplasty treatment for a painful hemangioma. Note the white dense PMMA cement material (*arrow*) inside the lesion.

the central canal, or the neural foramen. A small leak through end-plate fractures may be acceptable, but a large amount of leakage within the disk space may increase the future risk of adjacent fracture.[10] If the PMMA preferentially flows to undesirable areas, the needle can be repositioned, and the material already injected is allowed to harden. A coaxial technique is very helpful in such instances, as the cement-injecting needle can be taken out while keeping the access needle in place. This allows the cement already injected in the body to harden faster, as it is exposed to a body temperature that is higher than room temperature. Injection is then resumed in few minutes, with expectation of PMMA cement now filling in the desirable area. If the PMMA continues to flow in undesirable areas, further injection should be stopped.

Another useful tool that can allow safe injection of PMMA is plasma-mediated ablation. This can be especially helpful in treating lesions with posterior cortical disruption and large epidural extensions. Such lesions carry a higher risk of potential extraosseous extension of PMMA cement. The bipolar plasma-mediated radiofrequency-based device can be advanced through the vertebroplasty needle and placed inside the lesion. A plasma field is then created that has sufficient energy to dissolve soft tissue into molecules at relatively low temperature (40° to 70°C). This molecular dissociation converts the ablated tissue into gases that leave the body via the cannula.[11] Using this process, a cavity can be created inside the desired portion of the lesion with preferential flow of subsequently injected PMMA material into this void due to low resistance.

Postprocedure CT imaging should be routinely obtained in pathological fractures. This provides useful baseline information about the distribution of PMMA and demonstrates any suspected or unsuspected complications including cement leakage, changes in tumor position, procedure-related hematoma, and fracture.

Complications

The complication rates in various major series are 1.3% for osteoporosis, 2.5% for hemangiomas, and 10% for neoplastic disease.[12] The primary cause of a symptomatic complication is the leakage of cement beyond the confines of vertebral body. The cement can leak into epidural and paravertebral venous plexus or in adjacent spaces via existing fracture lines or cortical destruction. More often than not, small PMMA leakages are asymptomatic. However, PMMA material located within the epidural veins or foraminal veins can cause spinal cord or nerve root compression. A significant neurologic compromise may require immediate surgical intervention. Migration of small amounts of PMMA to the pulmonary veins is generally not clinically significant, but symptomatic pulmonary embolus and death have been reported.[12] Leakage within the disk space can increase the future risk of adjacent level fractures. Other complications include vascular or neural injuries from improper needle technique, iatrogenic fracture, infection, hematoma, and pneumothorax.[10]

Complications are best avoided by awareness of the factors that contribute to their occurrence. Following meticulous needle placement technique, close monitoring, and avoiding excessive amounts of PMMA injection especially in pathological fractures are strongly suggested.

▣ Preoperative and Therapeutic Embolization

Surgery of hypervascular spine tumors can be associated with significant blood loss and increased transfusion requirements. Excessive bleeding during surgery also prolongs operative time and increases complexity. Spinal tumor embolization is performed before the surgery to reduce intraoperative bleeding. By reducing intraoperative bleeding, it improves visualization of the operative field and reduces operation time.[13] Tumor embolization can also be used as palliative therapy for certain unresectable tumors. It reduces the mass effect on spinal cord or nerves by causing tumor necrosis and shrinkage. However, one should be aware of the possibility of immediate postembolization worsening of the mass effect due to edema that requires judicious use of short-term steroids. Curative embolization is occasionally used in patients with certain benign primary tumors, such as aneurysmal bone cysts and atypical hemangiomas.[14]

Preprocedural Imaging

An understanding of normal vascular anatomy, abnormal tumor feeding vessels, and potentially dangerous anastomoses is essential in performing safe and effective embolization of the vascular spinal tumors. Preprocedure cross-sectional imaging is necessary for appropriate planning of spinal angiography and embolization. Contrast-enhanced CT and MRI are very helpful in determining the location and full extent of the tumor.

Spinal Angiography

High-quality digital subtraction angiography is essential for the identification of the tumor feeding vessels and for localizing radiculomedullary arteries potentially contributing to the artery of Adamkiewicz. This procedure generally can be performed under moderate sedation. General anesthesia is used for children or uncooperative patients.

An arterial vascular sheath is first placed within the common femoral artery that provides vascular access for the procedure. Depending on the tumor level and intended therapy, certain vessels need to be selectively catheterized to better evaluate the blood supply and pertinent flow dynamics.

For the cervical and upper thoracic spine tumors, the vertebral artery, thyrocervical trunk, costocervical trunk, and superior intercostal arteries are selectively catheterized and evaluated. In addition, external and internal carotid arteries are evaluated for any blood supply and potentially dangerous anastomosis during embolization. For the lower thoracic and lumbar spine lesions, bilateral segmental arteries at the level of tumor as well as two adjacent segments above and below are evaluated. In addition, internal iliac, iliolumbar, lateral, and median sacral arteries are evaluated for lower lumbar and sacral lesions.[14]

The catheter is selectively placed inside each vessel under study, 3 to 5 mL of nonionic iodinated contrast is injected by hand, and real-time digital subtraction images are obtained. Tumor blush with the origin of tumor-feeding vessels and any associated radiculomedullary arteries

are evaluated. It is critical to identify anterior and posterior spinal arteries and their contributors to avoid unintentional embolization of these important arteries that can cause spinal cord stroke. A cone-beam volume study that can now be obtained with C-arm digital angiography system can provide more detailed anatomic information about the tumor-feeding arteries and potential contributors to the spinal arteries.

Embolization Procedure

The goal of tumor embolization is to selectively occlude the tumor-feeding arteries by delivering embolic agent. It is even more important not to embolize any vessel that can jeopardize normal function. The tumor-feeding arteries are selectively catheterized using a 3-French (F) microcatheter advanced through a 5F or 6F diagnostic catheter in coaxial fashion. A high-quality magnified preembolization angiogram is obtained to further delineate the tumor-feeding artery and to confirm that there are no branches contributing to the spinal artery (**Fig. 3.5**). This preembolization angiogram also provides important information about the rate at which

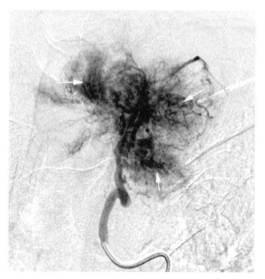
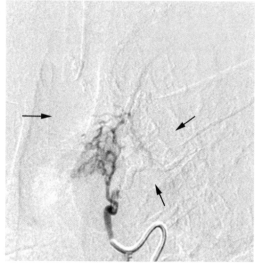

a

b

Fig. 3.5a,b Preoperative tumor embolization of a hypervascular spine tumor. **(a)** Selective angiogram of the radiculomedullary artery with a dense tumor blush (*arrows*). **(b)** Postembolization angiogram of the same vessel demonstrates occlusion of the tumor feeding arteries. Note the lack of contrast in the areas of tumor blush present in the preembolization angiogram (*arrows*).

the embolic material can be injected without any reflux into the normal circulation. If the tumor-feeding vessels are too small to be selectively catheterized, microcoils can be placed in the segmental artery beyond the origin of tumor vessels. This provides a preferential blood flow into the tumor vessels. The embolization agent is then delivered proximal to the origin of tumor vessels, and the preferential blood flow carries the embolic agent into the tumor vessels.

The commonly used agents for embolization include polyvinyl alcohol (PVA) particles, trisacryl microspheres, liquid N-butyl cyanoacrylate (NBCA), ethyl-vinyl alcohol copolymer (EVOH) onyx, Gelfoam pledgets, and microcoils. For optimal tumor embolization, the embolic agent should penetrate the tumor capillary bed and cause permanent vascular occlusion. Coils by themselves are not effective, as they occlude only the proximal tumor vessels, and tumor can rapidly recruit new blood supply from intersegmental collaterals. However, coils can play a useful role by providing preferential flow away from uninvolved distal vessels and dangerous intersegmental anastomoses.[13]

Liquid agents such as alcohol, NBCA, and onyx can provide rapid and permanent embolization, but their use requires experience and great technical expertise. Ethanol causes extensive tumor necrosis due to intimal sclerosis and intense inflammatory response. Selective catheterization and careful, slow infusion is required to avoid any reflux and complications with this agent. NBCA rapidly polymerizes into a solid material as it comes in contact with blood or saline. This requires fast, continuous, and precise injection for optimal embolization.[15] In contrast, onyx can be injected slowly and provides deeper penetration, with the ability to occlude multiple vessels from a single catheterization. Particulate agents are the most commonly used and are very effective for tumor embolization.[16] The ideal agent should be non-biodegradable with a size and shape that enable it to achieve distal penetration into tumor vessels and cause permanent occlusion. Smaller particles have better penetration into the tumor vessels. However, very small particles, especially of sizes less than 100 μm, have a higher risk of causing spinal cord ischemia and soft tissue necrosis. Generally, particles of sizes 300 to 500 μm are preferred and can provide adequate embolization with a lower risk of ischemic complications.[17]

Embolization can be risky if tumor-feeding vessels are arising from the same or an adjacent radiculomedullary artery that is also supplying the spinal artery. If there is sufficient distance between the two and the tumor-feeding vessels are distal to the origin of the radiculomedullary artery, one can judiciously attempt embolization by selectively catheterizing the feeding artery. The procedure should be immediately terminated on any suspicion of reflux of embolization material into the radiculomedullary artery or any change in neurologic status of the patient.

Embolization of cervical spine tumors is more technically challenging because of complex arterial anatomy. Selective catheterization of tumor-feeding arteries is critical to avoid brain and spinal cord stroke. If one is unable to selectively catheterize the tumor-feeding vessels, a temporary balloon can be inflated distally in the vertebral or carotid artery to avoid any intracranial reflux of the embolization material.

If there is tumor encasement of the vertebral or carotid artery, permanent occlusion of the artery using coils or detachable balloon enables en-bloc surgical resection. A balloon test occlusion is performed before proceeding with permanent occlusion to determine if the patient can tolerate such a procedure. During the balloon test occlusion, the main artery is temporarily occluded by inflating a balloon inside the lumen followed by appropriate neurologic testing to evaluate its effect. The parent artery can be sacrificed with relatively low risk if the patient does not develop any neurologic deficits during the temporary occlusion of the artery, including certain provocative measures such as reducing blood pressure during the temporary occlusion.[18]

A complete neurologic examination should be performed before and immediately after the embolization procedure to identify any complications. After embolization, patients are admitted to the intensive care unit for close monitoring of their neurologic status. Post-embolization necrosis and inflammatory response can cause tumor swelling and spinal cord compression. Short-term steroids are generally used to minimize this. Some patients experience the self-limiting postembolization syndrome, characterized by nausea, vomiting, low-grade fever, and pain. It can generally be managed with conservative therapy.

The embolization is ideally performed from 24 to 72 hours before the surgical resection to allow time for maximal thrombosis of the occluded vessels and to prevent any recanalization or recruitment of new blood supply via collaterals. In some cases where there is cord compression, it may be prudent to do surgery on the same day, after the embolization, to avoid worsening of compression due to tumor necrosis and swelling.[19]

Many studies have shown that intraoperative blood loss is significantly less in patients who underwent preoperative embolization than in those who did not. Additional benefits include shorter operating time and a reduced need for blood transfusion. There is evidence that a complete embolization results in significantly less intraoperative blood loss than an incomplete embolization. Complete embolization can generally be achieved in 50 to 86% of patients with spinal tumors.[20] Common causes of incomplete embolization include the presence of the adjacent radiculomedullary artery supplying the spinal artery, difficult anatomy precluding selective catheterization of feeding arteries, and dissection of the feeding arteries from the guidewire or catheter, limiting the access for embolization.

Embolization of a spinal tumor can occasionally be used as the primary therapeutic treatment. Certain benign tumors such as aggressive hemangiomas and aneurysmal bone cysts may respond to serial embolization. Palliative embolization can be used in patients with unresectable spinal tumors.

The most catastrophic complication of spinal tumor embolization is spinal cord and brain stroke. The other possible complications include paresthesias, transient paraparesis, and cord compression due to tumor necrosis and edema.

A high-quality diagnostic angiogram and careful evaluation of a preembolization angiogram is critical to identify and avoid embolization of radiculomedullary arteries contributing to spinal artery. Frequent angiograms should be obtained during the embolization procedure to identify any new collateral pathways that were not visible on the preembolization angiogram.

▓ Chapter Summary

Image-guided biopsy has emerged as a safe, effective, and accurate tool for the definitive diagnosis of spine tumors. In many institutions, it has become the first test in establishing the definitive diagnosis and has better patient tolerance, lower morbidity, and lower cost than conventional open surgical biopsy. Vertebroplasty and kyphoplasty are percutaneous vertebral augmentation procedures available for the treatment of painful tumor and associated pathological fractures. The primary goal of these procedures is to reduce pain and improve structurally stability. The clinical outcome of a vertebral augmentation procedure performed for spine tumors depends not only on the skills of the surgeon but also on the appropriate utilization of available tools and injectable materials. The judicious combined use of plasma-mediated ablation with vertebroplasty and thorough knowledge of the cement properties improves the safety and efficacy of these procedures. Preoperative embolization of vascular tumors of the spine significantly reduces intraoperative blood loss. A detailed understanding of the vascular anatomy of the spine is essential for safe and effective embolization. The recent development of newer embolic agents and improved imaging equipment enable a more complete devascularization of tumors.

As with any surgical procedure, interventional procedures are not without their complications. A thorough knowledge of anatomy and wise selection of the tools is crucial to the success of the procedure. Integration of image-guided interventions into a multidisciplinary team of experienced surgeons, radiation and medical oncologists, and pathologists is important for ensuring optimal patient care.

- ◆ Image-guided needle biopsy has become the definitive test in assessing spine tumors and has lower morbidity, better patient tolerance, and lower cost than open surgical biopsy.
- ◆ Knowledge of anatomy and available tools is crucial to the success of the procedure. Technique should be discussed with the treating surgeon. Proper technique and selection of the imaging guidance system are often key to obtaining adequate diagnostic biopsy samples.
- ◆ Coaxial biopsy technique in appropriate anatomic planes should be followed to avoid further spread of disease.
- ◆ The goal of vertebral augmentation procedure in pathological fractures is to improve pain and structural stability of the bone through the safe injection of stabilizing material.
- ◆ Plasma-mediated tumor ablation is a useful tool in tumors with large epidural extension to create

a cavity in the tumor that allows for judicious use of PMMA injection.
- ◆ Preoperative embolization of hypervascular tumors results in significant reduced intraoperative blood loss, shorter operating time, and less transfusion requirement.

- ◆ Complications are best avoided by awareness of the factors that contribute to their occurrence. Following meticulous needle placement technique, close monitoring, and avoiding an excessive amount of cement, especially in pathological fractures, are strongly recommended.
- ◆ A high-quality diagnostic spinal angiogram and careful evaluation of the preembolization angiogram are critical to identify and avoid embolization of any branches contributing to spinal artery.
- ◆ Frequent angiograms should be obtained during particle embolization procedure to identify any new collateral pathways that may not be visible on preembolization angiogram.

References

Five Must-Read References

1. Kornblum MB, Wesolowski DP, Fischgrund JS, Herkowitz HN. Computed tomography-guided biopsy of the spine. A review of 103 patients. Spine 1998;23: 81–85
2. Yaffe D, Greenberg G, Leitner J, Gipstein R, Shapiro M, Bachar GN. CT-guided percutaneous biopsy of thoracic and lumbar spine: A new coaxial technique. AJNR Am J Neuroradiol 2003;24:2111–2113
3. Rimondi E, Staals EL, Errani C, et al. Percutaneous CT-guided biopsy of the spine: results of 430 biopsies. Eur Spine J 2008;17:975–981
4. Tampieri D, Weill A, Melanson D, Ethier R. Percutaneous aspiration biopsy in cervical spine lytic lesions. Indications and technique. Neuroradiology 1991;33: 43–47
5. Gupta S, Henningsen JA, Wallace MJ, et al. Percutaneous biopsy of head and neck lesions with CT guidance: various approaches and relevant anatomic and technical considerations. Radiographics 2007; 27:371–390
6. Jensen ME, Evans AJ, Mathis JM, Kallmes DF, Cloft HJ, Dion JE. Percutaneous polymethylmethacrylate vertebroplasty in the treatment of osteoporotic vertebral body compression fractures: technical aspects. AJNR Am J Neuroradiol 1997;18:1897–1904

7. Barr JD, Barr MS, Lemley TJ, McCann RM. Percutaneous vertebroplasty for pain relief and spinal stabilization. Spine 2000;25:923–928
8. Janjan NA. Radiation for bone metastases: conventional techniques and the role of systemic radiopharmaceuticals. Cancer 1997;80(8, Suppl):1628–1645
9. Georgy BA, Wong W. Plasma-mediated radiofrequency ablation assisted percutaneous cement injection for treating advanced malignant vertebral compression fractures. AJNR Am J Neuroradiol 2007; 28:700–705
10. Lin EP, Ekholm S, Hiwatashi A, Westesson PL. Vertebroplasty: cement leakage into the disc increases the risk of new fracture of adjacent vertebral body. AJNR Am J Neuroradiol 2004;25:175–180
11. Pearce JA. Electrosurgery. New York: Wiley Medical, 1986
12. Murphy KJ, Deramond H. Percutaneous vertebroplasty in benign and malignant disease. Neuroimaging Clin N Am 2000;10:535–545
13. Berkefeld J, Scale D, Kirchner J, Heinrich T, Kollath J. Hypervascular spinal tumors: influence of the embolization technique on perioperative hemorrhage. AJNR Am J Neuroradiol 1999;20:757–763

14. Ozkan E, Gupta S. Embolization of spinal tumors: vascular anatomy, indications, and technique. Tech Vasc Interv Radiol 2011;14:129–140

15. Mindea SA, Eddleman CS, Hage ZA, Batjer HH, Ondra SL, Bendok BR. Endovascular embolization of a recurrent cervical giant cell neoplasm using N-butyl 2-cyanoacrylate. J Clin Neurosci 2009;16:452–454

16. Gore P, Theodore N, Brasiliense L, et al. The utility of onyx for preoperative embolization of cranial and spinal tumors. Neurosurgery 2008;62:1204–1211, discussion 1211–1212

17. Bendszus M, Klein R, Burger R, Warmuth-Metz M, Hofmann E, Solymosi L. Efficacy of trisacryl gelatin microspheres versus polyvinyl alcohol particles in the preoperative embolization of meningiomas. AJNR Am J Neuroradiol 2000;21:255–261

18. Bernstein A, Lasjunias P, TerBrugge KG. Tumors of the spinal column and spinal cord. In: Surgical Neuroangiography, vol 2. Berlin: Springer, 2004:874–877

19. Kai Y, Hamada J, Morioka M, Yano S, Todaka T, Ushio Y. Appropriate interval between embolization and surgery in patients with meningioma. AJNR Am J Neuroradiol 2002;23:139–142

20. Prabhu VC, Bilsky MH, Jambhekar K, et al. Results of preoperative embolization for metastatic spinal neoplasms. J Neurosurg 2003;98(2, Suppl):156–164

4

Radiation Therapy for Primary Bone Tumors

Brent Y. Kimball and Yoshiya (Josh) Yamada

▓ Introduction

Primary malignant bone tumors of the spine present significant treatment challenges with regard to achieving local tumor control while preserving neurologic function. The most common primary tumors involving the spinal column are chordomas, chondrosarcomas, and osteogenic sarcomas. Significant advances in both surgery and radiation are redefining their roles in the treatment of these lesions. Advanced surgical techniques for en-bloc resection of primary spine tumors improves the ability to achieve marginal or wide curative resections[1-3]; however, many tumors are not amenable to en-bloc resection. Conventionally fractionated radiotherapy is frequently used as an adjuvant to surgery. In most cases, conventional external beam radiation is not an effective primary therapy for many primary spine tumors. The poor long-term outcomes after conventional radiation therapy is likely related to the relatively low dose of radiation that can be given near the spinal cord. Concern about spinal cord tolerance has typically limited radiation doses to less than 54 Gy in standard fractions.[4,5] Low-dose areas within the irradiated field are the most likely to result in disease recurrence.[6]

Three radiation techniques are currently being used to increase the dose to the tumor while sparing normal tissue tolerance in an attempt to treat primary spine tumors: particle

beam treatment, such as proton beam therapy; brachytherapy; and high-dose conformal photon therapy, such as image-guided intensity-modulated radiation therapy (IMRT) or stereotactic radiosurgery (SRS). Although class 1 evidence is lacking, mounting research demonstrates the contribution of high-dose radiation to achieve local tumor control for various spine tumor pathologies. Recently, the ability to deliver SRS using image-guided IMRT has proven useful in the neoadjuvant and postoperative setting.

▓ Surgery

The role of en-bloc resection to achieve a marginal or wide resection is well established for extremity sarcomas.[7-9] Over the past 10 years, spine surgeons have developed techniques for en-bloc resection of primary spine tumors that improves cure rates compared with piecemeal, curettage techniques. These techniques are safe for patients with isolated vertebral body or posterior element disease. Boriani et al[10] published a surgical series regarding en-bloc spondylectomy for low-grade chondrosarcoma of the mobile spine in 22 patients. Of the 12 patients who underwent en-bloc excision, 9 (75%) maintained local control at a median follow-up of 81 months (range, 2 to 236 months). Of the three recurrences, two had contaminated margins at surgery from epidural disease. The remaining 10 patients underwent curettage resection and by definition had intralesional resections with positive histological margins. At a median follow-up of 36 months, the recurrence rate was 100%, and 80% died of disease.[10] Of note, in this group, three patients received conventional-dose external beam radiation and no patients received high-dose conformal radiation with proton beams or image-guided IMRT.

Although curative resections are feasible in some patients, many patients present with factors that may preclude en-bloc resection that achieves negative histological margins. En-bloc resection of the isolated vertebral body or posterior elements is technically feasible. However, according to the Weinstein–Boriani–Biagini (WBB) classification,[11] patients who present with epidural tumor, multilevel large paraspinal masses, or circumferential bone disease are not candidates for marginal or wide excisions (i.e., en bloc with negative margins). The feasibility of achieving a wide or marginal excision is limited by the risk of neurologic or adjacent structure injury. For example, resecting the dura en bloc with a specimen could possibly provide a margin on epidural tumor. Unfortunately, the loss of spinal fluid buffering the spinal cord increases the probability of injury to the spinal cord and complications of cerebrospinal fluid (CSF) leak. If tumor is spilled during resection, there seems to be a higher probability of intradural seeding as well.[12] In a series of 59 spine sarcomas reviewed using the radiographic criteria established by the WBB classification, approximately 15% of patients were candidates for en-bloc excisions that could achieve a wide or marginal margins. As noted in extremity sarcomas, once the tumor is violated, the risk of recurrence significantly increases.[7] However, the treatment of sarcomas at other sites has demonstrated the utility of adjuvant high-dose radiation in the setting of microscopic or gross residual disease post resection.[13]

▨ Radiation Therapy

Radiation therapy is an extremely important modality in the treatment of primary spine tu-mors. However, the relative radioresistance of these tumors requires doses well above spinal cord tolerance for durable local tumor control. From the paradigm of extremity sarcomas, radiation doses of greater than 60 Gy in 2-Gy fractions are required for control of positive microscopic margins and greater than 70 Gy for gross residual disease.[14] Traditional concepts of spinal cord tolerance using conventional radiation techniques establishes the $TD_{5/5}$ (the tolerance dose at which there is a 5% probability of a complication within 5 years) at 50 Gy in 1.2- to 2-Gy fractions above which there appears to be a significantly increased risk of developing radiation myelitis.[15] Toxicity to the spinal cord may also be associated with the length of cord irradiated. In addition to the spinal cord, toxicities to paraspinal structures, such as the bowel, the kidneys, and the esophagus, need to be considered. Unfortunately, the radiation tolerances of these organs range from 23 to 60 Gy. Thus, technologies and techniques that minimize the radiation dose to critical organs and allow high dose to the tumor are essential for meaningful radiation treatment of spine malignancies.

Proton Beam

Advances in radiation technology, including the introduction of hadrons (high-dose protons or charged particles, including carbon ions, helium, or neon), have led to higher doses of radiation being delivered to the target volume with reduced tissue injury and improved radiobiological effect.[16] There are many important similarities as well as differences between IMRT and proton beam radiotherapy. The rationale for using proton beams is the excellent dose distribution at the tumor target and virtually no exit dose beyond the target volume. The Bragg peak phenomenon characteristic of proton beam radiation results in an extremely steep dose falloff that can be measured over a course of millimeters (**Fig. 4.1**).

The biological impact of proton beam treatment and IMRT is relatively minor. The conversion factor commonly used to compare the effectiveness of proton beam treatment with photon radiotherapy is 1.1. Thus, 1 Gy of proton

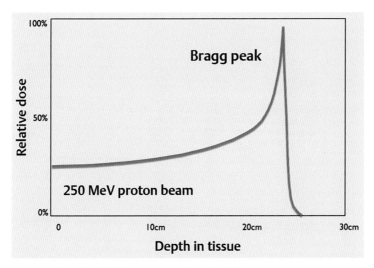

Fig. 4.1 The Bragg peak effect for 250-MeV protons. Note that there is no dose at a depth beyond the Bragg peak.

radiation is biologically equivalent to 1.1 Gy of radiation from a cobalt source, or 1.1 cobalt gray equivalents (CGE). The advantage of proton beam treatment does not lie in an enhanced effect of protons against tumor cells. Rather, the advantage lies primarily in the lack of exit dose after the Bragg peak (**Fig. 4.2**). If the Bragg peak occurs just before the spinal cord, then the spinal cord receives minimal radiation dose, in stark contrast to photon radiation, for which exit dose is significant. If manipulated properly, proton beams can deliver higher doses to a tumor in close proximity to the spinal cord while exposing the spinal cord to minimal radiation doses. IMRT always delivers higher radiation dose to spinal cord adjacent to a spinal tumor, because there is no Bragg peak effect with photons, and some photons will pass through the tumor into the spinal cord. IMRT can deliver radiation dose to the tumor up to what is considered the cord tolerance.

In most cases, doses of up to 74 Gy can be given to a vertebral body tumor while limiting the spinal cord to 50 to 54 Gy. Thus, IMRT is able to deliver similarly high doses of radiation to the tumor, but the spinal cord doses are potentially lower with the use of proton beams.[17] Proton beam radiation has a distinct disadvantage in patients with implanted spinal fixation hardware. The greater density of metallic im-

plants can affect the range of protons up to 10 mm and the dose greater than 10% in the high-dose region.[18] When the spinal cord may only be a few millimeters away from the high-dose region, the uncertainties associated with titanium implants are unacceptable. Monte Carlo simulation techniques are necessary to obtain accurate dosimetry in the setting of spinal instrumentation. On the other hand, photon radiation and IMRT dosimetry are minimally impacted by surgical hardware.

Heavy ions such as carbon ions provide biological, in addition to physical, advantages compared with photons or protons, in terms of their high relative biological effectiveness and reduced oxygen-enhancement ratio in the tumor region.[19] Hypofractionated carbon ion therapy is a promising treatment approach for large sacral chordomas.[20]

There has been considerable experience with the treatment of neuraxis tumors using proton beams to deliver fractionated therapy. Proton beam radiotherapy's main limitation is the high cost of building and maintaining such facilities. The cost/benefit ratio of proton beam treatment is extremely controversial, but the cost of proton therapy is expected to decrease rapidly. Currently it is approximately twice as expensive as IMRT.[21] Excellent results for uveal melanoma have been reported using proton

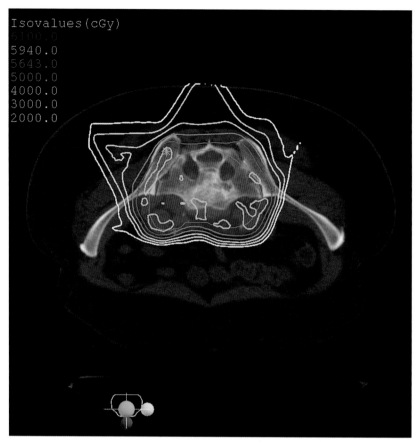

Isovalues(cGy)
6100.0
5940.0
5643.0
5000.0
4000.0
3000.0
2000.0

Fig. 4.2 Axial proton beam dose distribution for a sacral lesion entering posteriorly. Note the lack of exit dose into the pelvis.

beam therapy in a hypofractionated manner (median dose 70 CGE in five fractions),[22] but data reporting the use of single-fraction radiation with proton beam therapy for the management of tumors of the neuraxis is lacking.

Proton-beam therapy combined with wide en-bloc excision is the accepted treatment standard in the management of chordomas at a number of cancer centers, especially in patients with a primary tumor as opposed to disease recurrence.[16]

Hug[23] reported radiation results from 47 patients with primary or recurrent osteogenic and chondrogenic tumors treated with combined proton/photon therapy. The 5-year local control rates were 53% for chordoma, 50% for osteogenic sarcoma, and 100% for chondrosarcoma.[23] Of the six failures, five were in field recurrences and one out of field. A trend was

noted toward improved local tumor control in patients receiving greater than 77 CGE. The failures were seen primarily in patients with less than 77 CGE delivered to the tumor volume.

Austin et al[6] reported a case series of 141 patients treated for chordoma and chondrosarcoma of the skull base and cervical spine, using mixed proton/photon beam therapy at a median of 69 CGE. At a median follow-up of 3 years, 26 failures were noted. Of these failures, 23% received the prescribed tumoral dose. However, 77% of failures occurred in areas that received less than the prescribed tumoral dose, the majority of which were in regions constrained by normal tissue tolerance. All tumors that failed in the high-dose region had volumes greater than 75 cc. Patients with cervical spine disease had a higher rate of recurrence (10 of 26) and larger tumors (average volume of 102 cc) than those with base of skull disease (16 of 115) with an average volume of 63 cc. These studies underscores the challenges of delivering uniformity of prescribed dose and the treatment of large-volume tumors in close proximity to dose-limiting neural structures.[6]

Intensity-Modulated Radiation Therapy

Total doses in excess of 70 Gy can be routinely administered to paraspinal tumors using photon IMRT techniques while maintaining spinal cord doses at the same level achieved with proton beams (**Fig. 4.3**). Typically, five to seven radiation beams are utilized around a single isocenter. An inverse treatment planning algorithm is used to assign target doses to target volumes, and penalties are given to excessive doses to avoidance organs at risk. Multiple iterations of the number of beams, beam angles, and beam energies are utilized to arrive at a best possible solution that meets the dose goals for the target volumes and dose-sensitive nearby organs. Each individual beam intensity is modulated during treatment in a way that the sum total of all the beams results in a dose cloud that conforms to the three-dimensional characteristics of the target volume and typically requires very high dose gradients near the spinal canal and esophagus, in the case of cervical and thoracic lesions. Kidneys and bowel loops are common avoidance structures in the lumbar spine.

At Memorial Sloan-Kettering Cancer Center (MSKCC), we have reported the use of high-dose IMRT for the management of primary malignancies of the mobile spine. The actuarial

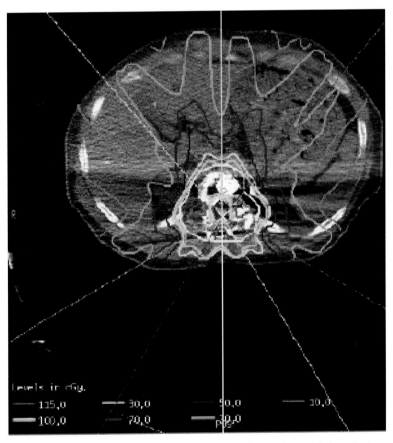

Fig. 4.3 Dose distribution for a T11 osteosarcoma that is circumferential around the spinal canal. The prescribed dose was 72 Gy and the maximum dose to the spinal cord was 54 Gy.

local control was found to be 75%, with follow-up extending to a maximum of 40 months. No patient experienced myelitis. The median dose was 6,600 cGy (range, 5,400–7,200 cGy).[24] We have treated seven chordomas and five chondrosarcomas, two of which were highgrade and the remaining intermediate or low grade. At a median follow-up of 18 months, the local control rate for chordomas was 86% and for chondrosarcomas was 80%, with the single failure occurring in a high-grade patient. The follow-up is too short to draw meaningful conclusions, but fractionated therapy using image-guided IMRT is possible at doses similar to those reported for proton beam therapy.[25]

Brachytherapy

Brachytherapy has also been used to treat primary tumors. Iodine 125 has commonly been used to treat positive microscopic disease or minimal residual gross disease following tumor resection. Good results have been reported in the treatment of paraspinal tumors and epidural disease.[26,27] Rogers et al[27] reported a series of 25 patients who were implanted intraoperatively with ^{125}I seeds. Twenty-two (88%) failed prior external beam radiation therapy. At a mean follow-up of 19.2 months, four patients demonstrated local failure and the 3-year actuarial control rate was 72.9%. No radiation toxicity was seen in this study. However, radiation myelitis has been reported 34 months following the routine administration of ^{131}I for metastatic thyroid cancer. The level of myelitis entailed significant epidural disease that was nearly circumferential, likely resulting in a high surface dose to the spinal cord over a short period of time.[28]

DeLaney et al[29] have developed applicators for the delivery of high-dose radiation using iridium 192 and yttrium 90.[29] ^{90}Y is a pure B-emitter and ideal for delivering high-dose radiation (e.g., 7.5 to 15 Gy) to the dura without toxicity to the spinal cord. The ^{90}Y dose penetrance is 29% at 2 mm and 9% at 4 mm. This provides an adequate margin on the spinal cord, if the gross tumor has been resected in the absence of a spinal fluid leak. In this series, seven of eight patients were treated for sarcoma, six of whom were controlled at a median of 24 months. No radiation myelitis has been seen to date. ^{90}Y may ultimately prove to be excellent as an adjuvant therapy for radioresistant tumors with epidural disease when combined with image-guided IMRT or proton beam therapy. Image-guided IMRT uses dose painting to lessen the dose at the spinal cord margin in order to spare spinal cord tolerance, potentially underdosing this area. ^{90}Y may improve the dose distribution for epidural disease and facilitate treatment planning and delivery of image-guided IMRT. The limitation of ^{90}Y is that the applicators are custom made for each patient and the isotope has a very short half-life. If the epidural tumor resection is more extensive than predicted by magnetic resonance imaging (MRI) or the case is delayed several days, the plaque may be wasted.

Memorial Sloan-Kettering Cancer Center is pioneering the use of a similar dural plaque application of intraoperative brachytherapy for the treatment of metastatic and primary spine tumors. In this type of brachytherapy a thin piece of silicone is coated with radioactive phosphorus (^{32}P). ^{32}P has a two week half life and is slightly less penetrating than ^{90}YT, both important advantages for ^{32}P. The plaque is temporarily inserted directly onto dura contaminated with tumor cells during surgery and removed before the operation is over (**Fig. 4.4**). Similar to the ^{192}Ir and ^{90}Y used by Delaney et al,[29] this allows delivery of high doses to the cord surface (25 Gy) while sparing the nearby spinal cord to doses typically less than 2 Gy.

High-dose-rate (HDR) brachytherapy can also be delivered to spine tumors using small catheters while the patient is under anesthesia. As with other forms of brachytherapy, this application may assist in the dosimetric planning challenges of radiotherapy.[30] ^{32}P has been used successfully for years as a local treatment for other types of tumors, but its safety and utility in the management of primary spinal axis tumors is still under investigation at MSKCC.[31]

Stereotactic Radiation

Stereotactic spine radiosurgery delivers an entire course of radiation in one to five fractions.

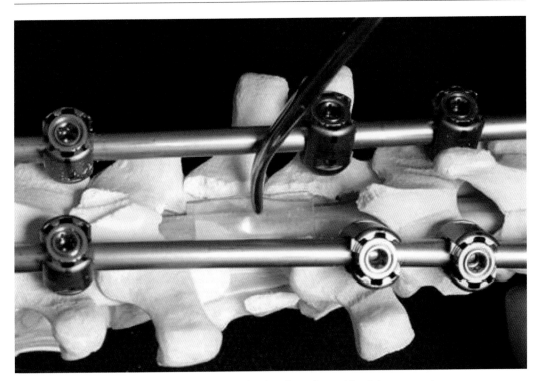

Fig. 4.4 The [30]P source is placed directly on the dural surface after epidural decompression.

Hence, the dose of radiation per fraction is much higher than with conventional radiotherapy, and extreme accuracy and precision is crucial. IMRT techniques are typically used to generate the necessary conformity to limit doses within safe levels to nearby organs at risk. Image-guided technology, such as on-board cone beam computed tomography (CT) scanners, which are integrated into the radiation delivery platform, provide three-dimensional imaging and spatial data to ensure that the radiation is given exactly to the right place in near real time. The role for stereotactic radiosurgery in the treatment of primary tumors is yet to be determined, and experience is limited compared to proton beam therapy. Theoretically, high-dose single-fraction therapy may improve local tumor control compared to standard fraction therapy. From a biological standpoint, tumor histologies with low α/β ratios, such as sarcomas, respond better to larger fraction sizes. Preclinical evidence suggests that single-fraction therapy greater than 8 to 10 Gy results in apoptosis of tumor cells based on the acid sphingomyelinase

pathway.[30] Microvascular damage in the tumor from high-dose fractions likely contributes to cell death.

The radiobiological benefit may be most pronounced in tumor types traditionally considered resistant to standard fractionated radiation therapy. A construct called the biological effective dose (BED) (**Table 4.1**) has become a widely accepted way to compare the potency of different radiation dose schedules.[32] Although the assumptions made for BED calculations based on linear quadratic formalism are not likely to be accurate at high doses per fraction, such as in radiosurgery,[33] a comparison of different dose schedules demonstrates the significant advantage of increasing the dose of radiation per fraction for radioresistant tumors ($\alpha/\beta = 2$) compared with relatively sensitive tumors ($\alpha/\beta = 10$). Thus increasing the fraction size is a form of biological dose escalation. Based on this simplified analysis, a course of proton beam radiotherapy giving 76 CGy in 2-Gy fractions would give the BED of 152 Gy for radioresistant tumors.

Table 4.1 Biologic Effective Dose (BED) Schedules

	24 Gy/12	24 Gy/8	24 Gy/6	24 Gy/4	240 Gy/2	24 Gy/1
$\alpha/\beta = 2$	48 Gy	72 Gy	96 Gy	120 Gy	168 Gy	312 Gy
$\alpha/\beta = 10$	29 Gy	31 Gy	34 Gy	38 Gy	53 Gy	81.6 Gy

Note: The schedules demonstrate the significant advantage of increasing the dose of radiation per fraction for radioresistant tumors ($\alpha/\beta = 2$) compared to relatively sensitive tumors ($\alpha/\beta = 10$).

In order for such high biological doses of radiation to be administered safely, it is critical that radiation be delivered in a very conformal manner with high accuracy and precision, to prevent the exposure of dose-sensitive normal tissues to high doses. Image-guided techniques[34] coupled with IMRT have provided the avenue for such treatment. The extremely high local control rates and very low toxicity associated with metastatic renal cell carcinoma spine lesions treated with high-dose single-fraction radiosurgery appears to support this paradigm.[35]

Stereotactic radiosurgery is currently being used as neoadjuvant therapy at MSKCC. For tumors such as chordoma, chondrosarcoma, and liposarcoma, neoadjuvant radiation may decrease the possibility of tumor dissemination from intralesional resection. This may also benefit patients who ultimately undergo en-bloc resection with negative histological resections in which tumor dissemination is sometimes found. Although it is feasible to use image-guided IMRT to give high-dose radiation in standard fractionation, many primary tumors of the spine may respond best to high-dose hypofractionated or single-fraction radiation. However, when administering such high-dose therapy, extreme care and caution are mandatory to minimize complications. From a surgical perspective, the advantage of using highly conformal delivery of radiation is the decreased soft tissue damage and consequent decreased risk of wound complications. Patients may safely undergo surgery within 2 weeks of image-guided IMRT.

The technique for spine radiosurgery[36] utilizes an inverse optimized treatment planning. Typically, five to seven radiation beams are focused around a single isocenter. Each beam's intensity is modulated with multileaf collimation using a sliding window technique similar to that for IMRT. All target volumes are generated based on International Commission on Radiation Units and Measurements (ICRU) report 50 and on the guidelines set by the International Stereotactic Radiosurgery Consortium.[37] The gross tumor volume (GTV) is defined as gross disease visualized on MRI and CT imaging. The clinical target volume (CTV) was defined as the GTV as well as areas of potential microscopic spread. The planning target volume (PTV) included the CTV with a 2- to 3-mm margin for setup uncertainty and potential patient motion. In cases of epidural disease, the CTV and PTV overlap in the region of the spinal canal in order to spare the spinal cord.

As part of the planning process, all volumes are reviewed by a team of radiation oncologists and neurosurgeons. Similarly, with anterior extraosseous disease around the esophagus, CTV and PTV overlap GTV to limit esophageal dose. The spinal cord, as defined on a simulation CT myelogram, is constrained to a maximum dose of 14 Gy to a single voxel, and no treatment plan should exceed this level. The esophagus is constrained to 14.5 Gy to 2.5 cc of esophagus, although this constraint can be exceeded at the discretion of the treating physician. The cauda equina is limited to maximum dose of 18 Gy. Bowel is constrained to allow no more than 5 cc to receive more than 16 Gy. In cases of significant bowel overlapping target volumes in the sacrum, saline may be infused between tumor and bowel during treatment to temporarily displace bowel away from the anterior aspect of the target volume.[38]

Sarcoma and Radiation Treatment

Conventional radiation treatment of sarcomas of the spine requires prolonged treatment courses and results in poor local control. Hypofractionated and single-fraction image-guided SRS (IG-SRS) may provide a more effective means of managing these radioresistant lesions.

Primary sarcomas, although uncommon, carry a high mortality burden—nearly 50%.[39] Metastatic disease in the spine is far more common, accounting for up to 70% of all metastases to bone and affecting up to 10% of all cancer patients.[40,41] Aggressive surgical and radiotherapeutic approaches are often required to prevent tumor-associated neurologic damage, establish local control, and potentially improve overall survival.[40,42]

Radiation therapy is essential in spinal lesions to optimize local tumor control.[43,44] Conventional external beam radiation therapy (C-EBRT) provides limited control, as spinal sarcomas are considered radioresistant.[42,45,46] Yet, SRS may produce local control rates greater than 90% with low risk of injury to nearby organs and the spinal cord.[40,47–49] High-dose single or hypofractionated IG-SRS has also been implemented in the postoperative setting with similarly good control rates.[50–52]

At MSKCC between 2005 and 2012, 147 primary (26.5%) and metastatic (73.5%) spinal sarcoma lesions were treated, 49 with hypofractionated SRS (mean 24 Gy in three fractions) and 98 with single-fraction SRS (24 Gy). Median follow-up was 14.1 months (range, 1–80.7 months); for patients with primary lesions the median follow-up was 19.1 months and for metastatic lesions the median follow-up was 12.5 months. Of the 147 lesions, 18 (12.2%) were previously irradiated; 49 (33.3%) of the lesions were treated with IG-SRS postoperatively, and 12 (8.2%) were treated with neoadjuvant SRS. Overall local progression-free survival at 12 months was 92.1% (95% confidence interval [CI], 86.9–97.3%); overall survival at 12 months was 70.7% (95% CI, 61.7–79.7%). Patients treated with single-fraction IG-SRS had a significantly better local progression-free survival than patients treated with hypofractionated IG-SRS, 88.2% (95% CI, 80.2–96.2%) versus 68.2% (95% CI, 47.8–88.6%) at 24 months (log-rank $p = 0.005$).

Sixty-one lesions in 58 patients were treated with neoadjuvant or adjuvant IG-SRS (i.e., radiation therapy before or after surgical manage-

ment); 49 lesions were irradiated postoperatively and 12 preoperatively. Overall survival and local progression-free survival at 1 year were 70.1% (95% CI, 57.5–82.7%) and 88.1% (95% CI, 78.9–97.3%), respectively. This cohort included both metastatic and primary patients; for the metastatic subset ($n = 32$ patients, 35 lesions), the overall survival and local progression-free survival at 1 year were 61.2% (95% CI, 43.6–78.8%) and 86.5% (95% CI, 73.9–99.1%), respectively; for patients with primary lesions ($n = 26$ patients, 26 lesions), overall survival and local progression-free survival at 1 year were 81.8% (95% CI, 65.4–98.2%) and 90.2% (95% CI, 77–100%), respectively. Overall survival and local progression-free survival were not significantly different (log-rank $p = 0.123$ and 0.442, respectively) for primary versus metastatic lesions.

Timing of the radiation with respect to surgery did not have a significant effect on local progression-free survival (log-rank $p = 0.170$); however, patients treated with preoperative IG-SRS did have improved overall survival (log-rank $p = 0.040$). Patients treated with surgery and single-fraction IG-SRS had significantly better overall and local progression-free survival than patients treated with hypofractionated IG-SRS (log-rank $p = 0.030$ and 0.013, respectively). Eighteen lesions in 17 patients were treated with salvage IG-SRS (i.e., radiation therapy with or without surgical management for a previously treated lesion); 15 (83.3%) were treated in the postoperative setting. Overall survival and local progression-free survival at 1 year were 42% (95% CI, 14.6–69.4%) and 100%, respectively. This cohort included both metastatic and primary patients; for the metastatic subset ($n = 9$ patients, 10 lesions), overall survival and local progression-free survival at 1 year were 34.6% (95% CI, 0–71.2%) and 100%, respectively; for patients with primary lesions ($n = 8$ patients, 8 lesions), overall survival and local progression-free survival at 1 year were 50% (95% CI, 9.2–90.8%) and 100%, respectively. Overall survival and local progression-free survival were not significantly different (log-rank $p = 0.197$ and 1, respectively) for primary versus metastatic lesions, which reinforces the utility of SRS in the treatment of primary spinal sarcoma.

Based on this study, hypofractionated and single-fraction IG-SRS provides excellent local control for primary/recurrent and metastatic sarcomas of the spine. Single-fraction IG-SRS seems to be significantly more effective than hypofractionated treatment and should be a consideration for first-line therapy in the management of sarcomas of the spine; a prospective trial is needed to demonstrate a comparable outcome.

DeLaney et al[53] report a series of 50 patients with spinal sarcomas, of which 86% (43/50) were either chordoma or chondrosarcoma. The other seven patients were single pathologies, including osteosarcoma, Ewing's sarcoma, giant cell sarcoma, angiosarcoma, liposarcoma, and malignant peripheral nerve sheath tumor spindle/round cell—further illustrating the challenges in differentiating the many sarcomatous histologies. DeLaney et al demonstrated 5-year actuarial local control of 78%. They delivered radiation using a "shrinking fields" technique: 50.4 CGE (Gy RBE [relative biological effectiveness]) to subclinical disease, 70.2 Gy RBE to microscopic disease in the tumor bed, and 77.4 Gy RBE to gross disease at 1.8 Gy RBE qd. The spinal cord dose was limited to 63/54 Gy RBE to surface/center. Intraoperative boost doses of 7.5 to 10 Gy could be given by dural plaque. This study found extremely high local control in 34 of 36 (94%) primary tumors and in 23 of 23 (100%) primary chordomas. This reinforces the importance of combined radiation and surgical therapy at the time of primary presentation.[54]

At MSKCC, Yamada et al reported a series of 14 patients with primary spine/paraspinal sarcomas treated with multifractionated stereotactic and image-guided IMRT coupled with noninvasive body frames.[24] Previously unirradiated patients received a median prescribed dose of 70 Gy (range, 59.4–70 Gy) with a median planning target volume receiving the prescribed dose of 90%. The median dose maximum to the cord was 68% of the prescribed dose for previously unirradiated patients. Of the primary lesions, 81% exhibited local control with 2 to 30 months of follow-up. No cases of radiation-induced myelopathy were encountered.

■ Chordoma

Chordoma is a rare and relentless disease of the skull, spine, and sacrum.[55] Similar to the majority of mesenchymal tumors, it is not considered sensitive to radiation treatment. Intralesional or marginal resections in the spine and sacrum have a high probability of recurrence[3]; thus, en-bloc resection to achieve wide margins has been advocated as the only cure for chordomas.[1] Despite major surgical advances, total en-bloc resection may only be achieved in approximately 50% of sacral chordomas, with much lower rates for lesions of the spine or skull base; therefore, recurrence is common without en-bloc resection.[56,57] In part this may be due to the lack of effective adjuvant therapies.[55] Radiotherapy has often been used as adjuvant as well as primary treatment for chordomas. Good control rates were achieved in some series after en-bloc excision of primary chordomas in combination with preoperative and postoperative high-dose radiation,[53] yet recurrence rates in excess of 50% have been demonstrated in other series with long-term follow-up.[58]

Because the tolerance dose of the spinal cord, brainstem, cranial nerves, and rectum is much lower than effective doses to treat chordomas, delivery of high doses is limited. For example, treatment of the sacrococcygeal region with high doses of photon radiation therapy (45–80 Gy) can be achieved because the region is less susceptible than the cervical spine, where myelopathy due to radiation injury is common.[59] Radiation doses > 70 Gy are required for gross disease at conventional fractionation schemas.[60]

Treatment with conventional radiation therapy at doses of 40 to 60 Gy has led to poor results, with 5-year local control of only 10 to 40%.[61–64]

The best reported local control rate with photons based on modern, fractionated stereotactic radiation therapy for lesions in the skull base is a 5-year actuarial rate of approximately 50%.[58] Over the years, radical en-bloc surgical resection and radiation dose escalation have been further explored to improve survival.

Pearlman and Friedman[65] suggested a possible dose–response effect, although it has been established that increasing radiation doses in excess of 70 Gy will lead to long-term tumor control.[9,66]

Image-guided technology coupled with intensity-modulated photon radiation has made it possible to deliver very high dose radiotherapy to the spine and sacrum in a single fraction. A series at MSKCC showed that single-fraction spine radiosurgery can provide long-term local control in greater than 90% of cases for metastatic tumors considered resistant to conventional radiation.[48] Single-session high-dose radiosurgery for skull base chordomas has shown promise.[34,67]

Recently, Yamada et al[55] reviewed their experience with single-fraction high-dose SRS for chordoma of the spine and sacrum, and demonstrated good tumor control with low treatment-related morbidity. This series reported 24 patients with chordoma of the sacrum and mobile spine after being treated with high-dose single-fraction SRS (median dose, 24 Gy). Twenty-one primary and three metastatic tumors were treated. Seven patients were treated for postoperative tumor recurrence. In seven patients SRS was administered as planned adjuvant therapy, and in 13 patients SRS was administered as neoadjuvant therapy. Although surgery was planned in most cases where single-fraction SRS was delivered as the initial treatment, the lack of symptomatic and radiographic progression after SRS resulted in several patients refusing surgery. Thus, only six of 13 patients who underwent neoadjuvant SRS proceeded to surgery. This cohort provides information about local tumor control with single-fraction SRS as the sole treatment of newly diagnosed chordomas. The overall median follow-up was 24 months. Of the 24 patients, 23 (95%) demonstrated stable or reduced tumor burden based on serial MRI. One patient had radiographic progression of tumor 11 months after SRS. Complications were limited to one patient who developed sciatic neuropathy and one with vocal cord paralysis.

The most optimistic results in the treatment of chordomas have been reported by proton therapy for the skull base, in general combining maximal surgical tumor resection with ad-juvant high-dose particle therapy. The primary advantage of a proton beam is the protons' physical feature of the Bragg peak, which provides excellent conformity of the irradiation field. Utilization of this modality has been pioneered at Massachusetts General Hospital in collaboration with the Harvard Cyclotron Laboratory. A technique called spot scanning was developed at the Paul Scherrer Institute and reported on 26 patients with extracranial chordomas and a median follow-up period of 35 months after proton therapy. In this study, a 3-year disease-free survival of 77% was documented.[68] Most of the data on chordomas are taken from skull bases reports. A review of this literature demonstrates local control rates ranging from 67% at 3 years to 98% at 5 years with doses ranging from 50 to 83 Gy RBE.[69–73]

Because chordomas are rare and because it is difficult to randomize patients to treatments other than standard of care, it is unlikely that phase 3 trials will be done to compare different types of radiation, making the differences in clinical effect difficult to interpret.[16] The use of radiotherapy as primary or adjuvant treatment for chordoma is still debated. In the past, stand-alone radiotherapy was proven to be ineffective when coupled with debulking or palliative therapy.[74] It is clear that with the adjunct of single-fraction SRS and modern proton beam schemas, the role of adjuvant, neoadjuvant, and stand-alone radiotherapy will continue to evolve in the management of spinal chordomas.

■ Chondrosarcoma

Chondrosarcoma is the third most common type of primary bone tumor (after myeloma and osteosarcoma) and accounts for 20 to 27% of all primary malignant osseous tumors.[75] Typically these lesions are low grade and can arise de novo or from a preexisting cartilage lesion such as an osteochondroma or enchondroma. Less than 10% of all chondrosarcomas occur in the spine. Due to their biology, low percentage of dividing cells, and poor vascularity, these tumors have a tendency to be chemo- and radiotherapy resistant. However, chondrosarcomas grow slowly and rarely metastasize.[76] Surgical resection remains the mainstay of treatment of chondrosarcomas. The extent of surgical resection and adjuvant therapy is dependent on the clinical and histological characteristics of the lesions. Although wide, en-bloc excision is ideal for intermediate- and high-grade chondrosarcoma, less aggressive approaches may be acceptable for low-grade chondrosarcoma.

Due to their similar management challenges, chordoma and chondrosarcoma treatment series are often combined. As with chordoma management, radiation of chondrosarcoma is considered after incomplete resection, aiming at maximal local control (curative) and in situations where resection is not feasible or would cause unacceptable morbidity (palliative). For curative intentions, doses > 60 Gy are required to achieve local control.[76] Due to the limitations of conventional radiotherapy, proton and photon radiotherapy in chondrosarcoma are utilized. As with chordomas, most of the data on chondrosarcoma are taken from skull base reports. The literature demonstrates local control rates ranging from 94% at 3 years to 73% at 5 years with doses ranging from 50 to 83 Gy RBE.[69–73]

Similar to chordoma treatment, the importance of an escalated dose is emphasized. Austin et al[6] reported 26 local relapses in 141 patients treated by proton irradiation for chordoma or chondrosarcoma of the cranial base or cervical spine. Among 26 relapses, only six were reported in an area that had received 70 Gy or more versus 15 relapses in areas receiving a lower dose. Often the shielding of critical anatomic structures adjacent to tumor boundaries is the cause of underdosing and local failure.[77] The skull base literature reinforces the relationship between dose inhomogeneity and risk of local failure.[78] Noël et al[77] demonstrated 3-year local control rates of 69% in chordoma and 91% in chondrosarcomas. Their results emphasize the importance of adequate coverage of the target volume at an "effective" dose. Another important finding by Noël et al is that the minimum dose correlates to local control, a variable that is determined by dose constraints

of normal structures. Still most authors of reports in the skull base literature believe that surgery is the mainstay of treatment for this pathology.[79,80] Published data demonstrate that local control is dependent on the size of the residual tumor at the time of radiation.[70]

Radiotherapy with carbon ions or other charged particles is another attractive radiation modality. The physical advantages of protons are combined with a higher radiobiological activity. Schulz-Ertner et al[81] reported the effectiveness and toxicity of carbon ion radiotherapy in chondrosarcomas of the skull base.

Chapter Summary

From available data, en-bloc resection achieving negative histological margins may have a good rate of local tumor control. For patients who are not candidates for marginal or wide resections, adjuvant radiation adds a measure of tumor control. Proton beam, intraoperative radioactive implants, and high-dose conformal photon therapy all play a role in local tumor control and possibly cure. Advances in stereotactic planning are overcoming many of the tissue tolerance issues with high-dose photon radiosurgery. The success of proton therapy depends on dosimetric factors, mainly those related to dose homogeneity within the target, rather than on the prescribed dose. However, high-quality surgical resection remains critical, because it can dramatically improve anatomic relations between tumor and adjacent anatomic structures, which is a prognostic factor of dose homogeneity.[77]

Pearls

♦ Understand the importance of multidisciplinary management for optimal treatment of primary spine tumors.
♦ Image-guided radiotherapy, including stereotactic radiosurgery, provides a level of precision of treatment delivery that enables much higher doses of radiation to be given safely to primary spine tumors.
♦ Hypofractionation is a strategy to increase the biological effectiveness of radiation and may be

an effective treatment strategy for primary spine tumors.

◆ Intraoperative dural brachytherapy is a method of delivering high-dose radiation to the dural margin without significantly increasing the dose of radiation received by the spinal cord.

◆ Proton beam radiation and other charged particle radiation will continue to play an important role in the management of primary spine tumors.

References

Five Must-Read References

1. Boriani S, Bandiera S, Biagini R, et al. Chordoma of the mobile spine: fifty years of experience. Spine 2006; 31:493–503

2. Tomita K, Kawahara N, Baba H, Tsuchiya H, Fujita T, Toribatake Y. Total en bloc spondylectomy. A new surgical technique for primary malignant vertebral tumors. Spine 1997;22:324–333

3. Yao KC, Boriani S, Gokaslan ZL, Sundaresan N. En bloc spondylectomy for spinal metastases: a review of techniques. Neurosurg Focus 2003;15:E6

4. Fuller DB, Bloom JG. Radiotherapy for chordoma. Int J Radiat Oncol Biol Phys 1988;15:331–339

5. Krochak R, Harwood AR, Cummings BJ, Quirt IC. Results of radical radiation for chondrosarcoma of bone. Radiother Oncol 1983;1:109–115

6. Austin JP, Urie MM, Cardenosa G, Munzenrider JE. Probable causes of recurrence in patients with chordoma and chondrosarcoma of the base of skull and cervical spine. Int J Radiat Oncol Biol Phys 1993;25: 439–444

7. Bell RS, O'Sullivan B, Liu FF, et al. The surgical margin in soft tissue sarcoma. Chir Organi Mov 1990;75(1, Suppl)126–130

8. Pisters PW, Leung DH, Woodruff J, Shi W, Brennan MF. Analysis of prognostic factors in 1,041 patients with localized soft tissue sarcomas of the extremities. J Clin Oncol 1996;14:1679–1689

9. Tanabe KK, Pollock RE, Ellis LM, Murphy A, Sherman N, Romsdahl MM. Influence of surgical margins on outcome in patients with preoperatively irradiated extremity soft tissue sarcomas. Cancer 1994;73: 1652–1659

10. Boriani S, De Iure F, Bandiera S, et al. Chondrosarcoma of the mobile spine: report on 22 cases. Spine 2000;25:804–812

11. Boriani S, Weinstein JN, Biagini R. Primary bone tumors of the spine. Terminology and surgical staging. Spine 1997;22:1036–1044

12. Bilsky MH, Boland PJ, Panageas KS, Woodruff JM, Brennan MF, Healey JH. Intralesional resection of primary and metastatic sarcoma involving the spine:

outcome analysis of 59 patients. Neurosurgery 2001; 49:1277–1286, discussion 1286–1287

13. O'Sullivan B, Davis AM, Turcotte R, et al. Preoperative versus postoperative radiotherapy in soft-tissue sarcoma of the limbs: a randomised trial. Lancet 2002; 359:2235–2241

14. DeLaney TF, Trofimov AV, Engelsman M, Suit HD. Advanced-technology radiation therapy in the management of bone and soft tissue sarcomas. Cancer Contr 2005;12:27–35

15. Emami B, Lyman J, Brown A, et al. Tolerance of normal tissue to therapeutic irradiation. Int J Radiat Oncol Biol Phys 1991;21:109–122

16. Walcott BP, Nahed BV, Mohyeldin A, Coumans JV, Kahle KT, Ferreira MJ. Chordoma: current concepts, management, and future directions. Lancet Oncol 2012;13:e69–e76

17. Panahandeh H, Spadea M, Oh K, Seco J. Dosimetric analysis of proton passive-scattering stereotactic body radiotherapy (SBRT) of treated spine lesions versus photon SBRT. Med Phys 2011;38:3694

18. Verburg JM, Seco J. Dosimetric accuracy of proton therapy for chordoma patients with titanium implants. Med Phys 2013;40:071727

19. Tobias CA, Blakely EA, Alpen EL, et al. Molecular and cellular radiobiology of heavy ions. Int J Radiat Oncol Biol Phys 1982;8:2109–2120

20. Imai R, Kamada T, Sugahara S, Tsuji H, Tsujii H. Carbon ion radiotherapy for sacral chordoma. Br J Radiol 2011;84(Spec No 1):S48–S54

21. Mohan R, Bortfeld T. Proton therapy: clinical gains through current and future treatment programs. Front Radiat Ther Oncol 2011;43:440–464

22. Austin-Seymour M, Munzenrider JE, Goitein M, et al. Progress in low-LET heavy particle therapy: intracranial and paracranial tumors and uveal melanomas. Radiat Res Suppl 1985;8(Suppl):S219–S226

23. Hug EB. Review of skull base chordomas: prognostic factors and long-term results of proton-beam radiotherapy. Neurosurg Focus 2001;10:E11

24. Yamada Y, Lovelock DM, Yenice KM, et al. Multifractionated image-guided and stereotactic intensity-modulated radiotherapy of paraspinal tumors: a preliminary report. Int J Radiat Oncol Biol Phys 2005; 62:53–61

25. Terezakis SA, Lovelock DM, Bilsky MH, Hunt MA, Zatcky J, Yamada Y. Image-guided intensity-modulated photon radiotherapy using multifractionated regimen to paraspinal chordomas and rare sarcomas. Int J Radiat Oncol Biol Phys 2007;69:1502–1508

26. Cheng EY, Ozerdemoglu RA, Transfeldt EE, Thompson RC Jr. Lumbosacral chordoma. Prognostic factors and treatment. Spine 1999;24:1639–1645

27. Rogers CL, Theodore N, Dickman CA, et al. Surgery and permanent 125I seed paraspinal brachytherapy for malignant tumors with spinal cord compression. Int J Radiat Oncol Biol Phys 2002;54:505–513

28. Murakami H, Kawahara N, Yahata T, Yokoyama K, Komai K, Tomita K. Radiation myelopathy after radioactive iodine therapy for spine metastasis. Br J Radiol 2006;79:e45–e49

29. DeLaney TF, Chen GT, Mauceri TC, et al. Intraoperative dural irradiation by customized 192 iridium and 90 yttrium brachytherapy plaques. Int J Radiat Oncol Biol Phys 2003;57:239–245

30. Garcia-Barros M, Paris F, Cordon-Cardo C, et al. Tumor response to radiotherapy regulated by endothelial cell apoptosis. Science 2003;300:1155–1159

31. Memorial Sloan Kettering Cancer Center. http://www .mskcc.org/cancer-care/adult/spine-tumors/radiation -therapy. Accessed October 1, 2013

32. Hall EJ, Giaccia AJ. Radiobiology for the Radiologist, 6th ed. Philadelphia: Lippincott Williams & Wilkins, 2006

33. Flickinger JC, Kondziolka D, Lunsford LD. Radiobiological analysis of tissue responses following radiosurgery. Technol Cancer Res Treat 2003;2:87–92

34. Martin JJ, Niranjan A, Kondziolka D, Flickinger JC, Lozanne KA, Lunsford LD. Radiosurgery for chordomas and chondrosarcomas of the skull base. J Neurosurg 2007;107:758–764

35. Gerszten PC, Burton SA, Ozhasoglu C, et al. Stereotactic radiosurgery for spinal metastases from renal cell carcinoma. J Neurosurg Spine 2005;3:288–295

36. Lovelock DM, Hua C, Wang P, et al. Accurate setup of paraspinal patients using a noninvasive patient immobilization cradle and portal imaging. Med Phys 2005;32:2606–2614

37. Cox BW, Spratt DE, Lovelock M, et al. International Spine Radiosurgery Consortium consensus guidelines for target volume definition in spinal stereotactic radiosurgery. Int J Radiat Oncol Biol Phys 2012;83: e597–e605

38. Folkert MR, Bilsky MH, Cox BW, et al. Outcomes for hypofractionated and single-fraction image-guided radiation therapy for primary and metastatic sarcomas of the spine. Connective Tissue Oncology Society 17th Annual Meeting, Prague, November 17, 2012

39. Siegel R, Naishadham D, Jemal A. Cancer statistics, 2012. CA Cancer J Clin 2012;62:10–29

40. Gerszten PC, Mendel E, Yamada Y. Radiotherapy and radiosurgery for metastatic spine disease: what are the options, indications, and outcomes? Spine 2009; 34(22, Suppl):S78–S92

41. Chao ST, Koyfman SA, Woody N, et al. Recursive partitioning analysis index is predictive for overall survival in patients undergoing spine stereotactic body radiation therapy for spinal metastases. Int J Radiat Oncol Biol Phys 2012;82:1738–1743

42. Bilsky MH, Gerszten P, Laufer I, Yamada Y. Radiation for primary spine tumors. Neurosurg Clin N Am 2008;19:119–123

43. Patchell RA, Tibbs PA, Regine WF, et al. Direct decompressive surgical resection in the treatment of spinal cord compression caused by metastatic cancer: a randomised trial. Lancet 2005;366:643–648

44. Hug EB, Fitzek MM, Liebsch NJ, Munzenrider JE. Locally challenging osteo- and chondrogenic tumors of the axial skeleton: results of combined proton and photon radiation therapy using three-dimensional treatment planning. Int J Radiat Oncol Biol Phys 1995;31:467–476

45. Merimsky O, Kollender Y, Bokstein F, et al. Radiotherapy for spinal cord compression in patients with soft-tissue sarcoma. Int J Radiat Oncol Biol Phys 2004; 58:1468–1473

46. Boriani S, Saravanja D, Yamada Y, Varga PP, Biagini R, Fisher CG. Challenges of local recurrence and cure in low grade malignant tumors of the spine. Spine 2009;34(22, Suppl):S48–S57

47. Bilsky MH, Yamada Y, Yenice KM, et al. Intensity-modulated stereotactic radiotherapy of paraspinal tumors: a preliminary report. Neurosurgery 2004; 54:823–830, discussion 830–831

48. Yamada Y, Bilsky MH, Lovelock DM, et al. High-dose, single-fraction image-guided intensity-modulated radiotherapy for metastatic spinal lesions. Int J Radiat Oncol Biol Phys 2008;71:484–490

49. Levine AM, Coleman C, Horasek S. Stereotactic radiosurgery for the treatment of primary sarcomas and sarcoma metastases of the spine. Neurosurgery 2009; 64(2, Suppl):A54–A59

50. Rock JP, Ryu S, Shukairy MS, et al. Postoperative radiosurgery for malignant spinal tumors. Neurosurgery 2006;58:891–898, discussion 891–898

51. Moulding HD, Elder JB, Lis E, et al. Local disease control after decompressive surgery and adjuvant high-dose single-fraction radiosurgery for spine metastases. J Neurosurg Spine 2010;13:87–93

52. Sahgal A, Bilsky M, Chang EL, et al. Stereotactic body radiotherapy for spinal metastases: current status, with a focus on its application in the postoperative patient. J Neurosurg Spine 2011;14:151–166

53. DeLaney TF, Liebsch NJ, Pedlow FX, et al. Phase II study of high-dose photon/proton radiotherapy in the management of spine sarcomas. Int J Radiat Oncol Biol Phys 2009;74:732–739

54. Chang UK, Cho WI, Lee DH, et al. Stereotactic radiosurgery for primary and metastatic sarcomas involving the spine. J Neurooncol 2012;107:551–557

55. Yamada Y, Laufer I, Cox BW, et al. Preliminary results of high-dose single-fraction radiotherapy for the management of chordomas of the spine and sacrum. Neurosurgery 2013;73:673–680, discussion 680 [Epub ahead of print]

56. Tzortzidis F, Elahi F, Wright D, Natarajan SK, Sekhar LN. Patient outcome at long-term follow-up after aggressive microsurgical resection of cranial base chordomas. Neurosurgery 2006;59:230–237, discussion 230–237

57. Fuchs B, Dickey ID, Yaszemski MJ, Inwards CY, Sim FH. Operative management of sacral chordoma. J Bone Joint Surg Am 2005;87:2211–2216

58. Debus J, Schulz-Ertner D, Schad L, et al. Stereotactic fractionated radiotherapy for chordomas and chondrosarcomas of the skull base. Int J Radiat Oncol Biol Phys 2000;47(3):591–596

59. Casali PG, Stacchiotti S, Sangalli C, Olmi P, Gronchi A. Chordoma. Curr Opin Oncol 2007;19:367–370

60. Staab A, Rutz HP, Ares C, et al. Spot-scanning-based proton therapy for extracranial chordoma. Int J Radiat Oncol Biol Phys 2011;81:e489–e496

61. Forsyth PA, Cascino TL, Shaw EG, et al. Intracranial chordomas: a clinicopathological and prognostic study of 51 cases. J Neurosurg 1993;78:741–747

62. Catton C, O'Sullivan B, Bell R, et al. Chordoma: long-term follow-up after radical photon irradiation. Radiother Oncol 1996;41:67–72

63. Cummings BJ, Hodson DI, Bush RS. Chordoma: the results of megavoltage radiation therapy. Int J Radiat Oncol Biol Phys 1983;9:633–642

64. Romero J, Cardenes H, la Torre A, et al. Chordoma: results of radiation therapy in eighteen patients. Radiother Oncol 1993;29:27–32

65. Pearlman AW, Friedman M. Radical radiation therapy of chordoma. Am J Roentgenol Radium Ther Nucl Med 1970;108:332–341

66. Tai PT, Craighead P, Bagdon F. Optimization of radiotherapy for patients with cranial chordoma. A review of dose-response ratios for photon techniques. Cancer 1995;75:749–756

67. Krishnan S, Foote RL, Brown PD, Pollock BE, Link MJ, Garces YI. Radiosurgery for cranial base chordomas and chondrosarcomas. Neurosurgery 2005;56:777–784, discussion 777–784

68. Rutz HP, Weber DC, Sugahara S, et al. Extracranial chordoma: outcome in patients treated with function-preserving surgery followed by spot-scanning proton beam irradiation. Int J Radiat Oncol Biol Phys 2007;67:512–520

69. Fuji H, Nakasu Y, Ishida Y, et al. Feasibility of proton beam therapy for chordoma and chondrosarcoma of the skull base. Skull Base 2011;21:201–206

70. Noël G, Habrand JL, Mammar H, et al. Combination of photon and proton radiation therapy for chordomas and chondrosarcomas of the skull base: the Centre de Protonthérapie D'Orsay experience. Int J Radiat Oncol Biol Phys 2001;51:392–398

71. Munzenrider JE, Liebsch NJ. Proton therapy for tumors of the skull base. Strahlenther Onkol 1999;175(Suppl 2):57–63

72. Austin-Seymour M, Munzenrider J, Goitein M, et al. Fractionated proton radiation therapy of chordoma and low-grade chondrosarcoma of the base of the skull. J Neurosurg 1989;70:13–17

73. Hug EB, Loredo LN, Slater JD, et al. Proton radiation therapy for chordomas and chondrosarcomas of the skull base. J Neurosurg 1999;91:432–439

74. Boriani S, Chevalley F, Weinstein JN, et al. Chordoma of the spine above the sacrum. Treatment and outcome in 21 cases. Spine 1996;21:1569–1577

75. Björnsson J, McLeod RA, Unni KK, Ilstrup DM, Pritchard DJ. Primary chondrosarcoma of long bones and limb girdles. Cancer 1998;83:2105–2119

76. Gelderblom H, Hogendoorn PC, Dijkstra SD, et al. The clinical approach towards chondrosarcoma. Oncologist 2008;13:320–329

77. Noël G, Feuvret L, Ferrand R, Boisserie G, Mazeron JJ, Habrand JL. Radiotherapeutic factors in the management of cervical-basal chordomas and chondrosarcomas. Neurosurgery 2004;55:1252–1260, discussion 1260–1262

78. Terahara A, Niemierko A, Goitein M, et al. Analysis of the relationship between tumor dose inhomogeneity and local control in patients with skull base chordoma. Int J Radiat Oncol Biol Phys 1999;45:351–358

79. al-Mefty O, Borba LA. Skull base chordomas: a management challenge. J Neurosurg 1997;86:182–189

80. Sen CN, Sekhar LN, Schramm VL, Janecka IP. Chordoma and chondrosarcoma of the cranial base: an 8-year experience. Neurosurgery 1989;25:931–940, discussion 940–941

81. Schulz-Ertner D, Nikoghosyan A, Hof H, et al. Carbon ion radiotherapy of skull base chondrosarcomas. Int J Radiat Oncol Biol Phys 2007;67:171–177

5

Medical Oncology Principles for the Spine Oncology Surgeon

Scott H. Okuno, Steven I. Robinson, and Shreyaskumar Patel

▓ Introduction

Primary tumors of the spine are rare and require a multidisciplinary approach to provide the patient with the best outcome. The members of the team bring their expertise and the underlying principles of their discipline. Medical oncologists have a solid understanding of the natural history and available systemic options for each tumor. Additionally, they are often able to develop a long-standing relationship with the patient and the family, thus providing the multidisciplinary team with insight on the goals and expectations of the patient, as well as their tolerance for treatment.

This chapter discusses five principles of medical oncology that we consider key for all spine oncology surgeons when caring for patients with primary and metastatic tumors of the spine:

1. Tissue is the issue
2. Staging
3. The role of adjuvant therapy
4. Understanding the toxicity of therapy
5. Understanding the preferences of the patient

These principles can be applied to the patient with localized or metastatic disease. This chapter also discusses common patient scenarios that illustrate and reinforce these principles. We do not cover each of the tumors in depth, as they are discussed in other chapters in this masters series.

It is vital, when dealing with a patient with cancer, that we have the correct diagnosis. Obtaining appropriate tissue facilitates not only making the diagnosis but also performing additional testing on the tumor sample to help determine prognosis and treatment options.

Advances in imaging, with present-day options including magnetic resonance imaging (MRI), computed tomography (CT), and positron emission tomography (PET) scans, have enabled more accurate staging. Understanding both disease biology and imaging modality limitations is essential in guiding the choice of the appropriate imaging studies to properly stage patients.

Adjuvant or neoadjuvant systemic therapy has improved the outcome of patients with primary bone tumors such as Ewing's sarcoma and osteogenic sarcoma. The role of systemic therapy in the adjuvant setting with other primary spine tumors is less clear. However, there are circumstances where the use of adjuvant systemic options may positively impact the surgical approach.

It is difficult to keep abreast of all the evolving therapeutic options and their associated side effects. These side effects, in particular, can have impact on the surgery and the postoperative course. The medical oncologist can be a valuable resource for information about these issues.

Ultimately, achieving the patient's goals is central to the care plan. As caregivers of patients with both curable and incurable cancers, we need to provide our patients with information about the potential benefits and side effects of any treatment we recommend, allowing them to be an active participant in the decision-making process.

Tissue Is the Issue

This first principle of medical oncology cannot be underestimated. Not only is tissue needed to make the diagnosis, but how we obtain the tissue and what additional testing can be done on that specimen has revolutionized the way we treat patients with cancer. In the past most of the biopsies that were needed to make the diagnosis were done with an open approach (open biopsy). The open procedure enabled the surgeon to obtain an adequate tissue sample to make the diagnosis and do any requisite ancillary testing. Additionally, the surgeon was able to control any bleeding that might have occurred during the biopsy procedure. The open biopsy often required the use of anesthesia and sutures. This added to the expense and recovery time. With the advancement of cross-sectional imaging, interventional radiologists are now able to perform percutaneous CT-guided biopsies on almost any tissue in any location. These tissue cores are for the most part enough to obtain a diagnosis and appropriate ancillary testing. This has reduced both recovery time and cost. The diagnostic accuracy for spine CT-guided biopsies can be has high as 97% with a low complication rate (see text box).[1–3]

Percutaneous CT–Guided Biopsy of the Spine: Accuracy in Diagnosis and Complication Rates

- ◆ Accuracy
  - ◦ 71–97%
- ◆ Complications
  - ◦ 0–21%
  - ◦ Pulmonary, neurologic, infectious, and bleed

Not only is tissue the issue to make the diagnosis, but it also provides tumor sample to

perform additional ancillary testing to help determine prognosis and therapeutic options. Although these additional tests at present have limited value for primary bone tumors, they do have significant impact for nonprimary bone tumors for which spine oncologist are frequently consulted. We highlight two common tumors, lung cancer and breast cancer, for which additional ancillary testing is important in the management of the patient (**Figs. 5.1** and **5.2**).

In the past, patients diagnosed with lung cancer were either classified as small cell lung carcinoma (SCLC) or non–small cell lung carcinoma (NSCLC). The NSCLC was further classified as squamous cell carcinoma, adenocarcinoma, large cell, or not otherwise specified (NOS). The lumping of all NSCLCs together despite the different histologies was largely due to the fact that our therapies were not that specific for the different histologies. With the increase in therapeutic options and improved subclassification of adenocarcinomas, we now know that all NSCLCs are not the same and their treat-

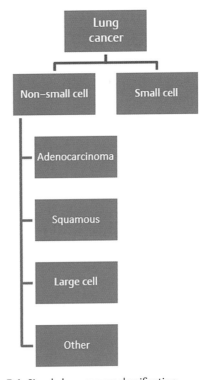

Fig. 5.1 Simple lung cancer classification.

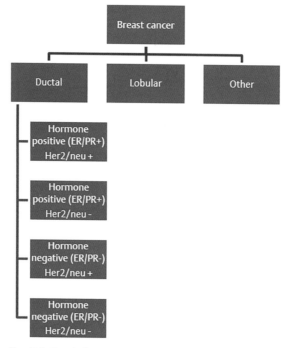

Fig. 5.2 Simple breast cancer classification.

ment and prognosis often differ. For instance, squamous cell carcinoma, which accounts for 20% of NSCLCs, occurs mainly in smokers, does not have mutations in the epidermal growth factor receptor, and is less responsive to the chemotherapy agent pemetrexed. When treated with a platinum-based doublet, patients with squamous histology who received cisplatin and pemetrexed had a 3-month decrease in their median overall survival compared to non–squamous cell histology, but had an almost 2-month improved median survival when they received cisplatin in combination with gemcitabine.[4,5] Thus treatment decisions can be better tailored for patients with squamous cell carcinoma.

For patients with adenocarcinoma NSCLC in addition to the histology, we now need to know the molecular characterization of the adenocarcinoma to better tailor treatment and provide prognosis (**Table 5.1**). The tissue samples of patients with adenocarcinoma NSCLC routinely undergo genotyping for epidermal growth factor receptor (EGFR) mutation, ALK (anaplastic

Table 5.1 Adenocarcinoma Non–Small Cell Lung Carcinoma (NSCLC): Subclassification by Molecular Testing and Implications

Adenocarcinoma NSCLC	Subclassification by Molecular Testing (% Incidence)	Prognosis	Targeted Therapy
EGFR mutation	15	Favorable	Erlotinib and gefitinib
ALK translocation	4	Favorable	Crizotinib
RAS mutation	20–25	In metastatic disease may help predict response or improve response to certain chemotherapy agents	None at this time

Abbreviation: EGFR, epidermal growth factor receptor.

lymphoma kinase) translocation, and *Ras* (rat sarcoma) mutations. The EGFR mutations occur in approximately 15% of adenocarcinoma NSCLC histology and generally occur in nonsmokers. These tumors are sensitive to EGFR oral tyrosine kinase inhibitors such as erlotinib or gefitinib. and patients have a more favorable prognosis. The *ALK* translocation similarly occurs in non-smokers, but in a smaller number of patients, occurring in less than 4% of patients with ade-nocarcinoma NSCLC. These tumors are sensitive to a new tyrosine kinase inhibitor, crizotinib, with improved prognosis. The *KRAS* mutation occurs in about 25% of adenocarcinoma NSCLC and is found in mainly smokers. The prognostic value of *KRAS* is limited, but therapeutic options and further studies are underway to determine if attacking the downstream target of *KRAS* might be helpful. Thus, in approaching patients with adenocarcinoma NSCLC, additional molecular testing can help with both prognosis and treatment options.

Another common cancer that metastasizes to bone is breast carcinoma. The two main histological classifications of breast cancer are lobular and ductal. The vast majority of breast cancer is ductal (> 75%) and, just like NSCLC, can be further classified based on additional ancillary tumor testing. The three most common ancillary tests are estrogen receptor (ER), progesterone receptor (PR), and Her2Neu (HER2). Knowing the status of these three tests, the oncologist can help provide the patient with information about their prognosis and direct therapeutic options. Patients with tumors that are ER and PR positive are sensitive to hormonal therapy and have a significantly favorable prognosis compared with patients whose tumors are ER and PR negative. The *HER2* oncogene is a member of the EGFR family and is also helpful in prognosis and tailoring treatment. Tumors that are HER2/neu positive are sensitive to drugs that target the HER2 receptor. Trastuzumab and pertuzumab are intravenously administered monoclonal antibodies that target HER2/neu, and lapatinib is orally administered and targets both EGFR and HER2. The addition of these drugs to standard treatment regimen improves the overall survival of patients with metastatic breast cancer.

Patients whose tumors are negative for ER, PR, and HER2/neu are classified as having triple negative breast cancer and, in the metastatic setting, have decreased survival.

Hence, tissue is the issue, having impact on the diagnosis, prognosis, and treatment decision making. Adequate tissue can be safely and accurately obtained by CT-guided biopsy to run the necessary ancillary tests.

◼ Staging

The second principle in medical oncology is staging—delineating the extent of the tumor. Historically, clinicians had to rely on physical examination findings or crude radiology imaging to get an idea of the exact location of the tumor and its extent within the body. Advances in radiology techniques have allowed us to stage the patient more accurately, but for certain tumors we still require additional testing. Moreover, we need to understand the pros and cons of each imaging modality.

The appropriate staging tests depend on the type of tumor (tissue is the issue—the first principle of medical oncology) and understanding of the expected pattern of metastases. For the two most common primary solid bone tumors of the spine, Ewing's sarcoma and osteogenic sarcoma, as well the common hematology primary bone tumors, lymphoma or multiple myeloma of the spine, staging studies differ (**Table 5.2**).

Ewing's sarcoma (or the Ewing family of tumors) is often evaluated initially with a plain X-ray of the affected bone. For suspicious lesions, CT imaging can help to determine the extent of cortical destruction, whereas MRI can better help to search for intramedullary disease (bone metastases) and soft tissue extension. Because Ewing's sarcoma has a predilection to metastasize to the lung, a CT scan of the chest is an integral part of the staging process. Technetium bone scan of the entire skeleton completes the imaging evaluation for the presence of synchronous bone metastases. Although fluorodeoxyglucose (FDG)-PET is often used for staging, there are limitations and benefits com-

Table 5.2 Staging Studies Differences Between Ewing's Sarcoma and Osteogenic Sarcoma

Staging Studies	Ewing's Sarcoma	Osteogenic Sarcoma
CT	Chest	Chest
MRI	Of the affected lesion including the whole bone	Of the affected lesion including the whole bone
Technetium bone scan	Can be done, but FDG-PET/CT gaining favor	Preferred
FDG-PET/CT	Can be done if all bones are included and a diagnostic CT chest is done	Limited by lack of sensitivity to pulmonary metastasis and detection of small bone lesions
Bone marrow biopsy	Bilateral bone marrow	Not indicated

Abbreviations: CT, computed tomography; MRI, magnetic resonance imaging; FDG-PET, fluorodeoxyglucose–positron emission tomography.

pared with the CT chest and bone scan. Many of the FDG-PET/CT scans are low resolution, which decreases their ability to detect pulmonary metastases. In addition, routine FDG-PET/CT scans do not image all the bone in the body, and unless there is collaboration with the radiologist to cover all the bones, the patient might not be completely staging. FDG-PET imaging, however, is better than bone scans in detecting small bone lesions. Bone marrow biopsies (bilateral) have been historically performed for the staging of Ewing's sarcoma because standard staging studies were not specific or sensitive enough to detect involvement of the bone marrow. The use of FDG-PET in addition to a diagnostic CT chest and screening MRI of the entire spine are becoming common staging studies for Ewing's sarcoma. Additional blood testing, including a complete blood count (CBC), creatinine, and liver function tests, is also routinely done, and further evaluation would be needed if these tests are significantly abnormal.

In contradistinction to Ewing's sarcoma, osteogenic sarcoma rarely metastasizes to bone marrow, so bilateral bone marrow biopsies are not part of the routine staging studies. The CT chest and bone scan, as with Ewing's sarcoma, are standard staging studies for osteogenic sarcoma given its predilection to metastasize to the lung and bone. The role of FDG-PET for osteogenic staging is limited by its lack of detection of small pulmonary metastases and less sensitivity in detecting bone metastases compared with technetium bone scans. The role of FDG-PET in more accurate assessment of response to preoperative therapy is evolving. Appropriate imaging of the local disease including the entire affected and adjacent bones with an MRI is part of the staging, as skip lesions can be detected.

The hematologic primary bone tumors lymphoma and multiple myeloma have different staging studies. Lymphoma can be classified broadly into Hodgkin's lymphoma (HL) and non-Hodgkin's lymphoma (NHL). Staging studies of HL include FDG-PET/CT, but bone marrow biopsies are unnecessary. For NHL, the standard staging is a CT of the chest, abdomen, and pelvis. In addition, because the bone marrow is involved 30 to 50% of the time, bilateral bone marrow biopsies are necessary to complete the staging. The use of FDG-PET is only for the aggressive histologies of NHL (tissue is the issue), such as diffuse large-cell NHL. Cerebrospinal fluid analysis is additionally included in the staging of central nervous system (CNS) lymphoma. Similar to Ewing's sarcoma and osteogenic sarcoma, routine CBC, creatinine, and liver function tests are obtained, but serum protein electrophoresis (SPEP) and β_2-microglobulin (indolent lymphoma) are also obtained for lymphoma.

Plasmacytoma/multiple myeloma is another common hematologic malignancy of the spine, and appropriate staging is helpful in guiding treatment options. Solitary plasmacytoma can occur in the bone, and staging is needed to exclude multiple myeloma. Staging studies include metastatic bone survey and FDG-PET or

MRI of the entire spine and pelvis. In addition, laboratory studies, including CBC, creatinine, chemistry group, SPEP (serum protein electrophoresis), SIEP (serum immunolectrophoresis), quantitative immunoglobulins, urinary PEP (protein electrophoresis), and a unilateral bone marrow biopsy should be obtained. If the imaging studies do not show any additional lytic lesions and the criteria for multiple myeloma are not met on the lab tests or bone marrow biopsy, then treatment is primarily radiation. The benefits of additional systemic therapy are unclear, but up to 50% or more progress to multiple myeloma and 11% have local relapse, so long-term follow-up is needed.

Staging is essential in determining the extent of tumor involvement and ultimately choice of management. Each tumor varies in its predilection for the site of metastasis as well as sensitivity for detection on the varied imaging modalities. Thus the process of staging is tissue specific.

▪ Adjuvant Therapy

The third medical oncology principle that all spine surgeons should know is the value of adjuvant therapy or neoadjuvant therapy. Adjuvant therapy is referred to as the additional therapy after the primary lesion has been completely removed. When therapy is used prior to resection of the tumor, this is referred to as neoadjuvant treatment. The main reasons oncologists use neoadjuvant/adjuvant therapy are to improve local control, preferably shrink/calcify the tumor to improve surgical morbidity, and to control any additional micrometastatic disease that might be present but not detected by conventional methods. The value of adjuvant/neoadjuvant therapy is most evident for primary tumors of the spine: Ewing's sarcoma and osteogenic sarcoma. Ewing's sarcoma is a systemic disease. Even though the tumor appears to be localized to one bone by appropriate staging studies, without chemotherapy, the risk of recurrent and metastatic disease is over 80%.[6] With the addition of adjuvant/neoadjuvant systemic chemotherapy, the cure rate

can approach 80%. Osteogenic sarcoma has a similar 80% rate of metastatic disease without adjuvant/neoadjuvant systemic therapy. With the addition of chemotherapy, the cure rates are around 60 to 70%.[7]

The selection of adjuvant versus neoadjuvant chemotherapy is often based on historical data, but there are additional reasons to select one approach over the other. In principle, the use of neoadjuvant therapy will enable a reduction in tumor size, thus potentially facilitating surgical resection with appropriate margins. This can be especially valuable for large tumors that are "borderline resectable" or where critical neurologic or vascular structures can be spared. Neoadjuvant therapy also enables the natural biology of the cancer to declare itself. This is especially helpful when the oncology team and patient are contemplating an aggressive life-changing surgery, and additional time prior to surgery is needed to see if metastatic disease will develop and obviate the need for a life-changing curative surgery. In this situation, neoadjuvant chemotherapy can be used to help determine if the tumor is responsive to chemotherapy and the likelihood of controlling the micro-metastatic disease. Another benefit of neoadjuvant chemotherapy is its prognostic value in estimating the percent of necrosis after chemotherapy (pathological response). For osteogenic sarcoma, after two to four cycles of neoadjuvant chemotherapy, tumors at the time of resection that have ≥ 90% necrosis have a favorable outcome compared with those with < 90% necrosis.[8,9] Whether adjuvant intensified chemotherapy for tumors with < 90% necrosis improves overall survival is not known, and the results of the completed EURAMOS study are eagerly awaited.[10]

There are times when neoadjuvant therapy, although preferred, is not administered. Such incidental discoveries of malignancy can occur with excisions of presumed benign tumors, or removal of lesions found during repairs of fractures. In these situations, there is evidence for both Ewing's sarcoma and osteogenic sarcoma that when all the normally planned chemotherapy is given postoperatively, overall survival is not compromised.[11,12] Another scenario where neoadjuvant therapy is withheld is in patients whose clinical status is insufficient to withstand or tolerate systemic chemotherapy until the primary tumor is removed. The one caveat is that patients with Ewing's sarcoma can have significant systemic symptoms and appear not to be chemotherapy candidates, but because Ewing's sarcoma is very sensitive to chemotherapy, these patients can have dramatic clinical response, so all efforts to administer neoadjuvant chemotherapy should be tried. Other reasons to go directly to surgery without neoadjuvant chemotherapy are if the tumor is causing significant clinical compromise, or if a minor increase in the tumor size could be catastrophic, precluding curative resection. In these situations, a solid understanding of the likelihood of shrinkage of the tumor with neoadjuvant chemotherapy is needed to justify delaying surgery. For instance, primary osteogenic sarcoma of the spine historically does not shrink with neoadjuvant chemotherapy. On the other hand, Ewing's sarcoma has a greater chance of responding both in tumor size and percent necrosis and thus justify neoadjuvant chemotherapy, with a delay in surgery. As with all these situations, active collaboration between the members of the multidisciplinary team is critical in helping to make the best decision for the patient.

Adjuvant therapy is also routinely given after neoadjuvant chemotherapy and surgery to continue to control any additional micrometastatic disease. As noted above, intensification of adjuvant therapy for poor responders (< 90% necrosis) for osteogenic sarcoma is not known to impact survival, but additional therapy should be administered. Significant delay in resumptions of systemic chemotherapy on an adjuvant basis can compromise overall survival. Good communication and coordination with the medical oncologist for timely resumption of chemotherapy is important when the patient has appropriately recovered.

Unfortunately, not all patients are able or willing to resume chemotherapy after surgery. Determining this prior to surgery could help guide the surgeon on how close the margins can be or how much function should be compromised if overall survival will be reduced without adjuvant chemotherapy. Although by definition it is not considered adjuvant therapy if given when gross disease remains or there are positive resection margins (R2 and R1 resection, respectively), knowing the histology of the tumor could enable appropriate R2 or R1 resection followed by postoperative therapy, especially if the tumor is sensitive to both chemotherapy and radiation. The dilemma is that the oncology team cannot always predict who will be unable to undergo adjuvant therapy or postoperative therapy.

For the primary bone tumors of the spine (Ewing's sarcoma and osteogenic sarcoma), the main approach is to administer both neoadjuvant and adjuvant systemic therapy with R0 resection when possible.

▪ Toxicity of Systemic Therapy

The fourth medical oncology principle is to understand the toxicities of therapy. The importance of this principle for the oncological spine surgeon is in determining the optimal timing for surgery in relation to chemotherapy and to appropriately manage the patient in the postoperative period. The vast majority of chemotherapy drugs used to treat Ewing's sarcoma and osteogenic sarcoma of the spine and bone are cytotoxic agents that can affect the bone marrow as well as the kidney and liver. Most of the toxicity is evident by the low counts for CBC, elevated creatinine for the kidney, and elevated liver function tests for the liver. One has to be aware that despite normal counts at the time of chemotherapy administration, there is a known nadir period for these drugs. Recovery can be as quick as 2 weeks but can be delayed due to cumulative toxicity. Some of these drugs can affect the kidney's ability to maintain electrolyte balance (Fanconi's syndrome) despite a normal creatinine.

For metastatic disease from other solid tumors, there are many new agents that target the vascular endothelial growth factor and predispose patients to bleed and clot. The agent bevacizumab should be stopped up to 4 weeks prior to elective surgery to reduce the risk of bleeding.[13] In some patients there is no time to delay surgery, and managing the bleeding will have to be done expectantly. Coordination and collaboration with the treating medical oncologist to select an appropriate time for surgery is ideal. There are many new orally administered tyrosine kinase inhibitors to vascular endothelial growth factor (VEGF) that have significantly short half-lives compared with bevacizumab, and most clinical trials recommend that these agents be stopped 1 week prior to surgery, but there are immerging data that some of these drugs can be stopped as short as 1 day prior to surgery.[14] The complication rate after discontinuation of a VEGF inhibitor is likely also related to the location and histology of the tumor, and continued caution should be practiced when operating after stopping a VEGF inhibitor.

Certain drug exposures are important in managing the perioperative period. The best known is the prior exposure of the patient to bleomycin. This drug accumulates in the lung and can cause lung damage when a high concentration of oxygen is used perioperatively. The newer targeted agents have a host of adverse events that are not typically seen with standard cytotoxic agents. These adverse events should be noted and managed accordingly (see text box).[15]

Common Adverse Events with Agents that Target VEGF

- Hypertension
- Thrombotic risk
- Hemorrhage
- Wound complications including fistulas
- Reversible posterior leukoencephalopathy syndrome
- Cardiomyopathy
- Proteinuria

Patient's Preferences

The final medical oncology principle is arguably the most important and by no means unique to oncology: determining the patient's preferences. The medical oncologist is often able to establish a relationship with the patient and the family. Through initial consultation and follow-up visits, the medical oncologist is able to get to know the patients and understand their wishes and desires. This offers the oncology team valuable insight that can help direct treatment options. The only pitfall is that the medical oncologist does not have expertise regarding the surgical options and all the nuances of the expected outcomes and limitations of the various surgical procedures. The surgeon's input is therefore vital in this regard, and the best overall outcome requires an interactive multidisciplinary approach.

For primary spine tumors, especially if there is known or expected spinal cord or nerve damage, the surgeon is the most appropriate member of the oncology team to explain the options to the patient and to solicit the patient's input on the potential degree of loss of function or functional impairment that is acceptable to the patient. Many patients with metastatic solid tumors to the spine have undergone several toxic therapies and are unwilling to undergo further treatment; they feel ready for supportive care alone. It takes time for the oncology team to understand the patient's preferences. The oncology team feels helpless when additional therapy can be given, such as more chemotherapy, more radiation, and more surgery, but the patient says no more therapy. It is important to take the time to understand the wishes of the patient.

▪ Chapter Summary

The medical oncology principles discussed in this chapter are useful for any provider who treats patient with a malignancy. The first principle, tissue is the issue, emphasizes that in order to appropriately treat the tumor we need to know the specific type of tumor, as treatments are tailored for specific tumors. Once we know what type of tumor we are dealing with, we then need to know the extent of the tumor with appropriate staging (principle 2). Once we know the type and extent of the tumor, we then can decide the value of any adjuvant or neoadjuvant therapy (principle 3) to improve outcomes for the specific tumor. Patients who are on chemotherapy often benefit from surgical interventions, and a good understanding of toxicities of therapy (principle 4) will help the surgeon plan the timing of the surgery and appropriately manage the patient postoperatively. In the end, our role is to help the patient whose fears are real. We need to spend the time to listen their wishes and concerns (principle 5) in order help guide them to make the right decision.

Pearls

♦ Tissue is the issue. An accurate diagnosis is essential to guide appropriate management.

Staging

♦ Staging. Before embarking on a long journey, you need to know the extent of disease.
♦ The role of adjuvant therapy is to improve both local and distant disease control. Tumor removal is only one essential part of the treatment plan.
♦ Understand the risks and benefits of systemic therapy. When is the right time to operate without compromising the oncological outcome?
♦ Understand the preferences of the patient; take the time to listen.

Pitfalls

♦ Not all medical oncologists have the necessary experience and expertise. Get to know your oncologist.
♦ Do not rush into surgery.
♦ Do not failure to understand the natural history of the tumor.

References

Five Must-Read References

1. Rimondi E, Rossi G, Bartalena T, et al. Percutaneous CT-guided biopsy of the musculoskeletal system: results of 2027 cases. Eur J Radiol 2011;77:34–42 10.1016/j.ejrad.2010.06.055
2. Rimondi E, Staals EL, Errani C, et al. Percutaneous CT-guided biopsy of the spine: results of 430 biopsies. Eur Spine J 2008;17:975–981 10.1007/s00586-008-0678-x
3. Yaffe D, Greenberg G, Leitner J, Gipstein R, Shapiro M, Bachar GN. CT-guided percutaneous biopsy of thoracic and lumbar spine: A new coaxial technique. AJNR Am J Neuroradiol 2003;24:2111–2113
4. Scagliotti GV, Parikh P, von Pawel J, et al. Phase III study comparing cisplatin plus gemcitabine with cisplatin plus pemetrexed in chemotherapy-naive patients with advanced-stage non-small-cell lung cancer. J Clin Oncol 2008;26:3543–3551 10.1200/JCO.2007.15.0375
5. Syrigos KN, Vansteenkiste J, Parikh P, et al. Prognostic and predictive factors in a randomized phase III trial comparing cisplatin-pemetrexed versus cisplatin-gemcitabine in advanced non-small-cell lung cancer. Ann Oncol 2010;21:556–561 10.1093/annonc/mdp392
6. Womer RB, West DC, Krailo MD, et al. Randomized controlled trial of interval-compressed chemotherapy for the treatment of localized Ewing sarcoma: a report from the Children's Oncology Group. J Clin Oncol 2012; 30:4148–4154 10.1200/JCO.2011.41.5703
7. Bacci G, Picci P, Ferrari S, et al. Primary chemotherapy and delayed surgery for nonmetastatic osteosarcoma of the extremities. Results in 164 patients preoperatively treated with high doses of methotrexate followed by cisplatin and doxorubicin. Cancer 1993;72:3227–3238
8. Huvos AG, Rosen G, Marcove RC. Primary osteogenic sarcoma: pathologic aspects in 20 patients after treatment with chemotherapy en bloc resection, and prosthetic bone replacement. Arch Pathol Lab Med 1977;101:14–18
9. Bacci G, Mercuri M, Longhi A, et al. Grade of chemotherapy-induced necrosis as a predictor of local and systemic control in 881 patients with non-metastatic osteosarcoma of the extremities treated with neoadjuvant chemotherapy in a single institution. Eur J Cancer 2005;41:2079–2085 10.1016/j.ejca.2005.03.036
10. Bacci G, Forni C, Ferrari S, et al. Neoadjuvant chemotherapy for osteosarcoma of the extremity: intensification of preoperative treatment does not increase the rate of good histologic response to the primary tumor or improve the final outcome. J Pediatr Hematol Oncol 2003;25:845–853
11. Bacci G, Picci P, Gitelis S, Borghi A, Campanacci M. The treatment of localized Ewing's sarcoma: the experience at the Istituto Ortopedico Rizzoli in 163 cases treated with and without adjuvant chemotherapy. Cancer 1982;49:1561–1570

12. Goorin AM, Schwartzentruber DJ, Devidas M, et al; Pediatric Oncology Group. Presurgical chemotherapy compared with immediate surgery and adjuvant chemotherapy for nonmetastatic osteosarcoma: Pediatric Oncology Group Study POG-8651. J Clin Oncol 2003; 21:1574–1580 10.1200/JCO.2003.08.165

13. Gordon CR, Rojavin Y, Patel M, et al. A review on bevacizumab and surgical wound healing: an important warning to all surgeons. Ann Plast Surg 2009;62: 707–709 10.1097/SAP.0b013e3181828141

14. Margulis V, Matin SF, Tannir N, et al. Surgical morbidity associated with administration of targeted molecular therapies before cytoreductive nephrectomy or resection of locally recurrent renal cell carcinoma. J Urol 2008;180:94–98 10.1016/j.juro.2008.03.047

15. Chen HX, Cleck JN. Adverse effects of anticancer agents that target the VEGF pathway. Nat Rev Clin Oncol 2009;6:465–477 10.1038/nrclinonc.2009.94

6

Spinal Osteoid Osteoma and Osteoblastoma

Mélissa Nadeau and Christian P. DiPaola

▥ Introduction

Osteoid osteoma and osteoblastoma are solitary lesions that comprise the osteoblastic benign primary tumors of the spine. Despite the fact that they are histologically extremely similar, osteoid osteomas are not known to progress to osteoblastomas. Their distinction is largely based on their respective size and differing biological behavior. Osteoid osteomas are typically less than 2 cm in diameter, whereas osteoblastomas are larger than 2 cm. With regard to their biological behavior, osteoid osteomas run a predictable benign course with an effective response to treatment.[1,2] Conversely, osteoblastomas exhibit a spectrum of behaviors from relatively latent to extremely aggressive, with occasional malignant transformation to low-grade osteogenic sarcomas or "malignant osteoblastomas" 12 to 25% of the time.[3] Both the likelihood of local recurrence and the treatment of osteoid osteomas and osteoblastomas differ dramatically. Osteoblastomas are one of the most challenging benign spine tumors to treat because of a high preponderance for local recurrence, difficulty in predicting their behavior, and the limited treatment options.

Osteoid osteomas are four times more common than osteoblastomas overall.[4] Osteoblastomas make up 10 to 25% of all primary osseous spine tumors.[2] Both types of lesion are seen mainly in the long bones; only 10 to 20% of osteoid osteomas and 40% of osteoblastomas

occur in the spine.[1,4–6] Osteoid osteomas are more prevalent in the lumbar spine, whereas osteoblastomas do not have a predilection for any particular spinal region.

Both lesions are seen more commonly in males than females (2–4.5:1) in their late teens to early 20s.[5,7–10] The most common age of presentation is in the second to decade of life. Eighty percent to 100% of patients present with neck or back pain, which is usually localized[4]; 25 to 62% of patients with an osteoid osteoma or an osteoblastoma have a scoliosis at the time of presentation (more common with osteoid osteoma),[7,8,11] and 45% of cervical cases present with torticollis.[9] These findings are both the result of an inflammatory effect on paraspinal muscles, causing asymmetric muscle spasms.[11] In the immature thoracic and lumbar spine, this leads to growth inhibition of the vertebral epiphysis and a rotational deformity, resulting in rapidly progressive curve at a high risk of becoming structural.[12] The vast majority of spinal osteoid osteomas and osteoblastomas affect the posterior elements.[4,10,13] Due to their larger size, osteoblastomas may extend into the anterior vertebral body and the spinal canal, thus potentially causing neurologic symptoms.[1,2,14]

Because of their different behaviors, prognosis, and treatments, it is critical to fully investigate these lesions with the appropriate imaging and biopsy in order to confirm the accurate diagnosis of osteoid osteoma, osteoblastoma, or osteosarcoma.

Staging and Terminology

Benign musculoskeletal neoplasms are classified according to the Enneking staging system, which has been shown to be reliable and valid in the spine.[15] This system helps the clinician assess tumor behavior and helps guide treatment. Enneking's surgical principles dictate which treatment is most appropriate for each stage (**Fig. 6.1**).

It is essential for the oncological spine surgeon to completely assimilate the original definitions of the terms as described by Enneking.[16,17] Terms used to describe margins include *intralesional* (some tumor left behind), *marginal* (dissection along the tumor capsule or reactive zone), or *wide* (cuff of healthy tissue around the tumor is removed), and they must be distinguished from the different surgical techniques used to achieve these margins. These typically include the piecemeal technique, where the tumor is removed in several different pieces (e.g., curettage), or en bloc, in which the tumor is removed in one piece, regardless of the surgical margins. Another im-

portant distinction is that of the surgical and histological margins. The surgical margins describe the surgeon's planned and gross impression of the extent of resection intraoperatively. In contrast, histological margins are obtained when the intraoperative sample is sent to the pathology lab, and a microscopic analysis serves as the final verdict for surgeons regarding their success at achieving the planned surgical margins (intralesional, marginal, or wide).[16,17]

Osteoid Osteoma

Osteoid osteomas account for approximately 10% of primary bone tumors.[18] They are bone-forming tumors with limited growth potential that range from 15 to 20 mm in diameter. Patients typically present with constant or episodic pain that increases at night or with physical activity. The pain is caused by the presence of nerve endings within the tumor, which are stimulated by vascular pressure and the production of prostaglandins.[14] Symptoms classi-

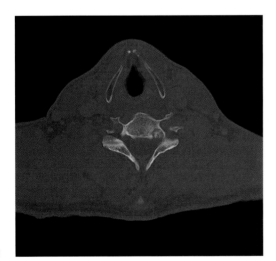
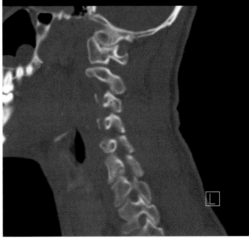

b

Fig. 6.1a,b A 40-year-old man presented with an insidious onset of left-sided neck pain radiating to his left scapular region, slowly progressive over 10 months. His pain was bothersome at night, and relieved with nonsteroidal anti-inflammatories. He denied any neurologic symptoms. Axial **(a)** and sagittal **(b)** computed tomography (CT) scans showed a well-circumscribed lesion with mineraliza-

tion in the nidus, radiolucent rim (representing the portion of the nidus that is not mineralized), and sclerotic rim. It measured 8 mm in diameter. Clinical and radiographic features were consistent with an osteoid osteoma, and the patient was therefore treated with radiofrequency ablation, resulting in a complete resolution of his symptoms.

cally respond to nonsteroidal anti-inflammatory drugs (NSAIDs), at least initially. Osteoid osteoma is the most common cause of painful scoliosis in adolescents.[18]

Imaging

On plain radiographs, osteoid osteomas may show an osteosclerotic lesion, with or without a visible radiolucent nidus, but they are often missed because of their location in the posterior elements and relatively small size (< 2 cm). On computed tomography (CT) scan, they are characterized by sclerosis surrounding a radiolucent nidus, and periosteal bone reaction is often seen. A central region of mineralization may be present. Magnetic resonance imaging (MRI) is best used to aid in preoperative planning to determine proximity to neurologic structures.[19] On T1- and T2-weighted images, the calcification within the nidus and surrounding sclerosis are both of low signal intensity. Enhancement of the vascular nidus with gadolinium may be seen. If neither of these imaging modalities depict a lesion, the most sensitive tool in the diagnosis of osteoid osteoma would then be a technetium bone scan, which shows intense radionucleotide uptake at the nidus, and a less intense larger area of uptake surrounding it.[20,21] If there is any doubt radiographically and clinically that this may be something other than an osteoid osteoma, a biopsy is indicated. This is further discussed in the osteoblastoma section of this chapter.

Treatment

Treatment options for osteoid osteoma consist of conservative treatment with NSAIDs, surgical excision (most commonly intralesional curettage or en-bloc excision), or percutaneous interventions. In adults, conservative management is the first line of treatment; if this fails, or if avoidance of long-term use of anti-inflammatories is preferred, surgical excision is indicated. In younger patients, surgical excision is generally recommended early, to prevent a scoliotic deformity. In cases where spinal deformity is already present, resection of the lesion can result in reversal of this deformity if

the lesion is resected within 15 months of its onset.[7,18]

Conventionally, the surgical excision of osteoid osteoma has been considered acceptable treatment for cure.[7,9,22–24] More recently, less invasive techniques, such as (ILP) and percutaneous radiofrequency ablation (RFA), initially employed in the appendicular skeleton, have begun to gain favor for use in the spine. These techniques have several advantages: they can be performed under local anesthesia, therefore simultaneous neurologic examination is possible; they cause minimal surgical trauma, and in turn patients experience less postoperative pain and have a decreased risk of impairment and infection; and they are associated with a shorter recovery period, shorter hospital stay, and thus lower cost.[14,25–27] On the other hand, the risk of causing local neural element injury with these techniques has been a significant concern in relation to their use in the spine.

Specifically regarding RFA, heating a needle tip to 90°C for 4 to 6 minutes in the nidus of a lesion raises concerns about thermal injury to nearby neural elements. However, an ex-vivo study has shown that there is no temperature increase within the spinal canal when an intact cortex separates neural structures from the needle tip, suggesting an insulating effect of cortical bone.[28] Furthermore, several recent studies have demonstrated the efficacy and safety of RFA when used in the spinal column.[29,30] Martel et al[29] treated 10 patients with 4 to 6 minutes of RFA aimed at the nidus of osteoid osteomas. The distance between the nidus and adjacent neural tissue was 2 to 12 mm (mean, 5 mm). There were no complications reported. Two patients (20%) required a second similar RFA treatment due to recurrence of pain at 2 months. Repeat treatment resulted in long-term symptom resolution. Vanderschueren et al[30] treated 24 patients with spinal osteoma with RFA. They reported a success rate of 79% (19/24) after a single treatment, and 96% (27/28) after a second treatment. There were no complications, and all patients were discharged from the hospital on the same day as the procedure. They concluded that CT-guided RFA should be the treatment of choice in lesions located at least 2 mm away from neural tissue, whereas surgical excision is advised for lesions adjacent (< 2 mm) to neural structures. Several other reports of a smaller number of patients with osteoid osteoma in the lamina, transverse process,[31] lumbar vertebral body,[27,32,33] pedicle,[28] and spinous processes[34] successfully treated with RFA support this as a treatment option for spinal osteoid osteoma lesions as well.

Osteoblastoma

Osteoblastomas are benign bone-forming neoplasms similar to osteoid osteomas. However, they have an unlimited growth potential, being larger than 2 cm by definition, and are clinically more aggressive. Patients with this type of lesion present with dull back pain or with symptoms of neurologic compression. In fact, 25 to 50% of patients present with a neurologic deficit.[7,35] In contrast to osteoid osteoma, symptoms typically are not different at night and respond poorly to NSAIDs. Scoliosis is also known to occur in spinal osteoblastoma, but less frequently than with osteoid osteoma.

Osteoblastomas can generally be categorized into two types: active and aggressive. The distinction between the two is critical, as it significantly impacts treatment and outcome. Unfortunately, this distinction is not easily made or well established in the literature, and therefore one must use a constellation of clinical and imaging findings. Investigators should use the Enneking staging system (**Table 6.1**) as a basis to categorize lesions; stage 2 lesions are labeled as active, and stage 3 as aggressive.[1,2]

Stage 2 lesions have well-defined borders, combined osteolytic and sclerotic features (often resembling osteoid osteoma where a sclerotic ring surrounds a lytic nidus), and no soft tissue involvement. Stage 3 lesions are more rapidly growing, usually exceeding 4 cm in diameter, and have a more destructive appearance on imaging. Their margins are poorly defined, they are primarily lytic, and they erode the cortex to invade the spinal canal and surrounding soft tissues. Some are very expansile, resembling an aneurysmal bony cyst.[2] The clinical course of both differ as well, with active lesions causing slowly progressive pain with or without spinal deformity secondary to muscle spasm, and aggressive lesions causing a faster progression of symptoms with possible early neurologic complaints. Another differentiating feature may be found histologically: aggressive osteoblastomas comprise large epithelioid osteoblasts, characterized by abundant eosinophilic cytoplasm twice the size of conventional osteoblasts.[36]

Imaging

On plain radiographs, 50% of osteoblastomas are lytic, 30% are sclerotic, and 20% are mixed[8]; 55% are found entirely in the posterior elements, 42% involve the posterior elements and vertebral body, and 3% involve the vertebral body exclusively.[36] Depending on whether they are active or aggressive, they have a different radiological appearance as described in the previous paragraph. Unlike osteoid osteomas, osteoblastomas are typically readily visible on plain radiographs. CT scanning is optimal preoperatively to precisely locate the tumor and

Table 6.1 Enneking Staging System for Benign Primary Spinal Neoplasms

Stage	Description	Margin for Control
1	Latent: usually asymptomatic	Intracapsular
2	Active: locally symptomatic	Marginal, or intracapsular + adjuvant therapy
3	Aggressive: symptomatic with local invasion and/or destruction of tissues with potential for metastasis	Wide, or marginal + adjuvant therapy

Source: Adapted from Enneking WF. A system of staging musculoskeletal neoplasms. Clin Orthop Relat Res 1986;204:9–24.

define the extent of bony involvement, whereas MRI is helpful in identifying intra- and extraosseous reactive changes, infiltration into surrounding soft tissues or spinal canal, and neurologic compression. The appearance of osteoblastoma on MRI, however, is generally nonspecific and may overestimate the size of the lesion due to local inflammation and edema.[18]

Histology

The differential diagnosis of osteoblastoma includes aneurysmal bone cyst, giant cell tumor, osteosarcoma, Ewing's sarcoma, cartilaginous tumors (enchondroma, osteochondroma, and chondrosarcoma), and osteomyelitis. Therefore, a biopsy is indicated prior to undertaking treatment.

Histological examination of osteoblastomas is characterized by a fibrovascular stroma and a nidus containing osteoblasts that produce osteoid tissue and woven bone. This is similar in osteoid osteomas, but, in addition, osteoblastomas commonly have large vascular spaces and reactive giant cells.[10,13] Aggressive (stage 3) osteoblastomas are more cellular, with swollen, plump osteoblasts,[13] and may have a multifoci growth pattern mimicking permeation. These features are also present in osteosarcoma; their foci are microscopically identical to those of aggressive osteoblastomas. However, true permeation of surrounding tissues and lack of "maturation" at the edges of the tumor are characteristic of osteosarcomas and can be used to differentiate osteosarcoma from aggressive osteoblastoma. This can easily be missed, and the review of the histology by an experienced musculoskeletal oncologist is recommended.[37]

Treatment

Osteoblastomas are managed surgically because of the recalcitrant nature of the pain they cause, as well as due to their locally aggressive behavior; their larger size leads to potentially significant bony destruction, deformity, instability, or neurologic compression.[18] Treatment options consist of intralesional curettage with bone grafting or cementation, or en-bloc resection. The former is recommended for active

(Enneking 2) osteoblastomas, and the latter for aggressive (Enneking 3) osteoblastomas; the spine's challenging structural and neurologic anatomy makes it extremely difficult to follow these guidelines.[2]

En-bloc resection with marginal or wide margins is more invasive and imposes greater morbidity on patients, but is justified by the high recurrence rate and possibility for malignant transformation of aggressive osteoblastomas when treated with a more conservative approach.[1,2] Schajowicz and Lemos[38] treated a series of aggressive osteoblastomas and recurrence rates were 100% (4/4) for the ones treated with intralesional curettage, 20% (1/5) for the ones treated with excision, and 0% (0/3) for the ones treated en bloc. In a clinically based systematic review done in collaboration with the Spine Oncology Study Group,[2] aggressive osteoblastomas were reported to recur at a rate of 50% when treated with subtotal resection, compared with 10 to 15% in less aggressive lesions. Despite weak evidence, the consensus expert opinion recommendation is to treat aggressive lesions with marginal or wide en-bloc excision, and nonaggressive lesions with intralesional curettage.[2]

Another factor that was found to affect the rate of recurrence is whether or not the lesions had been previously treated with intralesional curettage (and therefore were recurrent lesions) or had undergone an open biopsy. Boriani et al[1] showed that patients who had either an open biopsy or curettage had a recurrence rate of 67% (2/3 patients) after en-bloc resection, and 75% (3/4 patients) after a second intralesional curettage. This compares with a recurrence rate of 0% (0/10 patients) after en-bloc resection, and 7.1% (2/30 patients) after a second intralesional curettage in patients whose lesions were intact (no previous procedure at that site). Lucas et al,[36] in a review of 306 cases, found that there was recurrence after en-bloc only when the procedure was performed through a prior resection cavity. This highlights the importance of the correct diagnosis initially, including the differentiation of aggressive versus active lesions, and appropriate treatment based on this diagnosis, at the time of initial treatment.

Adjuvant Therapies: Radiation and Chemotherapy

The role of radiation and chemotherapy for incomplete surgical resection of osteoblastoma is not well defined. When aggressive lesions are not completely excisable due to anatomic (e.g., involvement of significant neural elements) or medical considerations, they have a higher likelihood of recurrence. If intralesional resection is the only option, postoperative radiation therapy is the most commonly used adjuvant therapy and is considered reasonable. Radiotherapy is also used in recurrent lesions, most often after repeat intralesional curettage. The benefit of this modality, however, is still very controversial, with the majority of cases showing no advantage and a minority of cases demonstrating some benefit.[6,39] Marsh et al[6] concluded, based on a review of 197 osteoblastoma cases, that radiation therapy does not alter the course of the disease and appears to be contraindicated. In contrast, Boriani et al[1] reviewed a series of 30 osteoblastoma cases and found that recurrences occurred in five of 22 patients treated with intralesional curettage alone, compared with no recurrences occurring in the 15 patients treated with both curettage and radiation (at 2-year follow-up).

Harrop et al,[2] in their systematic review, concluded that the evidence was again weak, but that radiotherapy in recurrent lesions or incompletely resected aggressive osteoblastomas should be considered as a treatment option.

The use of adjuvant chemotherapy is limited to anecdotal cases, and evidence to support its use is even weaker than for radiotherapy.[2] There are a limited number of case reports and anecdotes of recurrent osteoblastomas that underwent reexcision or radiation.[40-42] In all cases no further recurrence occurred when the chemotherapy was utilized; however, this success was often attributable to the surgical management only, with no demonstrated additional benefit of chemotherapy. Harrop et al[2] concluded in their systematic review that there is a limited role for chemotherapy in recurrent aggressive osteoblastoma. Further research is required to clarify the role of both these adjuvant treatments in the management of osteoblastoma.

▨ Clinical Cases

Pertinent clinical cases are presented in **Figs. 6.1, 6.2, 6.3, 6.4**.

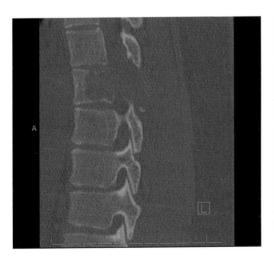

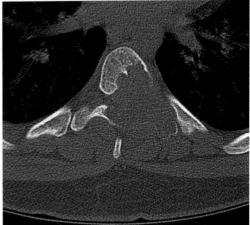

a   b

Fig. 6.2a–e A 17-year-old boy presented with a history of progressive midthoracic pain, radicular circumferential chest wall pain, and numbness from his feet gradually extending up to his abdomen. Examination revealed a sensory level at T6 and mild spasticity in his lower extremities. Sagittal **(a)** and axial **(b)** CT scans showed a large lytic lesion encompassing the bilateral laminas, left-sided transverse process and lateral mass, and almost half of the vertebral body. (*continued on next page*)

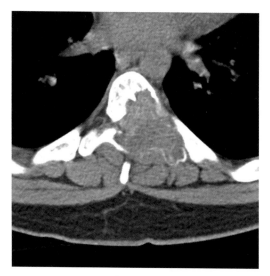

c

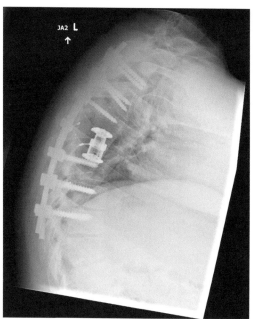

d

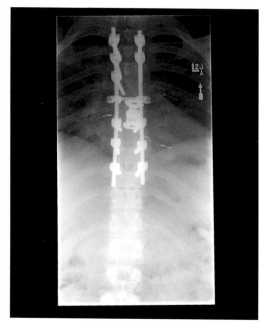

e

Fig. 6.2a–e (*continued*) **(c)** Soft tissue CT scan windows showed extension of the lesion into the spinal canal and compressing the cord. Biopsy confirmed the diagnosis of osteoblastoma. **(d,e)** Embolization of the tumor preceded an en-bloc resection with placement of an anterior cage, and a posterior instrumented fusion was performed. Pathology of the operative specimen revealed negative tumor margins. CT and magnetic resonance imaging (MRI) scans at 2 years showed no evidence of tumor recurrence.

▧ Chapter Summary

Osteoid osteoma and osteoblastoma comprise the osteoblastic benign primary tumors of the spine. Both tend to occur in young males and in the posterior spinal elements. Distinction is based on their respective size and different biological behavior. Osteoid osteomas tend to be symptomatologically well controlled with NSAIDs. Intralesional resection typically results in definitive cure. Less invasive techniques, most notably RFA, is becoming more accepted as a treatment option in spinal osteoid osteomas and has yielded excellent results in the literature.

Osteoblastomas are divided into active and aggressive lesions. The Enneking staging system, radiographic appearance, and histology on biopsy help determine whether a particular lesion is active or aggressive. Intralesional excision

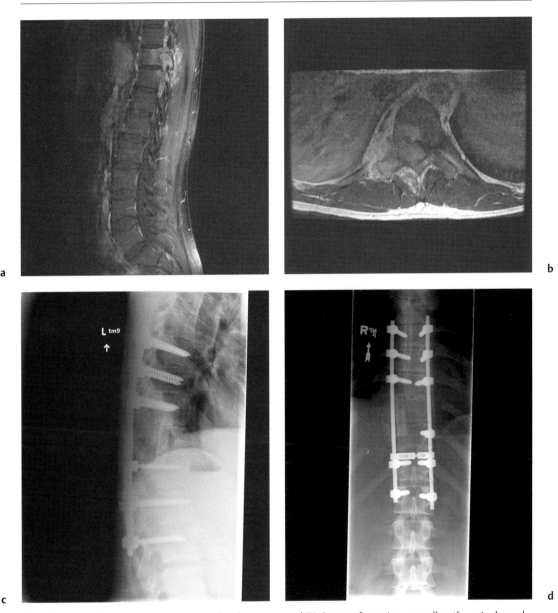

Fig. 6.3a–d A 21-year-old man presented with numbness and weakness in his legs. On exam he had a sensory level at T9, increased tone in his lower extremities, upper motor neuron signs, and pyramidal weakness. **(a,b)** Postgadolinium MRI showed an enhancing lesion at T10 and T11 involving the right posterior elements as well as the vertebral bodies. An epidural soft tissue mass was also evident and involving the right T9-10, T10-11, and T1-2 neuroforamina, as well as the spinal canal, where it caused cord compression. A CT scan (no images available) further delineated the extent of bony destruction. A CT-guided biopsy confirmed the diagnosis of osteoblastoma. **(c,d)** An en-bloc resection of the T10-T11 osteoblastoma was performed and stabilized with a fibular strut graft at the right T10 level and posterior instrumented fusion from T7 to L1.

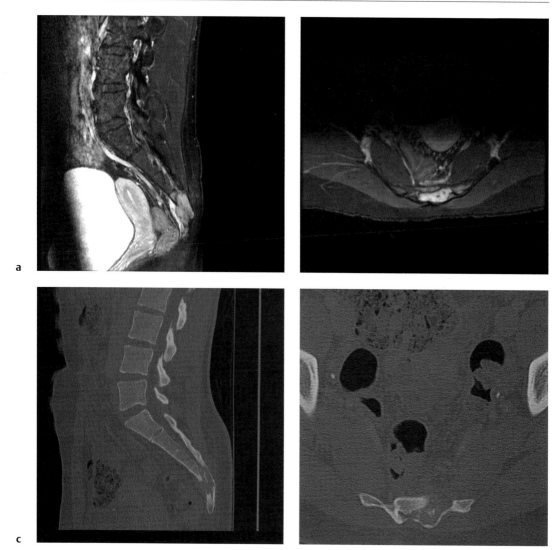

Fig. 6.4a–d A 24-year-old woman presented with a 1.5-year history of coccygeal region pain, and occasional left buttock radiating pain. Examination revealed tenderness to palpation over the sacral and coccygeal regions, but was otherwise normal. **(a,b)** CT scan showed an expansile lytic lesion within the fourth sacral vertebral body, expanding the left foramen as well. **(c,d)** Postgadolinium MRI showed an enhancing lesion involving the S4 and S5 vertebral bodies and posterior elements, with soft tissue extension into the canal and presacrally. A CT-guided biopsy confirmed the diagnosis of osteoblastoma. An en-bloc excision was performed from the S2-3 level down. The right S4 nerve root was sacrificed due to tumor involvement.

has proven to be effective in active lesions, whereas en-bloc resection is recommended for aggressive lesions, due to their relatively high rate of recurrence when treated intralesionally. Lesions that represent recurrences or that were partially resected (due to anatomic constraints) can be treated with radiation therapy, in addition to surgical treatment, in an attempt to minimize the rate of recurrence.

Osteoblastomas can become locally aggressive and can even become malignant. The different biological behaviors of osteoid osteoma, osteoblastoma, and osteosarcoma are of the utmost importance in treatment planning, as is recognizing the aggressiveness of the lesion. This chapter described the typical clinical presentation and imaging features of both types of lesions, as well as the advisable treatment for each.

Pearls

◆ Osteoid osteoma of the spine has never been reported to convert to osteoblastoma.
◆ Osteoid osteoma can be treated with minimally invasive techniques such as RFA.
◆ Osteoid osteoma can be treated with intralesional surgical resection if nonoperative measures fail.
◆ Not all osteoblastomas are equal; differentiating stage 2 active from stage 3 aggressive is critical because it influences treatment and prognosis.
◆ Aggressive osteoblastomas are generally large, lytic, and destructive, with broad zones of transition and soft tissue expansion. Histologically they comprise large epithelioid osteoblasts, characterized by abundant eosinophilic cytoplasm.
◆ Enneking stage 3 osteoblastomas have high recurrence rates when treated with subtotal resection. Therefore, the surgical goal should be a complete resection of the lesion with marginal or wide margins using an en-bloc surgical technique when anatomically possible. Where this is not feasible and positive margins must be left, radio-therapy is a reasonable consideration and may help decrease the rate of local recurrence.

Pitfalls

◆ Recognize the presentations of osteoid osteoma and osteoblastoma. They are a common cause of painful scoliosis in teenagers.
◆ Osteoblastomas typically occur in patients in their late teens (in males more commonly than females). However, there are reports of children developing these conditions at a younger age. Because these lesions can become locally aggressive and lead to spinal deformity or neurologic deficits, the clinician should be prepared to recognize these tumors and to pursue the appropriate investigations (imaging, biopsy).
◆ If standard imaging modalities (X-ray, CT scan, MRI scan) fail to identify a lesion, a technetium bone scan is the most sensitive tool for ruling out an osteoid osteoma.
◆ Avoid intralesional resection of Enneking stage 3 osteoblastomas if anatomically feasible.
◆ Do not underestimate the potential for malignant degeneration of osteoblastoma. Clinical behavior, timing of progression, neurologic involvement, and invasiveness all justify an aggressive treatment plan. Initial treatment has a significant impact on the recurrence rate.

References
Five Must-Read References

1. Boriani S, Amendola L, Bandiera S, et al. Staging and treatment of osteoblastoma in the mobile spine: a review of 51 cases. Eur Spine J 2012;21:2003–2010
2. Harrop JS, Schmidt MH, Boriani S, Shaffrey CI. Aggressive "benign" primary spine neoplasms: osteoblastoma, aneurysmal bone cyst, and giant cell tumor. Spine 2009;34(22, Suppl):S39–S47
3. Nishida K, Doita M, Kawahara N, Tomita K, Kurosaka M. Total en bloc spondylectomy in the treatment of aggressive osteoblastoma of the thoracic spine. Orthopedics 2008;31:403
4. Burn SC, Ansorge O, Zeller R, Drake JM. Management of osteoblastoma and osteoid osteoma of the spine in childhood. J Neurosurg Pediatr 2009;4:434–438
5. Jackson RP, Reckling FW, Mants FA. Osteoid osteoma and osteoblastoma. Similar histologic lesions with different natural histories. Clin Orthop Relat Res 1977;128:303–313
6. Marsh BW, Bonfiglio M, Brady LP, Enneking WF. Benign osteoblastoma: range of manifestations. J Bone Joint Surg Am 1975;57:1–9
7. Pettine KA, Klassen RA. Osteoid-osteoma and osteoblastoma of the spine. J Bone Joint Surg Am 1986;68:354–361
8. Nemoto O, Moser RP Jr, Van Dam BE, Aoki J, Gilkey FW. Osteoblastoma of the spine. A review of 75 cases. Spine 1990;15:1272–1280
9. Raskas DS, Graziano GP, Herzenberg JE, Heidelberger KP, Hensinger RN. Osteoid osteoma and osteoblastoma of the spine. J Spinal Disord 1992;5:204–211
10. Gasbarrini A, Cappuccio M, Bandiera S, Amendola L, van Urk P, Boriani S. Osteoid osteoma of the mobile spine: surgical outcomes in 81 patients. Spine 2011;36:2089–2093
11. Saifuddin A, White J, Sherazi Z, Shaikh MI, Natali C, Ransford AO. Osteoid osteoma and osteoblastoma of the spine. Factors associated with the presence of scoliosis. Spine 1998;23:47–53
12. Ransford AO, Pozo JL, Hutton PA, Kirwan EO. The behaviour pattern of the scoliosis associated with osteoid osteoma or osteoblastoma of the spine. J Bone Joint Surg Br 1984;66:16–20

13. Zileli M, Cagli S, Basdemir G, Ersahin Y. Osteoid osteomas and osteoblastomas of the spine. Neurosurg Focus 2003;15:E5

14. Beauchamp CP, Duncan CP, Dzus AK, Morton KS. Osteoblastoma: experience with 23 patients. Can J Surg 1992;35:199–202

15. Chan P, Boriani S, Fourney DR, et al. An assessment of the reliability of the Enneking and Weinstein-Boriani-Biagini classifications for staging of primary spinal tumors by the Spine Oncology Study Group. Spine 2009;34:384–391

16. Fisher CG, Saravanja DD, Dvorak MF, et al. Surgical management of primary bone tumors of the spine: validation of an approach to enhance cure and reduce local recurrence. Spine 2011;36:830–836

17. Enneking WF. A system of staging musculoskeletal neoplasms. Clin Orthop Relat Res 1986;204:9–24

18. Thakur NA, Daniels AH, Schiller J, et al. Benign tumors of the spine. J Am Acad Orthop Surg 2012;20:715–724

19. Hosalkar HS, Garg S, Moroz L, Pollack A, Dormans JP. The diagnostic accuracy of MRI versus CT imaging for osteoid osteoma in children. Clin Orthop Relat Res 2005;433:171–177

20. Azouz EM, Kozlowski K, Marton D, Sprague P, Zerhouni A, Asselah F. Osteoid osteoma and osteoblastoma of the spine in children. Report of 22 cases with brief literature review. Pediatr Radiol 1986;16:25–31

21. Iyer RS, Chapman T, Chew FS. Pediatric bone imaging: diagnostic imaging of osteoid osteoma. AJR Am J Roentgenol 2012;198:1039–1052

22. Fett HC Sr, Russo VP. Osteoid osteoma of a cervical vertebra; report of a case. J Bone Joint Surg Am 1959;41-A:948–950

23. Savini R, Martucci E, Prosperi P, Gusella A, Di Silvestre M. Osteoid osteoma of the spine. Ital J Orthop Traumatol 1988;14:233–238

24. Hermann G, Abdelwahab IF, Casden A, Mosesson R, Klein MJ. Osteoid osteoma of a cervical vertebral body. Br J Radiol 1999;72:1120–1123

25. Kaner T, Sasani M, Oktenoglu T, Aydin S, Ozer AF. Osteoid osteoma and osteoblastoma of the cervical spine: the cause of unusual persistent neck pain. Pain Physician 2010;13:549–554

26. Saccomanni B. Osteoid osteoma and osteoblastoma of the spine: a review of the literature. Curr Rev Musculoskelet Med 2009;2:65–67

27. Osti OL, Sebben R. High-frequency radio-wave ablation of osteoid osteoma in the lumbar spine. Eur Spine J 1998;7:422–425

28. Dupuy DE, Hong R, Oliver B, Goldberg SN. Radiofrequency ablation of spinal tumors: temperature distribution in the spinal canal. AJR Am J Roentgenol 2000;175:1263–1266

29. Martel J, Bueno A, Nieto-Morales ML, Ortiz EJ. Osteoid osteoma of the spine: CT-guided monopolar radiofrequency ablation. Eur J Radiol 2009;71:564–569

30. Vanderschueren GM, Obermann WR, Dijkstra SP, Taminiau AH, Bloem JL, van Erkel AR. Radiofrequency ablation of spinal osteoid osteoma: clinical outcome. Spine 2009;34:901–904

31. Cové JA, Taminiau AH, Obermann WR, Vanderschueren GM. Osteoid osteoma of the spine treated with percutaneous computed tomography-guided thermocoagulation. Spine 2000;25:1283–1286

32. Lindner NJ, Ozaki T, Roedl R, Gosheger G, Winkelmann W, Wörtler K. Percutaneous radiofrequency ablation in osteoid osteoma. J Bone Joint Surg Br 2001;83:391–396

33. Woertler K, Vestring T, Boettner F, Winkelmann W, Heindel W, Lindner N. Osteoid osteoma: CT-guided percutaneous radiofrequency ablation and follow-up in 47 patients. J Vasc Interv Radiol 2001;12:717–722

34. Laus M, Albisinni U, Alfonso C, Zappoli FA. Osteoid osteoma of the cervical spine: surgical treatment or percutaneous radiofrequency coagulation? Eur Spine J 2007;16:2078–2082

35. Cerase A, Priolo F. Skeletal benign bone-forming lesions. Eur J Radiol 1998;27(Suppl 1):S91–S97

36. Lucas DR, Unni KK, McLeod RA, O'Connor MI, Sim FH. Osteoblastoma: clinicopathologic study of 306 cases. Hum Pathol 1994;25:117–134

37. Bertoni F, Unni KK, McLeod RA, Dahlin DC. Osteosarcoma resembling osteoblastoma. Cancer 1985;55:416–426

38. Schajowicz F, Lemos C. Malignant osteoblastoma. J Bone Joint Surg Br 1976;58:202–211

39. Tonai M, Campbell CJ, Ahn GH, Schiller AL, Mankin HJ. Osteoblastoma: classification and report of 16 patients. Clin Orthop Relat Res 1982;167:222–235

40. Beyer WF, Kühn H. Can an osteoblastoma become malignant? Virchows Arch A Pathol Anat Histopathol 1985;408:297–305

41. Berberoglu S, Oguz A, Aribal E, Ataoglu O. Osteoblastoma response to radiotherapy and chemotherapy. Med Pediatr Oncol 1997;28:305–309

42. Camitta B, Wells R, Segura A, Unni KK, Murray K, Dunn D. Osteoblastoma response to chemotherapy. Cancer 1991;68:999–1003

7

Aneurysmal Bone Cyst and Giant Cell Tumor

Stefano Boriani, Stefano Bandiera, Riccardo Ghermandi,
Simone Colangeli, Luca Amendola, and Alessandro Gasbarrini

▩ Introduction

Many bone tumors include giant cells in their cytoarchitecture. Among them, aneurysmal bone cysts (ABCs) and giant cell tumors (GCTs) are the most frequently observed in the spine. Sometimes these tumors are difficult to differentiate from each other due to similar clinical findings, imaging findings, and debatable histological pattern. Therefore, this justifies the inclusion of these tumors in the same chapter.

▩ Aneurysmal Bone Cyst

Aneurysmal bone cysts were first described by Jaffe and Lichtenstein[1] in 1942, when it was differentiated from hemangiomas and other tumors containing giant cells. According to the World Health Organization (WHO), ABC is defined as a destructive, expansile, benign neoplasm of bone, composed of multiloculated blood-filled cystic spaces separated by connective tissue septa containing osteoclast-type giant cells, fibroblasts, and reactive woven bone.[2]

The ABCs represent about 1.0 to 1.4% of all primary bone tumors. The meta-epiphyseal regions of long bones are most likely to be affected, especially the femur and tibia.[1] Most cases of ABC are identified in the first two decades of life, and predominantly between 10 and 20 years of age. It rarely occurs after 30

years of age, even though it has been described in patients older than 50 years old. Approximately 10 to 30% of ABCs involve the mobile spine, most commonly in the thoracic and lumbar spine. The most common symptom is local pain. Swelling is frequent when an ABC arises from superficial bones, but this rarely occurs in the spine. ABCs mostly arise from the posterior elements, but frequently invade the pedicles, the epidural space, and the vertebral body, often resulting in pathological fractures and neurologic compromise. Radiographs typically show an expansile osteolytic cavity with strands of bone forming a bubbly appearance. The frequently observed "level" images are caused by the double density of the cyst's contents (blood and membranes) and may be considered pathognomonic of ABC. The cortex is often eggshell thin and blown out (**Fig. 7.1**). The lesion is often extremely vascular, but this feature is not often angiographically appreciated even though it is grossly apparent, mainly due to the large number of very thin feeding arteries. Spinal cord or nerve root compression associated with neurologic deficits can be the prominent initial symptom, as some lesions can present with very rapid growth and local aggressiveness.

Secondary ABC-like changes are seen in 10% of GCTs (**Fig. 7.2**), and less frequently in osteoblastomas, chondroblastomas, and fibrous dysplasias that have undergone hemorrhagic cystic changes. These hemorrhagic areas can be ob-

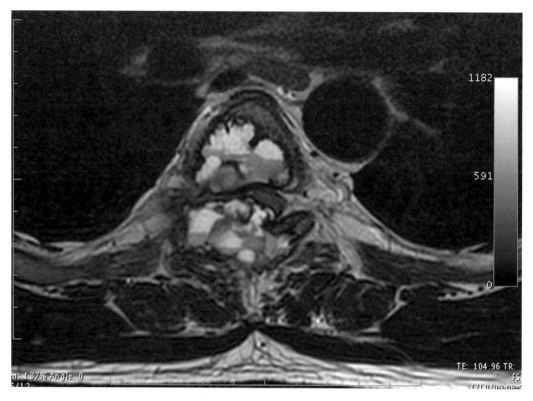

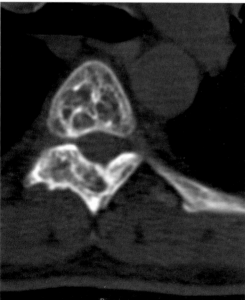

Fig. 7.1a,b An aneurysmal bone cyst at levels T5 and T6 in a 41-year-old man. **(a)** Typical magnetic resonance imaging (MRI) pattern demonstrating well-defined erosion of the posterior elements and part of the vertebral body and expanding into the soft tissue. There are multiple cystic images with double content of blood and membranes, invasion of the canal, and compression of the cord. The patient reported severe pain on the Visual Analogue Scale as well as lower limb weakness. **(b)** Five selective arterial embolizations (SAEs) were performed, with no surgical treatment. A computed tomography (CT) scan performed 2 years after treatment demonstrates shrinking and ossification of the cyst and complete bone remodeling. There is no soft tissue extension and no canal encroachment. Pain receded after the first SAE, and the patient gradually recovered his muscle strength. At the final follow-up he had no pain and normal muscle strength, and was able to perform his normal activities.

served also in primary malignant tumors (osteosarcoma, angiosarcoma) and even in metastases. Treatment and prognosis in these cases are similar to those of a solid tumor, and accuracy of histological diagnosis is mandatory for appropriate management.

Conversely, ABCs can contain variable amount of solid tissue, which is predominant in the so-called solid ABC tumor variant. Such mixture of solid and cystic pattern makes it sometimes extremely difficult to differentiate GCTs from ABCs, both giant cell–rich tumors. The ultimate differentiation can be done via immunohistochemical and molecular biology studies.

The ABCs sometimes have a self-limiting course, evolving to spontaneous healing characterized by disappearance of the double content and ending in ossification of the lytic areas. Turbulent courses, on the other hand, can be observed with huge masses and massive bone erosion. Pathological fractures or spinal cord or nerve compression can follow, sometimes requiring emergency surgery.

It is commonly accepted that intralesional excision (curettage) is the best treatment for primary ABCs. This procedure is frequently risky and sometimes complicated by significant interoperative hemorrhage, which can be

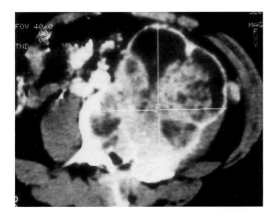

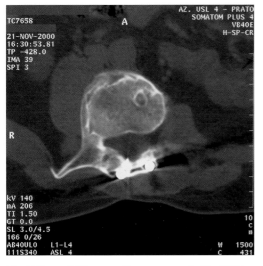

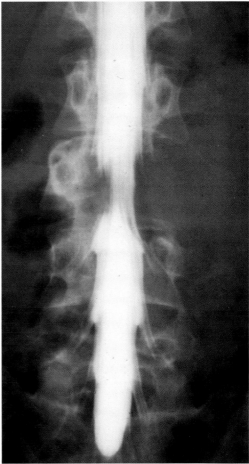

b

Fig. 7.2a–e A 26-year-old man presented in 1985 with a giant cell tumor (GCT) and a huge aneurysmal bone cyst (ABC). **(a)** The huge ABC-like mass is expanding into the abdomen. **(b)** A cauda equina is compressed by the epidural tumor growth, which was Enneking stage 3. An SAE was performed, which succeeded in reducing the mass, enabling a double-approach gross total excision, followed by conventional radiation therapy. **(c)** A CT scan 15 years later demonstrated no local recurrence.

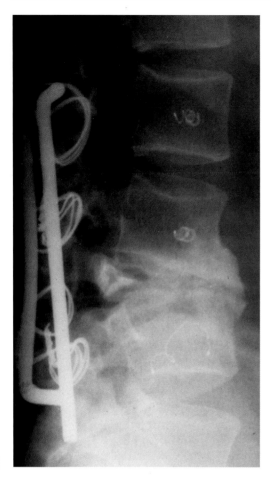

d

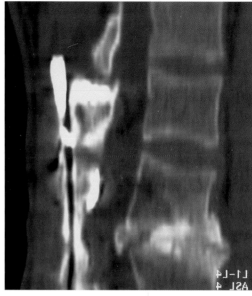

Fig. 7.2a–e (*continued*) **(d)** A standard radiogram 15 years later. **(e)** A CT scan sagittal reconstruction demonstrated loss of lordosis and fusion. The radiographic result is poor sagittal alignment, but the patient does not complain about pain and participates in sports activities, such as running. At a 25-year follow-up phone contact, the patient reported light back pain, full activity, and no tumor recurrence.

controlled by full removal of the cyst-lining wall at the time of surgery. In the spine, full surgical removal of the content of an ABC can be challenging and time-consuming, and may expose the patient to profuse bleeding. Many studies have attempted to reduce surgical morbidity and at the same time achieve full local control, with results indicating that preoperative selective embolization (with polyvinyl alcohol or absorbable gelatin or cyanoacrylate) can significantly reduce bleeding and become itself a treatment option.[3,4]

Recurrence rates for ABC in the spine have been reported in the range of 10 to 25%. ABC is considered radiosensitive,[5] and radiotherapy can be used as single treatment or adjuvant therapy, but radiation can also produce adverse effects on growth in children with consequent late deformities. Additionally, it may have delayed effects on the spinal cord (radiation-induced myelopathy) and increase the risk for sarcomas.

In some studies, more aggressive surgery such as en-bloc resection has been advocated as a possible option,[6] considering that an extralesional surgery is associated with less blood loss and with the highest local control rate. The required excision is frequently so destructive that instrumented fusion must be considered in the operative planning.

▦ Giant Cell Tumor

According to the WHO classification, GCT is a benign but locally aggressive primary tumor, composed of proliferation of mononuclear cells among which numerous macrophages and large osteoclast-like giant cells are scattered.[2] GCTs comprise 4 to 8% of all primary bone tumors, and it most commonly occurs between the second and fourth decade of life, with a slight female predominance.

Giant cell tumor is most commonly found in the juxta-articular metaphysis of long bones[7] and occurs rarely in the spine; the incidence in the mobile spine ranges from 1.4 to 9.4%. If the sacrum is included as part of the spine the incidence rises to 10%. GCT of the spine usually arises from the vertebral bodies, but multicentric simultaneous presentation has been documented.

Imaging patterns include a moth-eaten or irregular radiolucent erosive lesion (**Fig. 7.3**) with irregular thin sclerotic reaction, sometimes expanding the vertebral contour. Tumor expansion in the soft tissue or in the canal can cause destruction of the peripheral cortex (**Fig. 7.4**). Secondary ABC-like changes are seen in 10% of GCTs (**Fig. 7.2**).

Pain, mostly occurring during the night, is the most frequent symptom. Neurologic symptoms due to foramen or spinal canal encroachment by the tumor mass are less frequently reported, as are pathological fractures. However, the erosive activity of undetected GCT may ultimately lead to pathological fractures.

Ever since GCTs were identified, predicting their behavior has been challenging.[7] Various attempts to develop staging systems for the tumor have been unsuccessful.[8] According to the Enneking staging system,[9] GCT can be found as stage 2 active or stage 3 aggressive benign lesions. Active lesions are characterized by fully erosive patterns typically occurring in the vertebral body, with well-defined borders. Stage 3 aggressive lesions have indistinct margins eroding the cortex, expanding in the surrounding soft tissue, early invading the epidural space.

Prolonged disease-free survivals have been reported after curettage and radiotherapy, although some patients may require two or more additional procedures owing to local recurrence. On the other hand, en-bloc excision, when feasible, is curative.

Interestingly, GCTs can produce pulmonary metastases even without histological evidence

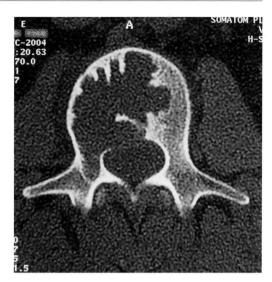

Fig. 7.3 A CT scan demonstrating a fully lytic change with thin osteosclerotic rim at the periphery in a 36-year-old man. The margins are well defined. No soft tissue mass is expanding outside the margin, and there is no epidural extension and no pathologic bone formation. This imaging is consistent with Enneking stage 2.

of malignancy. These metastases can be lethal in 25% of cases, but occasionally may regress spontaneously or be controlled by marginal excision. In 20 patients with lung metastases out of 671 patients with GCT observed at the Mayo Clinic, two patients died of the disease.

Selective arterial embolization (SAE) can decrease intraoperative bleeding and is therefore mandatory before intralesional excision. Radiation therapy must be considered only as an adjuvant after complete intralesional excision, but high-grade sarcomas are estimated to occur in 5 to 15% of cases treated by this modality.

Spinal GCTs have a considerably poorer prognosis than those in the appendicular skeleton, with recurrence rates of up to 80% after treatment. However, this high rate is possibly more related to the technically demanding surgery in the spine than to some intrinsic feature of GCT of the spine.

En-bloc resection is associated with the lowest risk of local recurrence, but this technique entails considerable morbidity and a not negligible mortality. Considering that the only

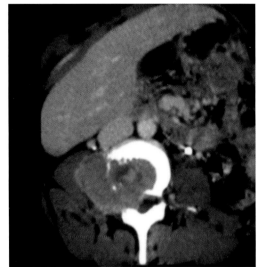

a

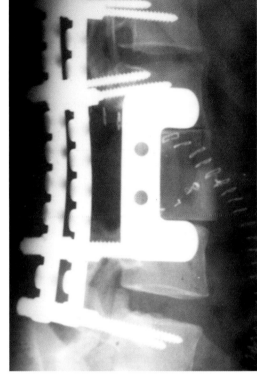

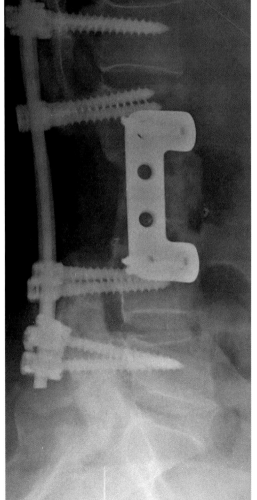

c

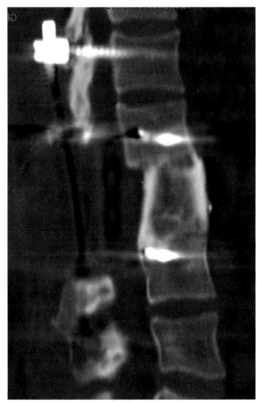

successful treatment seems to be en-bloc resection (which is not always feasible and is burdened by high morbidity and mortality), the possible role of local and systemic adjuvant therapies should be investigated. Currently, denosumab (a monoclonal antibody) is particularly promising.

Imaging findings include lytic changes both in ABCs and in GCTs. No pathological bone formation is detected. Reactive bone is frequently observed as a sclerotic border of variable thickness around the tumors, sometimes creating an effect of swollen vertebra. The tumor mass is sometimes large, and the erosive effect on the vertebra can be extensive. Magnetic resonance imaging (MRI) best defines the tumor extension, the amount of solid component, and the cystic areas.

Some patterns of ABC imaging are pathognomonic. Multiple bubble structures, each including double content (blood and membranes, whose interface changes orientation according to the gravity), with a variable amount of solid radiolucent tissue is frequently observed. Stage 2 GCTs (so-called active according to the Enneking staging system) have clearly defined margins, sometimes with an ossified border. Stage 3 GCTs (also called "aggressive benign") have typically fuzzy borders, early epidural invasion, and radiolucent erosion of the vertebra.

Even if imaging can be pathognomonic, histological diagnosis should always be performed due to the possibility that ABC is occurring as a secondary lesion in GCT or even in a malignant tumor. Diagnosis should always be achieved by histological and immunohistochemical studies. Biopsy should be performed by trocar under computed tomography (CT) scan control. This technique not only reduces morbidity and tumor contamination of surrounding soft tissues, but also enables taking the most representative sample for the pathologist, as the CT scan can identify the area of solid tissue where enough material for differential diagnosis will be found.

Considering that both spontaneous healing[10] and progression to malignancy[11] are reported in the literature, as well as secondary tumor, such as leukemia, occurring after treatment with radiation therapy, the decision-making process for selecting the most appropriate treatment should include a very careful evaluation of the risk–benefit ratio of each possible treatment.

Options for treating ABCs have included simple intralesional excision with or without fixation and bone grafting, gross total excision, en-bloc resection,[6] embolization,[4] intracystic injections,[12] radiation therapy,[5] or a combination of these methods. There is no evidence of a better outcome from any of the proposed treatments, but several complications were associated with more aggressive modalities of treatment, including massive bleeding, limitation of growth and range of motion in cases of arthrodesis, secondary malignancies after radiation, and even fatal events.

The treatment associated with the lowest recurrence rate is en-bloc resection,[6] but this treatment possibly exposes the patient to high surgical morbidity and theoretically must be considered as an overtreatment, considering the benign histological pattern. En-bloc resection should be performed only in very select cases, for example in posteriorly located lesions that are less technically demanding and that expose the patient to less blood loss compared with intralesional excision.

Fig. 7.4a–d (*opposite*) An Enneking stage 3 GCT at level L3 in a 37-year-old woman. **(a)** Lytic erosion of the vertebral body is seen, with soft tissue tumor expanding into the foramen, into the canal, and into the surrounding soft tissues. The patient reports back pain and weakness in the lower limbs. **(b)** An en-bloc resection was performed in 1994 by the double approach. The margins were defined as tumor free (marginal margin). Reconstruction was performed by allograft and anterior plate and posterior fixation with the hardware available at that time. **(c)** Standard radiogram at 16-year follow-up. The posterior system has been replaced due to screw failure. **(d)** A CT scan at 19-year follow-up shows no evidence of local recurrence and fusion of the graft.

Radiation therapy has also been used with good results, but due to the risk of radiation-induced sarcoma and cord myelopathy, this procedure should be considered only when all other treatments fail.[4,5]

In the literature, SAE was first used to reduce the intraoperative bleeding, and was palliative or curative in very select cases.[13] The first case fully treated with SAE was reported in 1990 by DeRosa et al.[3] Later, there were several reports of good results in patients treated only with SAE. In a recently published series of seven cases prospectively submitted to sequential embolizations,[4] no case required surgery and all evolved to full healing (**Fig. 7.5**). The technique included microcatheterization and infusion of embolic agents only into the feeding arteries via the microcatheter, thus sparing normal, uninvolved arteries. Most of these cases, however, required multiple sessions—sometimes as many as seven embolizations every 2 months. The longer time required to perform SAE and the exposure to radiation due to repeated angiographies and CT scanning must be considered in the decision-making process.

One of the limitations of SAE is the risk of embolization of the artery of Adamkiewicz. In case a feeding artery is detected as a branch of the artery to be embolized, the procedure must be aborted and converted to surgery.

An exhaustive literature review was performed in 2009 on 482 articles on ABC.[14] Only 94 articles pertained to the spine or vertebrae, mostly consisting of case reports and small case series. Based on such "very low quality" literature, therefore, a weak recommendation suggested selective arterial embolization as a stand-alone modality, whereas a strong recommendation could be given for selective arterial embolization as a preoperative adjuvant option, as it facilitates resection by reducing intraoperative blood loss. In contrast, radiation and chemotherapy were weakly recommended as additional therapy after incomplete resection and recurrence.

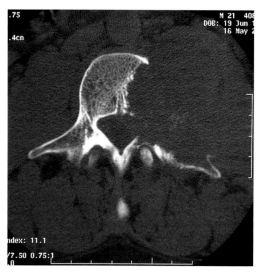 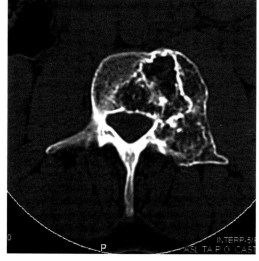

Fig. 7.5a,b An ABC at level L3 in a 21-year-old man. **(a)** Persistent and increasing anterior thigh pain suddenly evolved into severe motor weakness of the quadriceps. A CT scan at presentation shows the extension of the tumor in the soft tissues. The tumor is fully lytic, with a well-defined border in the vertebral body. **(b)** Sequential SAE was performed every 4 to 6 weeks. Pain disappeared after the second SAE and the patient's motor strength gradually recovered. A total of seven embolizations were performed. A CT scan performed 42 months after the last treatment session demonstrates shrinkage of the mass, full ossification, and no instability. The patient has had no recurrence, and enjoys full functioning.

The behavior of GCT is unpredictable based on currently available data. Rock[15] demonstrated the utility of the Enneking staging[9] in predicting local recurrences in the extremity, with Enneking stage 3 tumors having a higher local failure rate. A higher recurrence rate in patients under the age of 30 has been frequently reported.[16]

Although it is not clear from the data, it is possible that the more aggressive behavior noted in prepubertal subjects (**Fig. 7.6**) and in pregnant women may be connected with hormonal influences. However, gender is not considered as a risk factor for local recurrence. GCT can also occur in patients with Paget's disease, sometimes developing large and highly vascularized masses (**Fig. 7.7**) requiring accurate histological diagnosis in order to rule out secondary sarcoma.

In the literature, GCTs in the extremities have been treated surgically with en-bloc excision or by intralesional excision combined with local adjuvants such as phenol, hydrogen peroxide, and cryosurgery or with the margins extended by the use of a high-speed bur.[17]

Whether intralesional excision or an en-bloc wide excision is performed depends on the location of the tumor, its size, and the presence or absence of soft tissue involvement. A higher risk of recurrence has been reported with intralesional procedures as compared with wide resections, although Gitelis et al[17] reported similar local control rates with en-bloc procedures versus intralesional surgeries, which were moreover associated with fewer complications and better functional outcomes.

The recurrences of GCT of the limbs are usually successfully managed with further surgery, and this further supports the recommendation in favor of less aggressive surgery. However, in GCT of the spine, the treatment of the recurrence is not as safe and effective as in the limb, due to it being a more technically challenging treatment. In these cases, en-bloc resection may be a better option, as local control is a primary goal.[18] A study involving 49 patients found a rate of recurrence of 22% up to 60 months after index surgery.[16] En-bloc resection was associated with better local control with Enneking stage 3 tumors ($p = 0.01$) and intralesional resection provided adequate control of Enneking stage 2 tumors.

Although the mortality and morbidity of en-bloc resection in the spine are well known, the risks of en-bloc resection must be weighed against the risks of local recurrence and progression of malignancy. GCTs of the spine may be life-threatening, evidenced by a recent report of two patients who died from progression and lung metastases of their GCTs, and both of them had had a local recurrence.[16] The expected survival after pulmonary metastasis from GCT is around 17%. It is also remarkable that 80% of the pulmonary metastases are associated with a local recurrence.

Radiotherapy is still controversial. Excellent results are reported after megavoltage radiation therapy for axial or inoperable GCTs (with local control rates as high as 77%). Chakravarti et al[19] reported an 85% rate of progression-free survival in cases of inoperable GCTs following radiation treatment, and found no cases of malignant transformation after a median follow-up time of 9.3 years. Later, Caudell et al[20] advised caution using radiation for local control in previously treated patients. They reported a local control rate of 42%, contrasting with a local control rate of 82% in primarily radiated patients. The overall local control rate was 62% at 5 years. Miszczyk[21] reported on a series of GCTs treated either postoperatively with radiation or with radiation alone. The study reported a local control rate of 83% when radiation was used as an adjuvant and 69% when used alone. However, these differences were not statistically significant. In another study, conventional radiation did not improve the local control rate after intralesional excision compared with intralesional excision alone.[16]

The risk of postradiation sarcoma is of particular concern in patients with GCT. Studies from the Mayo Clinic[22] reported a 17% rate of secondary sarcoma arising in previously irradiated GCTs of the spine. In the previously reported review, one patient developed an osteogenic sarcoma 18 months after being treated with an intralesional resection and adjuvant radiation therapy (4,200 Gy).[16] Nonetheless, as

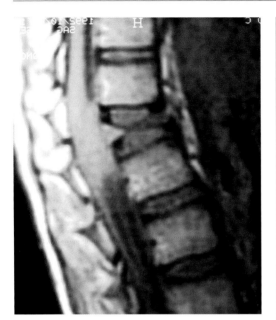

a

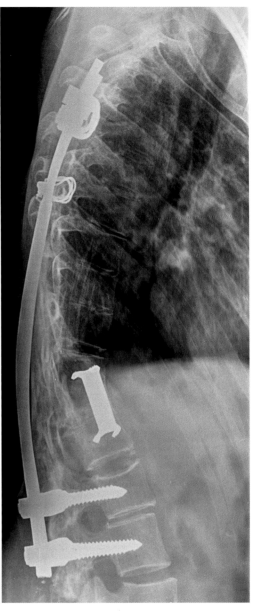

Fig. 7.6a,b A 12-year-old prepubertal girl was referred in 1992 with incomplete paraplegia that was formerly diagnosed as eosinophilic granuloma. **(a)** Early vertebral body collapse with soft tissue expansion in the canal. The canal encroachment is not consistent with the diagnosis of eosinophilic granuloma. The biopsy led to a diagnosis of GCT. An intralesional excision and fixation was performed. Her neurologic symptoms recovered, but five local recurrences followed, with two further episodes of motor and sensory paraplegia, requiring progressively more aggressive surgeries, including double-approach gross total excisions. Several complications occurred, including cerebrospinal fluid (CSF) leakage in the pleural cavity and failure of the posterior implant. Radiation therapy and a course of chemotherapy were performed after the last excision. **(b)** Radiographic image at 21-year follow-up (19 years after the last surgery) shows no evidence of disease.

Fig. 7.7a–e (*opposite*) A 54-year-old man presented in 2010 with a huge GCT evolving from Paget's disease (diagnosed 10 years earlier) in a 54-year-old man. **(a)** An MRI demonstrates a huge soft tissue mass expanding into the retroperitoneal and epidural space, with fuzzy margins. It is categorized as Enneking stage 3. **(b)** The mass extends over three vertebrae. **(c)** A CT-guided biopsy finds a benign GCT tumor. An SAE and a double-approach gross total excision are performed. A recurrence occurred after 8 months and was treated by a posterior-approach intralesional excision. Then denosumab was started in January 2011. **(d,e)** Scan at 3-year follow-up (July 2013). There has been no local recurrence, and the patient is still on Denosumab.

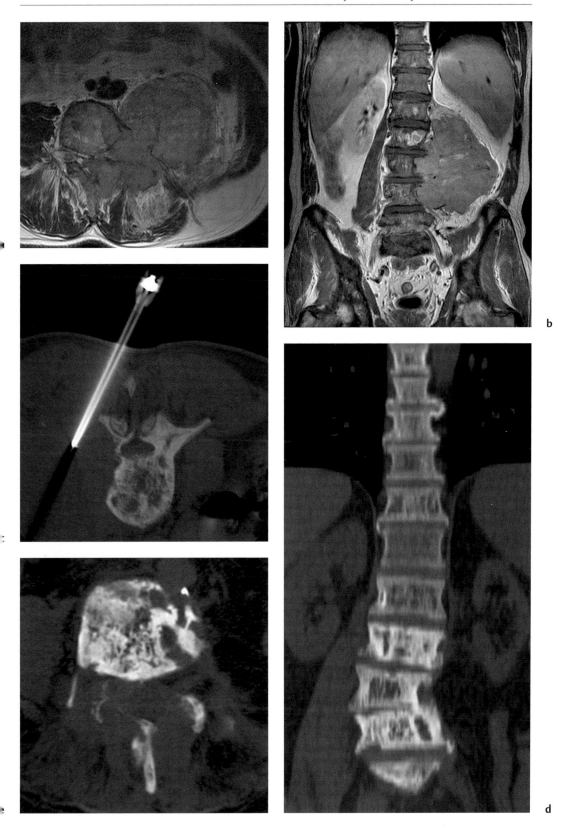

b

d

methods of radiation delivery have evolved, the risk of secondary sarcoma has diminished and will probably be even lower in the future, granting a relevant role to radiotherapy for inoperable lesions.

Embolization as a primary therapy has been recently proposed also for GCT, but only a few cases of sacral GCT have been reported yet.

Giant cell tumor is rich in osteoclast-like giant cells and contains mononuclear stromal cells that express RANK ligand (RANKL), a key mediator of osteoclast formation and activation. It is possible that the recruitment of osteoclast-like giant cells is related to stromal-cell expression of RANKL and that the giant cells are responsible for the aggressive osteolytic activity of the tumor. Thus, the most attractive actual perspective concerns the therapeutic role of denosumab, a human monoclonal antibody that specifically inhibits RANKL, thereby inhibiting osteoclast-mediated bone destruction. The preliminary results show a substantial reduction of the proportion of giant cell and a significant increase of mature bone.[22]

The satisfactory results initially obtained with denosumab in the treatment of GCT and the clear immunohistochemical similarity and relationship between GCT and ABC justify the hypothesis that denosumab may also have positive effects on ABC.[23]

An exhaustive literature review[14] was performed in 2009, finding 3060 articles on GCT. Only 178 articles pertained to the spine or vertebrae, mostly consisting of case reports and small case series. Only four articles were identified with case series larger than 10 patients. These abstracts were all very low quality literature, and no randomized or prospective literature was available. A strong recommendation (on very low quality evidence) can be made for en-bloc resection as the best treatment of GCT, when feasible based on staging, for both primary (Enneking stage 3) and recurrent GCT of the thoracic and lumbar spine.

A weak recommendation can be made for serial clinical and radiographic observation for residual tumor as the best strategy in managing incompletely resected GCT. A weak recommendation (based on very low quality evidence) can be made for radiation therapy as a treatment option for recurrent GCT.

▪ Problems to Avoid

Diagnosis

Planning the Treatment Without a Careful Histological and Immunohistochemical Diagnosis

Notwithstanding the pathognomonic elements reported describing imaging studies, histology is mandatory before planning treatment. A radiographically presumed ABC unresponsive to embolization could be a GCT on histological studies. A trocar biopsy from a cystic area in a GCT can mislead the pathologist into doing a histological analysis, resulting in the diagnosis of an ABC—or an ABC-like area within a GCT. More rarely, ABC-like areas can be found even in malignant tumors, associated with an even worse prognosis. Misdiagnosis or late diagnosis can threaten the life of the patient.

Treatment

Performing an Intralesional Excision of ABC and GCT Without Preoperative Embolization

This situation should be absolutely avoided, as both tumors are highly vascularized. Embolization is proven to significantly minimize the risk of intraoperative uncontrolled bleeding, which can be dangerous and life-threatening. Excessive bleeding may also prevent complete tumor resection particularly in the spine, where direct pressure is not always possible.

Intralesional Partial Excision of a GCT

This technique exposes the patient to a high risk of local recurrence, ranging from 20 to 30% (**Fig. 7.6**). Although the treatment of recurrences in the extremities is relatively safe, the treatment of a recurrence in the spine is difficult, less effective, and entails higher morbidity (epidural scar, dura almost impossible to release). The rate of further recurrence is not negligible.

En-Bloc Resection of ABC

This procedure exposes the patient to unnecessary morbidity. The rate of recurrence following en-bloc resection of an ABC is negligible, but mortality and morbidity of en-bloc resection should always be considered.

Not Considering Newest Options

The ABCs can successfully be treated by sequential embolization. Although exposure of the patient to radiation for multiple angiographies and frequent CT scans is not negligible, it seems less dangerous than intralesional excision, particularly if considering the risk of local recurrence and possible secondary damages to the spinal cord and the morbidity of surgery in previously treated patients.

Denosumab (a monoclonal human antibody, RANKL inhibitor) can be a viable option for recurrent GCT and ABC even though long-term results are still unclear. Its role could be also relevant as a preoperative adjuvant to reduce the tumor mass and to allow easier and more effective excision.

▨ Chapter Summary

Aneurysmal bone cysts and giant cell tumors are giant cell–rich tumors that may involve the spine. Both present as lytic lesions on X-rays and CT scans and can evolve into large destructive masses. Cystic areas filled with double content (blood and membranes) are typical of ABCs and possibly observed in about 10% GCTs. ABC-like areas can additionally be observed in a number of benign and malignant conditions ("secondary" ABC). Differentiation between these two tumors is sometimes difficult on imaging studies, and sometimes histology cannot clearly differentiate them. The definitive diagnosis is made via immunohistochemistry.

Selective arterial embolization is a valid technique for the treatment of ABCs, even if in most of the cases multiple procedures are required. It should be considered the first option because it has the best cost–benefit ratio. It is indicated in intact aneurysmal bone cysts, when diagnosis is certain, when it is technically feasible and safe (no feeding artery to the cord), and when no pathological fracture or neurologic involvement is found. If embolization fails, other options for treatment (mostly intralesional excision) would still be available.

Oncological and surgical staging are helpful for the deciding on the treatment of a GCT of the spine. Staging is based on CT and MRI scans, once a histological diagnosis is achieved by trocar biopsy under CT scan control. En-bloc resection should be considered for Enneking stage 3 GCTs of the spine. The choice of en-bloc resection must be balanced with the inherent risks of the procedure, including morbidity, mortality, and functional loss possibly required by the sacrifice of anatomic structures representing the margin. In cases of required intentional transgression or of accidental transgression, adjuvant therapies should be considered, starting with radiation therapy. Intralesional excision of Enneking stage 2 tumors usually provides adequate local control, and patients should be followed for at least 5 years because local relapse can occur late.

Denosumab (a human monoclonal antibody) can be an interesting option for GCT and ABC, but there are concerns about the progression of the tumors after stopping the treatment. Its role could be also relevant as a preoperative adjuvant to reduce the tumor mass and to allow easier and more effective excision.

Pearls

- ◆ The outcome of ABCs and GCTs can be heavily affected by a late or incorrect diagnosis or by inadequate treatment.
- ◆ Although 75% of ABCs occur in the first two decades of life, 85% of GCTs occur in patients older than 19.
- ◆ ABCs most commonly arise from the posterior vertebral elements, whereas GCTs are typically a tumor of the vertebral body.
- ◆ ABCs are characterized by a double-filled cystic pattern, whereas GCTs are mostly solid. Both occur more frequently in females.

Pitfalls

◆ Planning the treatment without a careful histological and immunohistochemical diagnosis
◆ Performing intralesional excision of ABCs or GCTs without preoperative embolization
◆ Intralesional partial excision of a GCT
◆ En-bloc resection of ABCs
◆ Not considering newest options
◆ Not considering newest options

Acknowledgment
The authors are indebted to Carlo Piovani for design, archive research, and image and editorial assistance.

References
Five Must-Read References

1. Jaffe HL, Lichtenstein L. Solitary unicameral bone cysts: with emphasis on the roentgen picture, the pathologic appearance and the pathogenesis. Arch Surg 1942;44:1004–1025
2. Fletcher CDM, Bridge JA. Hogendoorn PCW, Mertens F. WHO Classification of Tumours of Soft Tissue and Bone. Lyon, France: International Agency for Research on Cancer (IARC), 2013
3. DeRosa GP, Graziano GP, Scott J. Arterial embolization of aneurysmal bone cyst of the lumbar spine. A report of two cases. J Bone Joint Surg Am 1990; 72:777–780
4. Amendola L, Simonetti L, Simoes CE, Bandiera S, De Iure F, Boriani S. Aneurysmal bone cyst of the mobile spine: the therapeutic role of embolization. Eur Spine J 2013;22:533–541
5. Maeda M, Tateishi H, Takaiwa H, Kinoshita G, Hatano N, Nakano K. High-energy, low-dose radiation therapy for aneurysmal bone cyst. Report of a case. Clin Orthop Relat Res 1989;243:200–203
6. Zileli M, Isik HS, Ogut FE, Is M, Cagli S, Calli C. Aneurysmal bone cysts of the spine. Eur Spine J 2013;22: 593–601
7. Jaffe HL, Lichtenstein L, Portis RB. Giant cell tumor of bone: its pathologic appearance, grading, supposed variant and treatment. Arch Patol 1940;30:993–1031
8. Campanacci M, Giunti A, Olmi R. Giant cell tumor of bone: a study on 209 cases with long term follow-up. In 130. Ital J Orthop Traumatol 1975;1:249–277
9. Enneking WF. A system of staging musculoskeletal neoplasms. Clin Orthop Relat Res 1986;204:9–24
10. Malghem J, Maldague B, Esselinckx W, Noel H, De Nayer P, Vincent A. Spontaneous healing of aneurysmal bone cysts. A report of three cases. J Bone Joint Surg Br 1989;71:645–650
11. Kyriakos M, Hardy D. Malignant transformation of aneurysmal bone cyst, with an analysis of the literature. Cancer 1991;68:1770–1780
12. Adamsbaum C, Mascard E, Guinebretière JM, Kalifa G, Dubousset J. Intralesional Ethibloc injections in primary aneurysmal bone cysts: an efficient and safe treatment. Skeletal Radiol 2003;32:559–566
13. Koci TM, Mehringer CM, Yamagata N, Chiang F. Aneurysmal bone cyst of the thoracic spine: evolution after particulate embolization. AJNR Am J Neuroradiol 1995;16(4, Suppl):857–860
14. Harrop JS, Schmidt MH, Boriani S, Shaffrey CI. Aggressive "benign" primary spine neoplasms: osteoblastoma, aneurysmal bone cyst, and giant cell tumor. Spine 2009;34(22, Suppl):S39–S47
15. Rock M. Curettage of giant cell tumor of bone. Factors influencing local recurrences and metastasis. Chir Organi Mov 1990;75(1, Suppl):204–205
16. Boriani S, Bandiera S, Casadei R, et al. Giant cell tumor of the mobile spine: a review of 49 cases. Spine 2012;37:E37–E45
17. Gitelis S, Mallin BA, Piasecki P, Turner F. Intralesional excision compared with en bloc resection for giant-cell tumors of bone. J Bone Joint Surg Am 1993;75: 1648–1655
18. Stener B, Johnsen OE. Complete removal of three vertebrae for giant-cell tumour. J Bone Joint Surg Br 1971;53:278–287
19. Chakravarti A, Spiro IJ, Hug EB, Mankin HJ, Efird JT, Suit HD. Megavoltage radiation therapy for axial and inoperable giant-cell tumor of bone. J Bone Joint Surg Am. 1999 Nov;81(11):1566-1573
20. Caudell JJ, Ballo MT, Zagars GK, et al. Radiotherapy in the management of giant cell tumor of bone. Int J Radiat Oncol Biol Phys 2003;57:158–165
21. Miszczyk L, Wydmanski J, Spindel J. Efficacy of radiotherapy for giant cell tumor of bone: given either postoperatively or as sole treatment. Int J Radiat Oncol Biol Phys 2001;49:1239–1242
22. Thomas D, Henshaw R, Skubitz K, et al. Denosumab in patients with giant-cell tumour of bone: an open-label, phase 2 study. Lancet Oncol 2010;11:275–280
23. Lange T, Stehling C, Frohlich B, et al. Denosumab: a potential new and innovative treatment option for aneurysmal bone cysts. Eur Spine J 2013;22:1417–1422

8

Chordoma

Jackson Sui, Patricia L. Zadnik, Mari L. Groves, and Ziya L. Gokaslan

▩ Introduction

Chordomas are a rare, benign tumor arising from remnant notochordal cells. These lesions occur most commonly in the clivus and sacral spine, at the embryological end points of the notochord. Chordomas are most often locally invasive and aggressive; however, metastases to the lungs and other sites are not uncommon. Further, tumors in the sacral spine may grow to large sizes within the pelvis and abdomen, disrupting the bowel and bladder, and motor and sexual function. Although some drug therapies are under investigation, chordomas are classically resistant to chemotherapy and conventional radiation, and en-bloc surgical excision or gross total resection with subsequent radiotherapy offers the best outcomes for patients.[1–4]

Chordomas occur most frequently in middle-aged men. According to the Surveillance, Epidemiology, and End Results (SEER) database, which reviewed the outcomes of 414 chordoma patients, the average patient age is 59.9 years, with a slight majority (62.8%) of patients being male.[5] Chordomas are rare in the pediatric population. Classically, patients with local disease do well after surgery, with a median survival of 75 months reported in recent literature.[5,6] Patients with metastatic disease have significantly decreased survival (median 24 months), compared to a prolonged median survival for primary spinal chordoma patients.[7]

Based on natural history data, 5- and 10-year survival rates for chordoma patients are 62 to 67% and 40 to 45%, respectively.[5] However, for patients treated in modern case series with en-bloc resection and adjuvant radiotherapy, 5-year overall survival (OS) has been reported even higher for spinal chordomas.[8–11] This chapter reviews the diagnosis and treatment of spinal chordoma, as well as the histological and genetic characteristics that facilitate diagnosis and are driving novel therapeutics. Current literature and classes of evidence supporting the use of en-bloc resection and adjuvant therapy are reviewed.

▩ Clinical Presentation

Clinically, patients with chordoma most often present with pain. For patients with cervical spine chordoma, pain on neck flexion or rotation is most common. Myelopathy may be present if there is spinal cord compression. Thoracic and lumbar chordoma patients classically have local mechanical pain. Among all chordomas, sacral chordomas are the most common followed by lumbar chordomas. For patients with sacral chordoma, bowel or bladder dysfunction, saddle anesthesia, and foot drop or other gait abnormalities commonly occur, accompanied by local sacral pain. Neurologic compromise is less common for tumors in this region. Chordomas in the sacral spine grow slowly, gradually compressing the abdominal viscera, and patients may complain of chronic urinary retention, constipation, or pain that has progressively worsened over several months or years. For patients with large tumors, a mass may be palpable around the buttock. Further, sciatic type pain is not uncommon, radiating down the back of the leg to the bottom of the foot.

In a middle-aged patient presenting with sacral pain and symptoms of cauda equina, computed tomography (CT) and magnetic resonance imaging (MRI) should be performed to investigate the presence of a mass. On imaging, a chordoma may have a heterogeneously calcified appearance on plain radiographs. CT scans are more effective at capturing bony remodeling and destruction associated with chordoma growth, and evidence of widened foramina or thinning of cortical bone may be evident. Overall, MRI is the preferred imaging modality for exploring soft tissue extension associated with chordoma. Unlike other tumors of the spine, chordomas invade the disk spaces (**Fig 8.1**). On T1-weighted images, chordomas appear hypo-

to isointense to the vertebral bodies, and masses are likely to extend to adjacent levels and into the paraspinal musculature. Chordomas appear iso- to hyperintense to the bone on T2-weighted images (**Fig. 8.1a**) due to a high content of mucin or chondroid matrix, and these lesions may have moderate to robust contrast enhancement. Fat-suppressed MRI may be helpful to better delineate tumor margins (**Fig. 8.1b**).

Case Illustration

A 57-year-old man presented with a history of thoracic chordoma extending from the C7-T1 junction to the T3-4 disk space (**Fig 8.1**). He was initially informed that this was unresectable due to its location, and he was treated with traditional external beam radiation therapy and stereotactic radiosurgery; however, he continued to have progressive myelopathy.

The patient was then offered staged surgery for en-bloc resection of the tumor. A posterior incision was made from C1 to T9 and subperiosteal dissection was completed from C2 to T8. Extensive dissection was made beneath the

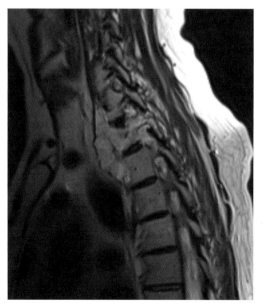
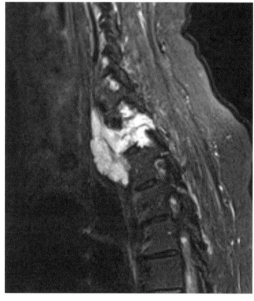

a   b

Fig 8.1a,b A heterogeneously hyperintense tumor was noted on T2-weighted **(a)** and fat-suppressed **(b)** imaging to extend from the C7-T1 junction to

the T4 disk space with significant paraspinal extension. The lesion was proven to be a chordoma on biopsy.

scapula bilaterally to visualize 7 cm from the midline. Cervical lateral mass screws were placed at C3-C6, with a rod inserted across the spinous process of C2 (**Fig 8.2a**). Thoracic pedicle screws were placed at T5-T8 and the ribs were dissected circumferentially and disarticulated at T2-T4 bilaterally. Care was taken to leave the tumor intact. Bilateral total laminectomy of C7-T4 was performed, as well as removal of the C7 lateral mass and the C7-T1 joint. The T1-T3 nerve roots were ligated and

transected. Additional dissection of the esophagus and vessels was made and these structures were protected, and a Tomita saw was introduced at the T3-T4 disk space (**Fig. 8.2a**). Two contoured, tapered rods were placed bilaterally with connectors.

For the second stage of the procedure the following day, an anterior cervical incision was made and extended through the cervicothoracic junction. The C7-T1 disk space was exposed and the disk excised, disconnecting the

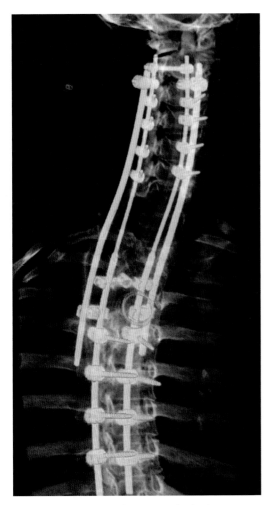

a

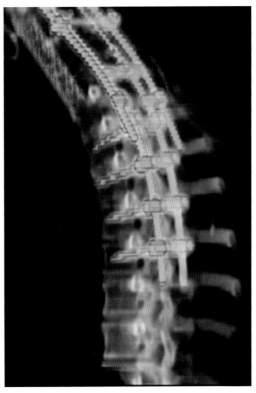

b

Fig 8.2a,b A computed tomography (CT) reconstruction of instrumentation following cervicothoracic chordoma resection. (a) Cervical lateral mass screws were placed at C3-C6, with a rod inserted across the spinous process of C2. Bilateral total laminectomies were performed at C7-T4. Thoracic pedicle screws were placed at T5-T8. A Tomita saw

can be seen at the T3-T4 disk space. Two contoured, tapered rods were placed bilaterally with connectors. (b) Postoperative view of instrumentation with the cage visible anteriorly. The T3-T4 disk space was transected with the Tomita saw, and a C7-T1 discectomy facilitated en-bloc removal of the mass. A cage was packed with allograft bone from C7-T4.

cervical and thoracic spines. The patient was then placed in the left lateral decubitus position with his head in a Mayfield three-point fixator. The posterior midline incision was opened and the latissimus dorsi muscle and scapula were reflected to visualize the chest wall. Thoracic surgery assisted with the chest wall exposure, with a thoracotomy between the fourth and fifth ribs, to visualize the lung. The lung was retracted caudally and the parietal pleura was incised to access the wires of the Tomita saw. The T3-T4 disk space was then transected. The tumor was dissected from the surrounding structures without violating the tumor capsule, and the tumor was removed en bloc. Reconstruction with a titanium mesh cage packed with demineralized bone matrix from C7-T4 was performed (**Fig. 8.2b**). The posterior fusion was completed using decorticated laminar bone from T4-T8, and two chest tubes were placed. Plastic surgery assisted with the closure of the chest wall and musculature. The patient remained in intensive care for 4 days, and was discharged to inpatient rehabilitation 2 weeks after surgery.

At 1 year after surgery, the patient had returned to full-time work. He had 5/5 strength in all extremities, with normal gait and fine motor skills in his hands. There was no evidence of residual tumor. He is alive 2½ years after surgery.

▦ Diagnosis

Biopsy of the lesion should be conducted under CT guidance to avoid open biopsy and contamination of tumor margins. This consideration must be balanced with the pathologist's need for tissue. At the time of biopsy, the skin incision should be carefully marked and excised en bloc in subsequent surgical procedures to prevent tumor seeding along the surgical tract. If a patient presents with a suspected chordoma, referral to a tertiary academic center is recommended for the biopsy to ensure the appropriate pathological diagnosis and treatment.

Chordomas may present in a variety of histological subtypes, and due to the rarity of this lesion, pathologists may have trouble distinguishing chordoma from other tumor types. Conventional chordoma is characterized by cells with a lobulated architecture and abundant myxoid matrix. On histopathological examination, chordoma tissue is often arranged in a lobular arrangement known as physaliphorous with intracytoplasmic "bubbles."[1] Tumors are more aggressive if histological tumor necrosis or Ki-67–positive staining is found. Anaplastic features, including marked nuclear atypia or a sarcomatoid pattern and solid architecture, correlate with high proliferation, metastasis, and a poor prognosis. Tumors with increased amounts of chondroid matrix are known as chondroid chordoma. Cellular based lesions are atypical chordomas and those with high-grade spindle-cell differentiation are dedifferentiated chordoma, which is often highly aggressive and presents with increased risk of metastasis. With dedifferentiated chordoma, the lesion may transform to a high-grade lesion, typically fibrous histiocytoma, fibrosarcoma, or, less often, osteosarcoma or rhabdomyosarcoma. Outcome data for patients with dedifferentiated chordoma are limited to case reports and small cohort studies. A case study of four patients with dedifferentiated chordoma reported survival of 63 and 76 months for two patients following surgical resection, and two deaths at 7 and 9 months.[12]

The genetics of chordoma have been studied extensively in recent years. The transcription factor T (brachyury) is overexpressed in chordomas. In animal models, members of our group generated a novel chordoma cell line, JCH7, from a 61-year-old woman with sacral chordoma, and silenced the *brachyury* gene using shRNA (small or short hairpin RNA).[13] This resulted in a 20 to 25% decrease in cell viability and cell size, as well as an arrest of cell growth and loss of the characteristic physaliferous cytoplasm. In a study using whole-exome and Sanger sequencing of brachyury in patients with chordomas and ancestry-matched controls, a common single nucleotide polymorphism (SNP) was associated with chordoma risk.[14] In a review of chordoma genetics and therapeutic targets, our group identified other chromosomal abnormalities, including deletions in 1p and 9p that are associated with uncontrolled cellular proliferation.[15] These genes may serve as targets for novel therapies in the future.

▥ En-Bloc Resection

En-bloc resection refers to a surgical technique of removing a tumor in one piece without violating the tumor margins; however, it is the final margins reported by the pathologist that are of prognostic significance. The margins can be intralesional, marginal, or wide. Classically, a wide surgical margin involves en-bloc resection of the tumor without disruption of the tumor capsule and sacrifice of adjacent soft tissue. Although surrounding tissues may appear macroscopically uninvolved, locally invasive disease may be present at a cellular or microscopic level. Thus, wide margins provide the most thorough resection of the lesion. Other considerations, such as the proximity of the spinal cord and bowel, can limit the feasibility of wide marginal resection for spinal chordomas, unless functional impairment is accepted.[16] Marginal resection involves the en-bloc removal of the tumor with dissection along the tumor capsule, which runs the risk of satellite tumor cells being left behind. In contrast, intralesional resection involves curettage and piecemeal resection of the tumor. Violation of the tumor capsule increases the risk of local tumor spillage and seeding along surgical margins, and almost always leaves residual tumor behind.

En-bloc resection, with marginal or wide margins, unequivocally provides better long-term survival. The Spine Oncology Study Group (SOSG) issued a strong recommendation based on moderate-quality evidence and consensus expert opinion that en-bloc resection should be undertaken for surgical treatment of spinal chordoma.[2] This was the result of a systematic review and ambispective multicenter cohort study by the SOSG.[2] However, the language used in the chordoma literature is inconsistent. The terms *gross total, radical,* and *en-bloc resection* are often used interchangeably, with considerable variability based on the surgeon's preferred terminology. In a literature review of peer-reviewed, PubMed-indexed, English-language articles from 1996 to 2011 with full text available, reporting data for en-bloc resection for chordoma, among studies with 94% or more patients undergoing en-bloc resection, the mean disease-free survival was 70 to 84.2 months (**Table 8.1**).

Surgical resection of the spinal tumor also varies by tumor location. Specifically, chordomas in the cervical spine present a unique challenge due to complex and functionally critical

Table 8.1 Literature Review of Reported Mean Disease-Free Survival

Source	Sample Size	Male (%)	En Bloc (%)	Margin Type (W, M, I)[a]	Mean Follow-Up (Months)	Mean Disease-Free Survival (Months)
Hsieh et al, 2011	5	60	100	W and M	54.7	84.2
Cloyd et al, 2009	2	50	100	M	21	NA
Ahmed et al, 2009	18	56	94	W, M, and I	132	70
Barrenechea et al, 2007	7	57	0	I	59	NA
Boriani et al, 2006	52	71	19	W, M, I, no resection	NA	NA
Fuchs et al, 2005	52	65	40	W, M, and I	94	70
Boriani et al, 1996	29	45	97	W, M, and I	30	NA

Note: Among studies with 94% or more patients undergoing en-bloc resection, mean disease-free survival was 70 to 84.2 months. Inclusion criteria for this review included Pubmed-indexed articles in English from 1996 to 2011, with full text available. Articles were reviewed for data reporting outcomes following en-bloc resection of chordoma.

[a]Margin type: W, wide; M, marginal; I, intralesional.

anatomy. In esophagus, trachea, carotid, and vertebral arteries, C5 through T1 limit the possibility of truly wide surgical margins. Location at the craniocervical junction, or extension of a skull base chordoma into the cervical spine, is associated with worse outcome.[17] When en-bloc resection is not possible, intralesional resection with subsequent stereotactic radiation has been reported to provide improved survival. This method has shown a 46% control rate at 5 years for tumors of the cervical spine.[18-20] In recent years, advances in surgical techniques have enabled more aggressive resection in patients with cervical spine chordoma, often through multistage operations.[17,21] This has led to mean a disease-free survival of 84.2 months for tumors of the cervical spine following en-bloc resection in one cohort study.[10]

Proper surgical planning through imaging has enabled the majority of chordomas of the thoracolumbar spine to be removed en bloc with disease-free margins. Using multiple surgical approaches is common, with a posterior approach being used in nearly every thoracolumbar chordoma surgery. The addition of an anterior approach may be performed as dictated by a tumor growing ventrally beyond the vertebra. This has been shown to improve disease-free survival.[8]

Case Illustration

A 45-year-old woman presented with back pain after a fall. Imaging revealed a lesion at L4 (**Fig. 8.3a,b**), and a percutaneous biopsy was consistent with chordoma. She was offered a staged procedure for en-bloc resection of the tumor. Stage one involved a posterior approach with L2, L3, and L5 laminectomies and en-bloc removal of the posterior elements of L4 using a Tomita saw. Posterior instrumentation was placed from T11 to the pelvis, with pedicle screws at T10-L1 and S1, and bilateral iliac screws. A Silastic sheet was placed between the thecal sac and instrumentation, and the wound was closed in a multilayered fashion. The next day, the iliopsoas and lumbar plexus was mobilized and dissected, from the posterior approach, and Tomita saws were placed posterior to the L2-L3 disk space and the L5-S1

disk space. Two days later, a vascular surgeon assisted in an anterior transabdominal and retroperitoneal exposure of the L3-L4, L4-L5, and L5-S1 interspaces, with mobilization of the abdominal aorta. The Tomita saws were advanced and the tumor was removed en bloc from the field; however, pathological review of the specimen demonstrated tumor within 1 mm of the anterior margins of the specimen. Anterior reconstruction from L2-S1 was performed using a distractable titanium case and a transvertebral screw in the L2 vertebral body, with titanium cabling to the posterior rod/screw construct (**Fig 8.3c**).

Postoperatively, the patient experienced *transfusion-related acute lung injury* (TRALI) and remained intubated following the second posterior operation. She was discharged to inpatient rehabilitation with 5/5 motor strength in all extremities. She received postoperative proton beam radiation. Two years after surgery, loosening of the iliac screws was noted and she underwent revision for replacement of bilateral iliac screws and addition of allograft fibular struts for posterior arthrodesis. She had no evidence of recurrence of disease at 2 years of clinical follow-up, and is alive 2½ years after surgery.

▓ Sacral Chordoma

Sacral chordomas pose unique challenges for surgeons, as they can grow to massive sizes. Potential problems include massive blood loss, soft tissue defects, and a high risk of wound infection. Procedures are posterior or staged anterior and posterior. Lumbopelvic reconstruction is rarely required after the procedure unless a total or high sacrectomy is required; reconstruction adds considerable complexity to the case. The best available evidence suggests that wide margins should be achieved during the resection.[3,8,9,22] Sacrectomy level is dictated by the nerve roots involved with the tumor. Fourney and colleagues,[9] correlating the level of resection with the postoperative motor, bowel, and bladder deficits, proposed a classification scheme. Neurologic deficits can lead to

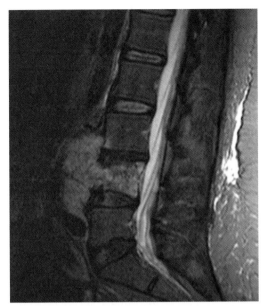

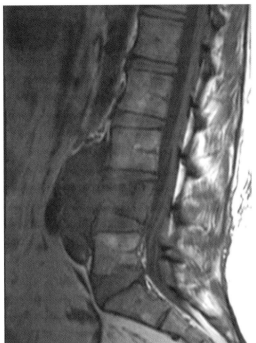

b

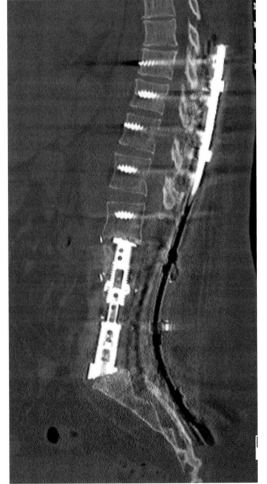

Fig. 8.3a–c Sagittal T2-weighted fat-suppressed **(a)** and T1-weighted **(b)** magnetic resonance imaging (MRI) demonstrating a lumbar chordoma at L4 with ventral extension from L3-L5. There is a loss of vertebral body height at L4. **(c)** Postoperative sagittal CT demonstrates anterior/posterior instrumentation.

profound morbidity, and, when possible, even unilateral preservation can permit satisfactory function. Although preservation of bilateral L5 nerve roots is necessary for satisfactory ambulation, unilateral preservation of S2-S5 permits satisfactory bowel control and possible maintenance of bladder and sexual function. Bilateral preservation of S2 with unilateral S3 results in almost normal bowel/bladder and sexual function. For patients with complete deficits prior to surgery, it is unlikely that surgery will restore the deficit.

Surgical resection of sacral chordoma classically involves a staged anterior and posterior resection, although more aggressive posterior-only procedures are now being done. In a large case series described at our institution, a posterior-only approach was safely used for en-bloc sacrectomy to limit the morbidity associated with anterior approaches.[23] The trade-off, however, is large soft tissue defects. When an anterior approach is done first, a pedicled flap reconstruction with a vertical rectus abdominis musculocutaneous (VRAM) flap is simple and readily available once the second-stage posterior approach is completed. With lone posterior approaches only, local gluteal muscle flaps along with an acellular dermal matrix to prevent bowl herniation are available. Sometimes the local gluteal muscle is not enough and free flaps must be used. These wounds commonly become infected, and rates up to 40% have been reported.[22] Patients should be informed of this likely complication.

Extensive lumbopelvic reconstruction is required when more than half of the sacroiliac joint is resected. A femoral strut or transiliac rod, lumbar posterior instrumentation, and iliac or S2 screws with cross-connectors should be used to effectively rejoin the lumbar spine and pelvis following total sacrectomy. Resection of the caudal sacrum up to the lower half of the sacroiliac joint may be performed without compromising stability.

Case Illustration

A 66-year-old man presented with sacral pain, loss of bowel and bladder control, right-sided foot drop, and a palpable mass in the buttocks.

Imaging revealed a massive tumor, and biopsy was consistent with chordoma (**Fig. 8.4a,b**). On questioning, the patient was aware of the tumor for several years. A multidisciplinary, staged surgical approach was offered to the patient, consisting of, on the first day of the operation, mobilization of the iliac vessels from the lumbosacral junction and ligation of the internal iliac vessels by the vascular team, a colostomy by the gastrointestinal surgery service, and a partial L5 corpectomy.

On the second day, harvesting of the left-sided rectus abdominis pedicle flap (fed by the inferior epigastric vessels) was completed by the plastic surgery team, and a posterior approach was initiated by the neurosurgical team. A T-shaped incision was made, extending between the greater trochanters and vertically to expose the lumbar spine to L3. The sacral nerve roots were ligated and posterior laminectomies were completed at L4 and L5, as an extensive dissection was made to remove all soft tissue from the tumor. The L5 spondylectomy was completed with sparing of the L5 nerve root, and the tumor was removed en bloc with the entire sacrum. Pedicle screw instrumentation followed in L2-L5, followed by iliac screw placement, and rod placement between the ilia (**Fig. 8.4c–e**). A contoured rod was placed vertically and connected to the iliac rod with J-shaped connectors. Then a femur shaft was cut in halves and was fitted into the defect extending from one ilium to the other side. This was wired in place using a titanium wire. Then, the dorsal aspect of the spinal column was decorticated, extending from L2 all the way down to the pelvis bilaterally. An allograft bone graft was mixed with ostium and demineralized bone matrix, and the bone graft was packed tightly, extending L2 all the way down the pelvis bilaterally and down to the femur shaft (**Fig. 8.4c–e).**

The patient experienced a drop in oxygen saturation and blood pressure in the operating room; however, he was successfully resuscitated and the plastic surgery team completed the complex wound closure the following day. He continued to improve and was discharged to inpatient rehabilitation 1 month after surgery. He is alive 2 years after surgery.

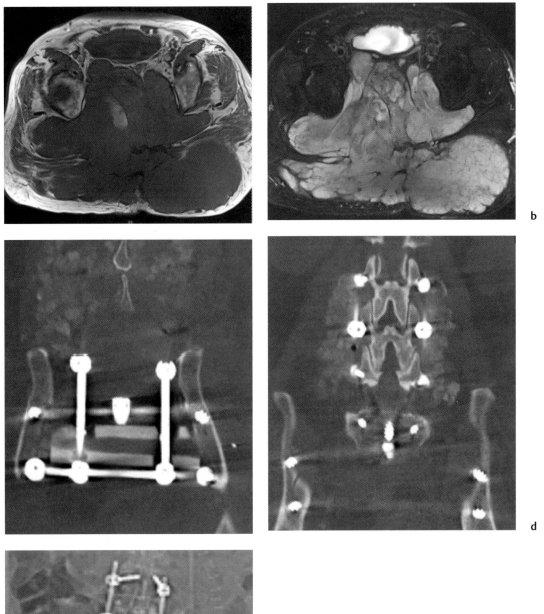

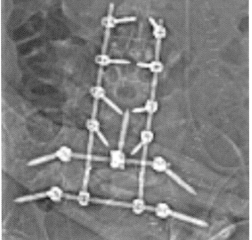

Fig. 8.4a–e Axial T1-weighted **(a)** and T2-weighted fat-suppressed **(b)** MRI of a massive sacral chordoma. The patient presented with sacral pain from a known lesion of several years. **(c,d)** Lumbopelvic reconstruction on postoperative CT scan. **(c)** Femoral strut with iliac screws and rods. **(d)** En-bloc sacrectomy is evident, seen as a complete absence of the bony sacrum. **(e)** CT scout image illustrating the full extent of lumbopelvic reconstruction, including bilateral iliac screws.

▦ Adjuvant Therapy

Radiation Therapy

Classically, chordoma has been considered a radioresistant lesion, requiring either high-dose fractionated photon or proton therapy; however, no class I evidence exists to guide the administration of radiotherapy. The SOSG issued a weak recommendation based on low-quality evidence that radiation therapy of 60- to 65-Gy equivalents or higher should be administered following incomplete or intralesional resection of chordoma.[2] This was the result of a systematic review and ambispective multicenter cohort study by the SOSG.[2]

In the literature, high-dose conformal conventional radiotherapy has been used in case reports and cohort studies to deliver directed therapy for chordoma following incomplete surgical resection or prior to surgical resection to reduce the violation of contaminated tumor margins[11,19]; however, incidental radiation to the spinal cord and paraspinal structures is a serious concern. Stereotactic radiosurgery has been proposed in some small case series for patients with spinal chordoma and in larger cohorts with skull base chordoma, and has demonstrated safety and efficacy with a 5-year OS of 74.3%.[24] Alternatively, proton therapy has emerged as yet another therapeutic option for chordoma.[11,25] In contrast to photon therapy, protons have limited scatter and can target tumors located in deep tissues without depositing radiation to structures behind or deep to the tumor. This is particularly advantageous for chordomas arising within the skull base or vertebral column that abut the delicate structures of the nervous system.

Radiation as an adjuvant therapy following surgical resection for chordoma has historically demonstrated improved progression-free survival (PFS) and OS.[19,26] Radiotherapy as a salvage therapy following multiple resections is demonstrably less effective. In a retrospective analysis of 27 patients with sacral chordoma who received surgery and proton ± photon radiation, patients with primary tumors had a 92.9% 5-year overall survival, whereas patients with recurrent tumors had a 66.7% 5-year OS.[11]

Notably, radiation doses were high in this cohort, ≥ 53 Gy in 24-42 fractions.

In the literature, many studies of high-dose proton/photon therapy as a definitive single therapy are limited to skull base or craniocervical junction chordomas, as these lesions are less amenable to en-bloc resection. In contrast, few studies have been published on the outcomes for proton/photon therapy alone for the treatment of spinal chordoma. In a retrospective review of 24 patients with primary unresectable chordoma of the spine who did not undergo surgical resection, local PFS and OS were 79.8% and 78.1% at 5 years, respectively.[25] In this study, the mean dose of proton/photon therapy was 77.4 Gy RBE (Gy RBE is defined as the proton dose unit, equal to Gy × the relative biological effectiveness).[25] In a small cohort of six patients who received high-dose proton or photon radiation only for primary or recurrent chordoma, four patients received high-dose radiation at ≥73 Gy equivalents, and three of these patients had local control at 2.9, 4.9, and 7.6 years.[11]

Chemotherapy

In a review of the current therapeutic options for chordoma, members of our group summarized the use of chemotherapy as an adjuvant for chordoma.[15] No class I evidence currently exists to drive the treatment of chordoma; however, regimens reported in small case-cohort studies include anthracycline, cisplatin, alkylating agents, and camptothecin. In a phase II prospective trial of imatinib, a tyrosine kinase inhibitor used for chronic myelogenous leukemia, 56 patients with platelet-derived growth factor (PDGF)-positive chordoma were given 800 mg of imatinib per day until tumor progression.[27] Overall tumor response rate, as defined by the *Response Evaluation Criteria In Solid Tumor* (RECIST), was recorded. A 64% clinical benefit rate was found, including patients with complete response, partial response, or stable disease for ≥ 6 months.[27] Recent trials of the epidermal growth factor receptor (EGFR)-inhibitor erlotinib have shown a good response with a 12-month uninterrupted use of the drug in a single patient,[28] and other EGFR inhibitors have been reported in a limited number of case reports. Similarly, one group reported response in recurrent disease with pulmonary metastases with the combined therapy cetuximab/gefitinib over a 9-month follow-up period.[29]

data have isolated the *brachyury* gene as a possible future target for therapy. In the future, randomized controlled prospective clinical trials will be helpful to determine the ideal treatments for patients with chordoma within the spinal column.

■ Chapter Summary

Patients with spinal chordoma have the potential for excellent long-term survival when given the proper care. Treatment starts at the first clinical encounter, with referral to a tertiary care center with high-volume experience in chordoma management. Open biopsy is not recommended, and CT-guided or fine-needle aspiration is appropriate with marking of the biopsy tract for later inclusion in the en-bloc resection. Pathological confirmation of physaliferous cells, as well as preoperative imaging hyperintensity on T2 and fat-suppressed images, in a tumor crossing the disk space or invading in to the paraspinal musculature strongly suggests a diagnosis of chordoma. The SOSG issued a strong recommendation for en-bloc resection and a weak recommendation for high-dose radiotherapy following incomplete or intralesional resection. A recent phase II trial of imatinib demonstrated modest clinical benefit based on the RECIST. Surgical resection and postoperative adjuvant therapy are dictated by the level of the tumor, and cervical and sacral tumors pose unique challenges for en-bloc resection and postoperative reconstruction. Genetic studies involving animal and human

Pearls

◆ The Spine Oncology Study Group (SOSG) issued a strong recommendation on moderate-quality evidence that en-bloc resection should be attempted in spinal chordoma.
◆ The SOSG offered a weak recommendation based on low-quality evidence that radiation therapy greater than 60 to 65 Gy equivalents is indicated following incomplete resection.
◆ Chemotherapy recommendations are based on mostly class II and IV evidence.
◆ One prospective, phase II trial reported a moderate clinical benefit based on the RECIST using imatinib in a subset of chordoma.
◆ For patients with sacral chordoma, en-bloc resection will result in a large soft tissue defect, and coordination of care with a plastic surgeon is recommended.

Pitfalls

◆ Open biopsy seeds the biopsy site with tumor and precludes later en-bloc resection.
◆ Surgical planning involves excision of the biopsy tract.
◆ En-bloc total or high sacrectomy can result in massive blood loss.
◆ Removal of greater than 50% of the sacroiliac joint requires lumbopelvic reconstruction.
◆ Wound infection rates are high following sacrectomy for sacral chordoma, and patients should be warned of this likely complication.

References
Five Must-Read References

1. Bjornsson J, Wold LE, Ebersold MJ, Laws ER. Chordoma of the mobile spine. A clinicopathologic analysis of 40 patients. Cancer 1993;71:735–740
2. Boriani S, Saravanja D, Yamada Y, Varga PP, Biagini R, Fisher CG. Challenges of local recurrence and cure in low grade malignant tumors of the spine. Spine 2009;34(22, Suppl):S48–S57
3. Sciubba DM, Cheng JJ, Petteys RJ, Weber KL, Frassica DA, Gokaslan ZL. Chordoma of the sacrum and verte-

bral bodies. J Am Acad Orthop Surg 2009;17:708–717
4. Walcott BP, Nahed BV, Mohyeldin A, Coumans JV, Kahle KT, Ferreira MJ. Chordoma: current concepts, management, and future directions. Lancet Oncol 2012;13:e69–e76
5. Mukherjee D, Chaichana KL, Gokaslan ZL, Aaronson O, Cheng JS, McGirt MJ. Survival of patients with malignant primary osseous spinal neoplasms: results

from the Surveillance, Epidemiology, and End Results (SEER) database from 1973 to 2003. J Neurosurg Spine 2011;14:143–150

6. McMaster ML, Goldstein AM, Bromley CM, Ishibe N, Parry DM. Chordoma: incidence and survival patterns in the United States, 1973-1995. Cancer Causes Control 2001;12:1–11

7. Mukherjee D, Chaichana KL, Adogwa O, et al. Association of extent of local tumor invasion and survival in patients with malignant primary osseous spinal neoplasms from the surveillance, epidemiology, and end results (SEER) database. World Neurosurg 2011; 76:580–585

8. Boriani S, Bandiera S, Biagini R, et al. Chordoma of the mobile spine: fifty years of experience. Spine 2006; 31:493–503

9. Fourney DR, Rhines LD, Hentschel SJ, et al. En bloc resection of primary sacral tumors: classification of surgical approaches and outcome. J Neurosurg Spine 2005;3:111–122

10. Hsieh PC, Gallia GL, Sciubba DM, et al. En bloc excisions of chordomas in the cervical spine: review of five consecutive cases with more than 4-year follow-up. Spine 2011;36:E1581–E1587

11. Park L, Delaney TF, Liebsch NJ, et al. Sacral chordomas: Impact of high-dose proton/photon-beam radiation therapy combined with or without surgery for primary versus recurrent tumor. Int J Radiat Oncol Biol Phys 2006;65:1514–1521

12. Hanna SA, Tirabosco R, Amin A, et al. Dedifferentiated chordoma: a report of four cases arising "de novo." J Bone Joint Surg Br 2008;90:652–656

13. Hsu W, Mohyeldin A, Shah SR, et al. Generation of chordoma cell line JHC7 and the identification of Brachyury as a novel molecular target. J Neurosurg 2011;115:760–769

14. Pillay N, Plagnol V, Tarpey PS, et al. A common single-nucleotide variant in T is strongly associated with chordoma. Nat Genet 2012;44:1185–1187

15. Bydon M, Papadimitriou K, Witham T, et al. Novel therapeutic targets in chordoma. Expert Opin Ther Targets 2012;16:1139–1143

16. Boriani S, Weinstein JN, Biagini R. Primary bone tumors of the spine. Terminology and surgical staging. Spine 1997;22:1036–1044

17. Yasuda M, Bresson D, Chibbaro S, et al. Chordomas of the skull base and cervical spine: clinical outcomes associated with a multimodal surgical resection combined with proton-beam radiation in 40 patients.

Neurosurg Rev 2012;35:171–182, discussion 182–183

18. Barrenechea IJ, Perin NI, Triana A, Lesser J, Costantino P, Sen C. Surgical management of chordomas of the cervical spine. J Neurosurg Spine 2007;6: 398–406

19. Boriani S, Chevalley F, Weinstein JN, et al. Chordoma of the spine above the sacrum. Treatment and outcome in 21 cases. Spine 1996;21:1569–1577

20. Noël G, Habrand JL, Jauffret E, et al. Radiation therapy for chordoma and chondrosarcoma of the skull base and the cervical spine. Prognostic factors and patterns of failure. Strahlenther Onkol 2003;179:241–248

21. Cloyd JM, Chou D, Deviren V, Ames CP. En bloc resection of primary tumors of the cervical spine: report of two cases and systematic review of the literature. Spine J 2009;9:928–935

22. Ruggieri P, Angelini A, Ussia G, Montalti M, Mercuri M. Surgical margins and local control in resection of sacral chordomas. Clin Orthop Relat Res 2010;468: 2939–2947

23. Clarke MJ, Dasenbrock H, Bydon A, et al. Posterior-only approach for en bloc sacrectomy: clinical outcomes in 36 consecutive patients. Neurosurgery 2012;71:357–364, discussion 364

24. Henderson FC, McCool K, Seigle J, Jean W, Harter W, Gagnon GJ. Treatment of chordomas with CyberKnife: Georgetown University experience and treatment recommendations. Neurosurgery 2009;64(2, Suppl):A44–A53

25. Chen YL, Liebsch N, Kobayashi W, et al. Definitive high-dose photon/proton radiotherapy for unresected mobile spine and sacral chordomas. Spine 2013;38: E930–E936

26. Thieblemont C, Biron P, Rocher F, et al. Prognostic factors in chordoma: role of postoperative radiotherapy. Eur J Cancer 1995;31A:2255–2259

27. Stacchiotti S, Casali PG, Lo Vullo S, et al. Chordoma of the mobile spine and sacrum: a retrospective analysis of a series of patients surgically treated at two referral centers. Ann Surg Oncol 2010;17:211–219

28. Launay SG, Chetaille B, Medina F, et al. Efficacy of epidermal growth factor receptor targeting in advanced chordoma: case report and literature review. BMC Cancer 2011;11:423–2407

29. Hof H, Welzel T, Debus J. Effectiveness of cetuximab/gefitinib in the therapy of a sacral chordoma. Onkologie 2006;29:572–574

9

Chondrosarcoma

Stefano Boriani, Stefano Bandiera, Riccardo Ghermandi, Simone Colangeli, Luca Amendola, and Alessandro Gasbarrini

▓ Introduction

Chondrosarcoma (CHS) is the third most common primary malignant bone tumor after osteosarcoma and Ewing's sarcoma. According to the World Health Organization's (WHO) accepted definition,[1] the term *chondrosarcoma* refers to "a group of locally aggressive or malignant tumors producing cartilaginous matrix, with different morphological features and clinical behavior." This family of tumors includes several subtypes: central, peripheral, mesenchymal, clear-cell, and dedifferentiated.

Central CHS arises centrally in bone and then expands, infiltrating the trabeculae and being partially countered by some thin reactive bone (**Fig. 9.1**). It then erodes the cortex and invades the epidural space (**Fig. 9.2**) and the surrounding soft tissues. Peripheral CHS takes the form of cartilaginous and myxoid masses that slowly grow and invade the surrounding soft tissues (**Fig. 9.3**).

Mesenchymal CHS is rare, comprising 0.7% of malignant tumors observed at the Mayo Clinic.[2] Usually, but not always, low-grade CHS includes cartilage and undifferentiated small round cells, sometimes bearing striking similarity to those in Ewing's sarcoma. Fortunately, they can be differentiated by areas of chondroid matrix, which do not occur in Ewing's sarcoma. Mesenchymal CHS in the spine is extremely rare.[3]

Clear-cell CHS is rarely observed in the spine. It is typically arranged in patterns of cartilage lobules. Benign giant cells are usually found throughout the tumor, either in small clusters or individually. This tumor is described as expansile and destructive, often with soft tissue extension and lack of mineralization. Its course is more aggressive and it is associated with a worse prognosis if it is underestimated and submitted for intralesional excision, whereas en-bloc resection is more successful.[4] Clear-cell CHS, however, can recur as long as 10 to 15 years after resection, and it can metastasize.

Dedifferentiated CHS is a highly vascularized, high-grade sarcoma that is extremely rare in the spine.[5] Its cartilage component has a low-grade appearance in contrast to the high-grade cartilaginous portions that are often found in osteosarcomas. This CHS variant requires aggressive surgery (en-bloc resection) combined with chemotherapy. Histological grading of all CHSs range from 1 to 3; a grade 4 CHS corresponds to dedifferentiated CHS.

The maximum incidence of CHS is found in patients 30 to 70 years of age. Rarely does CHS occur before the age of 20 years, and only exceptionally is it found before puberty. It occurs approximately twice as often in men as in women.

Spine CHSs represent only 10% of all CHS. Most cases of CHS observed in the spine are central and peripheral, both possibly arising from

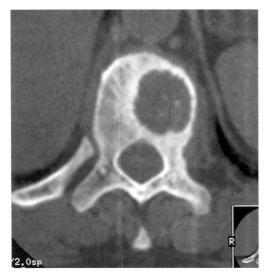

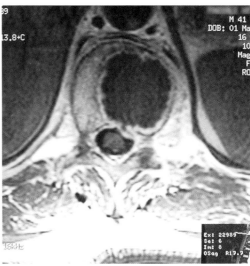

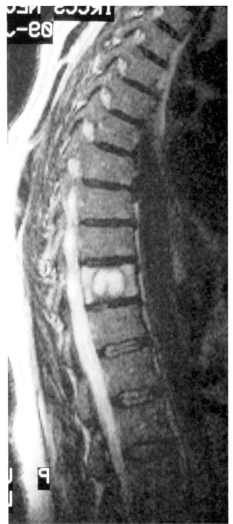

Fig. 9.1a–c A central chondrosarcoma (CHS) in a 54-year-old man. **(a)** A computed tomography (CT) scan demonstrates a lytic area arising in the vertebral body of T10, fully encased in the vertebral body, with well-defined margins, osteosclerotic reaction, and scattered rounded calcifications inside the tumor mass. **(b)** T1-weighted magnetic resonance imaging (MRI) demonstrates that the tumor has low intense signal. The tumor border is well defined. **(c)** T2-weighted MRI demonstrates that the tumor has a high-intensity signal and is surrounded by high-intensity cancellous bone signal related to edematous reaction.

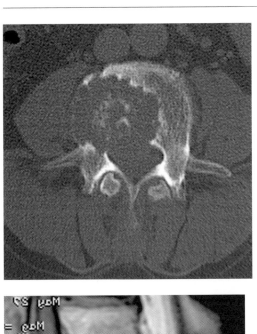

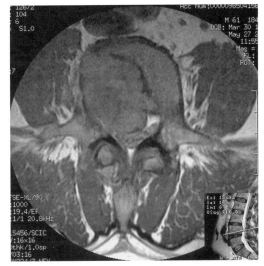

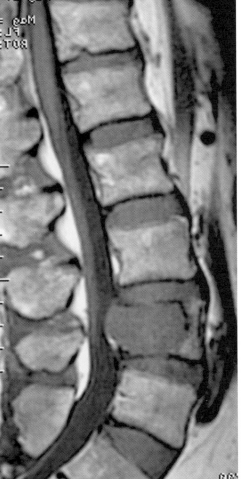

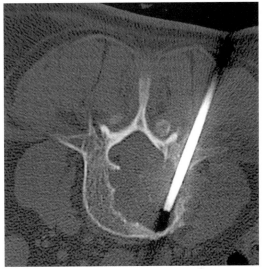

Fig. 9.2a–h A central CHS invading the canal, earlier than might be expected, in a 42-year-old woman. **(a)** CT scan demonstrates that a thin osteosclerotic border is limiting the tumor anterolaterally. There is a well-defined limit to the cancellous bone. Scattered calcifications are seen within the tumor mass. **(b,c)** MRI demonstrates better definition of the epidural extension **(d)** CT-guided trocar biopsy. (*continued on next page*)

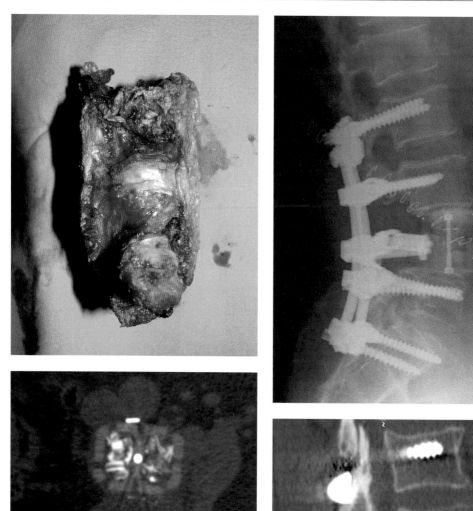

Fig. 9.2a–h (continued) **(e)** On the resected specimen the epidural extension is fully contained by the longitudinal ligament. **(f)** Reconstruction after the en-bloc resection. A carbon-fiber cage is filled with chips of autogenous graft. **(g,h)** At 5-year follow-up, there is no local recurrence. Bone in-growth of the graft is seen inside the carbon-fiber cage, with fusion to the contiguous end plates.

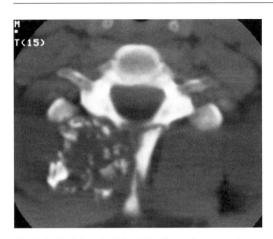

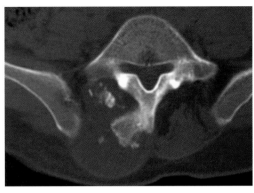

Fig. 9.4 Peripheral CHS secondary to exostosis of the spinous process of L5 in a 23-year-old woman. The image demonstrates the implant of the exostosis, typically characterized by continuity of the cortical bone and ingrowth of cancellous bone from the host bone. The cartilaginous cap is larger than 2 cm, thus confirming the diagnosis of CHS.

Fig. 9.3 Peripheral CHS arising from the posterior elements of C4 without any evidence of preexisting osteochondroma (exostosis) in a 28-year-old man. A huge radiolucent soft tissue mass is seen, with scattered round calcifications.

a precursor lesion such as an enchondroma, osteochondroma, or exostosis. These cases are referred to as "secondary" CHS (**Fig. 9.4**).

The CHSs in the spine are typically slow-growing tumors, and diagnosis is usually made later in their clinical course. Pain is the most frequent complaint of patients with central CHS in the mobile spine, as it provokes a dull, aching pain unrelated to activity and frequently nocturnal. Sacral CHSs are most commonly incidental tumors, owing to the large area where the tumor can develop before causing symptoms of compression (**Fig. 9.5**). When the posterior vertebral arches are involved, a fixed, hard, and nontender mass can be found (**Figs. 9.3** and **9.6**). Very rarely does a spinal CHS initially manifest with spinal cord or nerve root compression (**Fig. 9.6**).

Radiographically, central CHS of the spine is primarily a lytic lesion that arises centrally in the vertebral body (with or without a peripheral periosteal reaction), and sometimes sclerotic margins can also be visualized. In other cases, heavily calcified lobulated masses arise from the cortical margins. Later on, lytic bone destruction without mottled calcification can be seen, either as a soft tissue mass invading the epidural space (**Fig. 9.2**) or as a soft tissue mass with flocculating calcifications. As the tumor grows in size, the amount of reaction of surrounding bone evolves into massive permeative destruction of the underlying bone.

Computed tomography (CT) scan with magnetic resonance imaging (MRI) best demonstrates the extent of the lesion and the relationship with the surrounding anatomic structures, and it evaluates spinal cord compression (**Fig. 9.2b,c**).

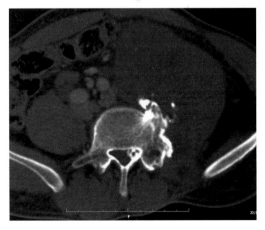

Fig. 9.5 Peripheral CHS secondary to exostosis of L5, growing in the abdomen without provoking pain, in a 36-year-old man. A painless mass was noted on physical examination.

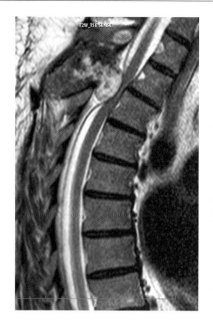
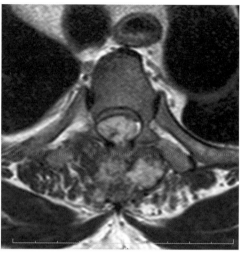

a

b

Fig. 9.6a,b A T4 CHS in a 59-year-old man. The patient gradually developed a gait impairment due to pyramidal symptoms. He experienced no pain; thus, the symptoms were underestimated until imaging was performed. **(a,b)** A huge chondroid low-vascularized mass is seen, arranged in lobules arising from and replacing the posterior elements, with severe cord compression.

The most difficult differential diagnosis is between low-grade CHS and benign, active, cartilaginous lesions. Classically, the imaging of peripheral CHS can be distinguished from an osteochondroma (exostosis) by the thickness of the cartilaginous cap. The size limit between osteochondroma (exostosis) and CHS has been established at 2 cm; a cap that is thicker than 2 cm is considered pathognomonic of CHS (**Fig. 9.4**).

Primary peripheral CHSs can be additionally distinguished from osteochondroma (exostosis) because CHSs consist of calcified cartilage, whereas most of the mass of an osteochondroma (exostosis) consists of pure bone. Furthermore, CHS can be distinguished from other malignant bone tumors of the spine because it frequently arises from the posterior elements, in contrast to osteosarcoma, Ewing's sarcoma, multiple myeloma, and the majority of bone metastases.

Central CHS is radiographically less distinguishable. It is characterized by radiolucent permeative destruction of the vertebral body (similar to chordoma) mixed with calcified areas.

The calcifications in the low-grade tumors have the characteristic ringed pattern. In high-grade lesions the calcifications are not the dominant radiographic pattern, and there are few radiological clues reminiscent of the cartilaginous histogenesis of the tumor: poorly defined margins, permeative destruction, and inconsistent bone reaction. Furthermore, high-grade lesions that have little or no calcifications may show unexpectedly as "cold" lesions on isotope scan, much like myeloma. Angiography is even less valuable than isotope scan because of the little vascularity of CHSs. These negative findings are helpful in determining the diagnosis when they are associated with aggressive images on the MRI.

The management of CHSs of the limbs is clearly established and commonly accepted. There is extensive evidence, dating back many years, that the prognosis is dependent on the histological grade of malignancy and on the surgical treatment.[6–9] CHSs historically have been considered resistant to most protocols of radiation therapy and chemotherapy.

According to Campanacci et al,[9] intralesional excision can be considered a valid option in grade 1 CHS of the appendicular skeleton, resulting in a low rate of resectable recurrence versus more effective but significantly more aggressive en-bloc resection.

However, in the spine local adjuvants such as phenol and cryosurgery are less commonly used. Recurrent CHS is frequently associated with malignant progression, worsening the prognosis. Local recurrences in the spine are debilitating and aggressive, sometimes provoking serious neurologic deficits and leading to difficult palliation and eventually to death after revision surgery, owing to its high morbidity. Thus, it would be feasible to say that with CHSs of the spine, there is a direct correlation between the success of the first surgery and the ultimate prognosis.

The role of en-bloc resection in the treatment of CHS has been accepted since the pioneering work by Stener,[10] who also described how to plan these surgical procedures based on the tumor extension and the local anatomy. Because of the difficulties associated with en-bloc surgery in the spine, and because spine surgeons use various oncological criteria (**Fig. 9.7**), lesions of the vertebral column have had a poor prognosis independent of the histological grade.[11-14]

An exhaustive literature review based on the best available evidence and clinical expertise concluded that the optimal surgical management for CHS of the spine is en-bloc surgical resection with wide or marginal margins,[11] as evidenced by a decrease in local recurrence, longer disease-free survival, and, ultimately, a reduction of death related to disease (strong recommendation, moderate-quality evidence). Furthermore, radiation is not indicated for the primary treatment of chondrosarcoma of the spine (strong recommendation, very low quality evidence). However, radiation therapy of at least 60 to 65 Gy equivalents is indicated as an adjuvant treatment when there has been incomplete resection or an intralesional margin (weak recommendation, low-quality evidence).

Because CHSs grow slowly, local recurrence and metastases may occur more than 10 years after removal of the tumor; the 5-year survival is not a significant criterion for cure. All reports with shorter follow-ups have a lesser validity

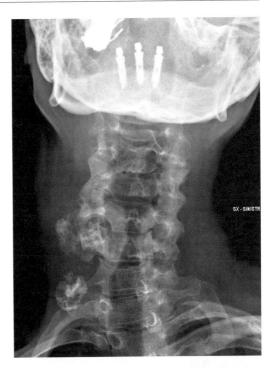

a

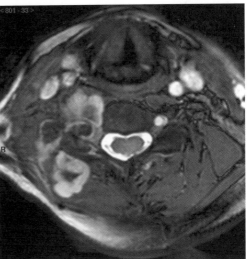

b

Fig. 9.7a–f A C5–C7 recurrent CHS in multiple exostoses in a 56-year-old woman, who submitted to five previous surgeries that were planned to remove piecemeal the exostosis without any concern about histological diagnosis or the criteria of surgical oncology, aiming only to preserve function. **(a)** Conventional radiogram demonstrates ossifications in the soft tissues. **(b)** MRI demonstrates a peripheral CHS involving the right lateral vertebral body, including the vertebral artery and the foramen, and expanding into the soft tissues. (*continued on next page*)

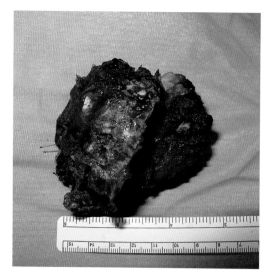

c

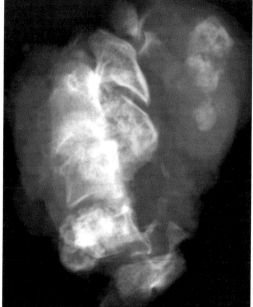

d

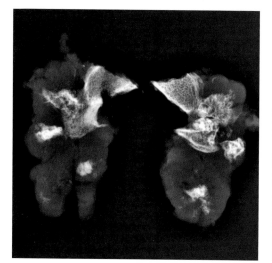

e

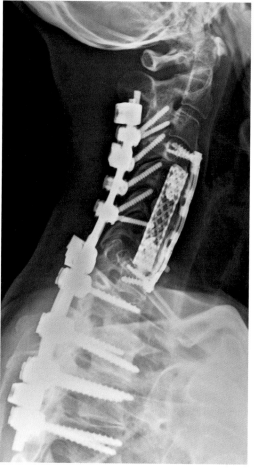

f

Fig. 9.7a–f (*continued*) **(c)** The specimen after en-bloc resection, confirmed by a pathologist to be a marginal margin tumor-free resection. The sacrifice of the C5-C6-C7 right nerve roots was required for achieving such an oncological result. The sagittal section of the vertebral body and the canal are seen. **(d,e)** Radiograms of the resected specimen. **(f)** Full circumferential reconstruction after sagittal en-bloc resection of three vertebral bodies.

when comparing paradigms of treatment. Moreover, due to the frequent underestimation of CHS, the overall rate for cure is less than that for osteosarcoma at 5 years.

Technique

Diagnosis

To carefully determine the variety of CHS (central, peripheral [primary or secondary], mesenchymal, clear cell, or dedifferentiated) and its grade of malignancy, the pathologist needs an adequate amount of appropriate and significant tissue. The surgeon or the interventional radiologist must be able to "read" the imaging and find the most representative specimen for this purpose. CT-guided biopsy should be performed by a trocar thick enough (12 or 16 gauge) to provide an adequate amount of material. The trocar must be directed to an area of cartilage, avoiding necrotic areas or mature bone. This is particularly relevant when the imaging studies suggest a secondary CHS. All tissue possibly belonging to the primitive benign lesion should be avoided, and it would be best to perform the biopsy from the cartilaginous cap, possibly taking out a carrot of all its thickness. The most aggressive and infiltrative portion of the tumor is the best location for taking a biopsy specimen.

Grossly, CHSs are mostly myxoid and diffluent. They are significantly less vascularized and prone to bleeding than other malignancies, but the tumor has an intrinsic pressure that expels the soft, viscous, jelly-like material, which quickly flows into the surrounding spaces. Open biopsy can spread tumor in extracompartmental areas, such as the epidural space, dramatically reducing the effectiveness of a resection even if it is performed with an appropriate margin. Even minor contamination of the soft tissues by spilling of the myxoid contents of the tumor can worsen the prognosis, and not even a trocar biopsy can prevent it. En-bloc resection without biopsy can be considered, as suggested by Stener,[10] in selected cases where imaging is pathognomonic and en-bloc resec-tion is feasible. However, this is rarely feasible even for highly experienced tumor surgeons.

Treatment

Some prognostic factors have been significantly related to poor local control and disease survival. The outcome of CHS seems to be affected by the size of the lesion, the histological grade,[12] the incisional biopsy and inadequate surgical margins,[1] primary surgery out of a tumor center, and older patient age.[11–15] On the other hand, en-bloc resection with tumor-free margins is associated with the best results,[13–16] whereas most patients with recurrent tumors die of the disease.[15,16]

A large multicenter study reported findings similar to those of the systematic review,[15] and provided moderate-quality evidence supporting en-bloc resection in the management of CHSs of the spine. There was a statistically significant increase in mortality in patients who developed a local recurrence. Mortality was also directly related to the margins, with a significant increase in mortality in patients undergoing intralesional surgery.

Once it is accepted that en-bloc resection is the best option for the treatment of CHS of the spine, as in CHS in the limbs, two major issues arise: (1) when planning an en-bloc resection, the decision-making process should consider the possibility of functional loss related to the extension of the resection, and (2) a strategy should be established in cases where en-bloc resection is not feasible or is not able to achieve full tumor-free margins.

Common Problems

Margins and Anatomic Sacrifices

One of the challenges in treating spinal tumors is the close proximity of the tumor margins to important structures such as the spinal cord, nerve roots, and large arteries and veins. It is important for the surgeon to inform the patient that it may be necessary to sacrifice some of these structures when attempting an en-bloc resection in order to minimize the risk of recurrence and improve the prognosis. There are specific surgical techniques for tumor resection in the dura mater,[17] the cauda equina, the aorta,[18] and even the spinal cord. In case of extracompartmental CHS in the spine, an en-bloc resection could include neighboring structures such as the thoracic wall, which could represent the oncological margin.

En-bloc resection of cervical CHSs is seldom possible and technically demanding; most of the time one or more cervical nerve roots need to be sacrificed (**Fig. 9.7**) with consequent functional loss. In cases of sacral CHSs, when the tumor grows above the level of S3, en-bloc resection has been associated with loss of sphincter control.[16]

Inappropriate Oncological Excision

The surgeon may decide against doing an en-bloc resection, or the patient may refuse permission, for several reasons:

- Tumor-free margins cannot be achieved because of invasion of both pedicles or in cases of large extracompartmental tumors, or for other reasons.
- The surgery is technically demanding (for example, a high cervical spine tumor).
- The surgery-related morbidity is deemed to be excessive (for example, sacral tumors in patients over 80 years of age).
- The surgery entails excessive functional loss (for example, sacral tumors in young patients).

In the decision-making process, the treatment team should consider and discuss the higher morbidity that may be associated with the lowest risk of local recurrence, the need further surgeries and treatments, and the possible progression of malignancy that eventually may lead to the patient's death.

Performing either a gross total excision or an en-bloc excision with intralesional margins, for intentional or accidental margin violation, will leave residual tumor requiring local adjuvants. The impact that the addition of radiation or local adjuvant therapy has on local recurrence and survival should be carefully considered. Alternative treatments should be sought when en-bloc resection is not feasible or when the patient refuses to give permission. Radiation therapy for CHS, whether as a primary or adjunct therapy, has changed significantly in recent years, as it has been suggested that doses higher than 50 Gy may be beneficial.[19]

Incorrect Diagnosis

The most frequent misdiagnoses entail confusing low-grade CHS with enchondroma or osteochondroma, or confusing dedifferentiated CHS with osteosarcoma. The solution is to perform a trocar biopsy under CT scan control, to obtain a representative specimen for pathological analysis, and to avoid areas of necrosis as well as the peripheral part of the tumor. When a cartilaginous cap is noted, it is advisable to obtain a full sample of the total height.

Incorrect Biopsy Technique

Open biopsy of a CHS will contaminate all adjacent tissues. When this occurs in the spine, where including all the contaminated tissues in the resected specimen is difficult or impossible, it will negatively affect the prognosis. Even worse is to perform an intralesional excision or a cord decompression without first having done biopsy. A full imaging workup should always be performed; a careful analysis of a radiographic detail can raise the suspicion of a CHS. A decompression performed in a CHS presuming the diagnosis of metastasis can improve neurologic function, but it exposes the patient to tumor progression and can preclude doing the appropriate surgery. This can result in recurrence, progression of malignancy, and eventually death. In cases where the diagnosis or treatment is in doubt, the patient should always be referred to an experienced tumor center. A biopsy performed in an inexperienced center or an inappropriate intralesional excision can have a negative impact on the prognosis.

Undertreatment

Performing an intralesional excision in a case where en-bloc excision is feasible exposes the patient to a poorer local and systemic prognosis. Thus, surgeons should obtain appropriate oncological training before treating primary spine tumors. The criteria for en-bloc resection have been proposed based on the Weinstein–Boriani–Biagini (WBB) staging system,[13] but they are also discussed in cornerstone papers by Roy Camille, Tomita, and, primarily, Stener,[10] who brilliantly described how to plan en-bloc resections in the spine.

Patients may deem the functional sacrifices entailed in this type of major surgery to be unacceptable. But it would be a mistake to recommend an intralesional surgery to these patients if an en-bloc resection is feasible, as it is the best standard of care.

Errors in the Decision-Making Process

The opposite mistake would be to perform en-bloc resection in a grade 1 CHS of the sacrum without first having a candid discussion with the patient. In this case, a major sacrifice of genitourinary function must be carefully explained to the patient. Patients understandably may refuse to accept surgery than entails such a sacrifice, even in the case of a late recurrence after adjuvant high-dose radiotherapy of an intralesional margin to save function (intentional transgression).

Incongruous Selection of Nonsurgical Treatments

Conventional radiotherapy as an adjuvant and chemotherapy in low-grade CHS are notoriously ineffective. New radiotherapy techniques and experimental medical oncology protocols are opening new pathways. A multidisciplinary approach is mandatory to offer patients a wider spectrum of therapeutic options.

▦ Chapter Summary

Chondrosarcoma is the third most frequent malignant primary bone tumor, after osteosarcoma and Ewing's sarcoma, but it is the most frequent malignant tumor in the spine (10% of all CHSs occur in the spine). CHSs occur mainly in adults, particularly elderly men. Radiographically, CHSs present as scattering round ossifications within a lytic area or as a mass expanding the soft tissue.

The management of CHS of the spine is challenging. It is a slow-growing tumor, often extensive at presentation, that involves complex anatomy. It responds partially to adjuvant therapies and tends to recur if it is inadequately managed. The condition tends to be lethal after a long disease course. Progression of malignancy or dedifferentiation also has been described in long-surviving patients and is mostly observed in recurrent tumors.

The course of the disease depends on the aggressiveness of the tumor, on its size, and on the feasibility of performing an en-bloc resection. A literature review suggests that en-bloc surgery, as pioneered in CHS by Stener[10] in 1971, can give the patient the best chance of survival and the lowest rate of local recurrence, when it succeeds in removing the whole tumor mass together with a continuous, even thin (marginal margin), shell of healthy tissue, and when its expected morbidity outweighs the risk of disease-related morbidity or death. Careful preoperative planning for surgical tumor removal and spine reconstruction is mandatory and must be based on oncological and surgical staging.

Intralesional excision (performed because of the anatomic extension or size of the CHS, or because the patient refused to undergo an en-bloc procedure) and en-bloc resection with intralesional margin (because the tumor mass came apart, with consequent contamination) seem to be effective only in slowing the tumor growth and do not prevent even a late (3 years or more) local recurrence. No chemotherapy protocol has been validated to improve the control of the disease in these cases, but intralesional excision can be combined with megavoltage or proton-beam therapy or other radiation therapy techniques to deliver high doses (> 70 Gy) to residual tumors.

Recent trials utilizing new technologies are promising, as they reduce the surgery-related morbidity, particularly when anatomic relevant structures can be resected, allowing the same local and systemic control that until now has been available only from surgical procedures.

Pearls

Diagnosis
- Open biopsy can spread tumor in extracompartmental areas.
- Computer tomography–guided biopsy should be performed with a trocar from an area of cartilage (from the cartilaginous cap of a peripheral CHS) and should avoid necrotic areas or mature bone, possibly taking out a carrot of all its thickness to provide an adequate amount of material.

Treatment
- En-bloc resection with tumor-free margins is associated with the best results.
- Prognosis is affected by many factors: histological grade, size of the lesion, increasing patient age, incisional biopsy, primary surgery out of a tumor center, but the most important is inadequate surgical margin.
- To achieve appropriate margins, demanding surgery that entails morbidity may be necessary, and functional sacrifices may be required.
- Intentional or incidental transgression of oncological principles may require adjuvant treatment. The role of radiation therapies is still unclear.

Pitfalls

Incorrect Diagnosis
- The most frequent misdiagnoses are low-grade CHS versus enchondroma or osteochondroma, and dedifferentiated CHS versus osteosarcoma.

Incorrect Biopsy Technique
- Open biopsy of a CHS will contaminate all adjacent tissues.
- Intralesional excision performed for cord decompression without previous biopsy exposes the patient to a high risk of local recurrence.

Undertreatment
- Performing an intralesional excision in a case where en-bloc excision is feasible exposes the patient to a worse local and systemic prognosis.

Inaccurate Decision-Making Process
- Performing en-bloc resection in a grade 1 CHS of the sacrum without accurate discussion with the patient and careful explanation of the loss of genitourinary function would be a mistake.

Incongruous Selection of Nonsurgical Treatments
- Conventional radiotherapy and chemotherapy in low-grade CHS are not effective. New radiotherapy protocols (including high doses of radiations and accelerated particles) and experimental medical oncology protocols are opening new pathways.

Acknowledgment
The authors are indebted to Carlo Piovani for design, archive research, and image and editorial assistance.

References
Five Must-Read References
1. Fletcher CDM, Bridge JA, Hogendoorn PCW, Mertens F. WHO Classification of Tumours of Soft Tissue and Bone. Lyon, France: International Agency for Research on Cancer (IARC), 2013
2. Unni KK, Inwards CY. Dahlin's Bone Tumors, 6th ed. Philadelphia: Lippincott Williams & Wilkins, 2010
3. Matsuda Y, Sakayama K, Sugawara Y, et al. Mesenchymal chondrosarcoma treated with total en bloc spondylectomy for 2 consecutive lumbar vertebrae resulted in continuous disease-free survival for more than 5 years: case report. Spine 2006;31:E231–E236
4. Hsu W, McCarthy E, Gokaslan ZL, Wolinsky JP. Clear-cell chondrosarcoma of the lumbar spine: case report and review of the literature. Neurosurgery 2011;68: E1160–E1164, discussion 1164
5. Littrell LA, Wenger DE, Wold LE, et al. Radiographic, CT, and MR imaging features of dedifferentiated chondrosarcomas: a retrospective review of 174 de novo cases. Radiographics 2004;24:1397–1409
6. Enneking WF. Musculoskeletal Tumor Surgery, vols I and II. Edinburgh, New York: Churchill Livingstone, 1983
7. Ozaki T, Lindner N, Hillmann A, Rödl R, Blasius S, Winkelmann W. Influence of intralesional surgery on treatment outcome of chondrosarcoma. Cancer 1996;77:1292–1297
8. Mankin HJ, Cantley KP, Lippiello L, Schiller AL, Campbell CJ. The biology of human chondrosarcoma. I. Description of the cases, grading, and biochemical analyses. J Bone Joint Surg Am 1980;62:160–176
9. Campanacci DA, Scoccianti G, Franchi A, et al. Surgical treatment of central grade 1 chondrosarcoma of the appendicular skeleton. J Orthop Traumatol 2013; 14:101–107

10. Stener B. Total spondylectomy in chondrosarcoma arising from the seventh thoracic vertebra. J Bone Joint Surg Br 1971;53:288–295

11. Boriani S, Saravanja D, Yamada Y, Varga PP, Biagini R, Fisher CG. Challenges of local recurrence and cure in low grade malignant tumors of the spine. Spine 2009;34(22, Suppl):S48–S57

12. Bergh P, Gunterberg B, Meis-Kindblom JM, Kindblom LG. Prognostic factors and outcome of pelvic, sacral, and spinal chondrosarcomas: a center-based study of 69 cases. Cancer 2001;91:1201–1212

13. Boriani S, De Iure F, Bandiera S, et al. Chondrosarcoma of the mobile spine: report on 22 cases. Spine 2000;25:804–812

14. Schoenfeld AJ, Hornicek FJ, Pedlow FX, et al. Chondrosarcoma of the mobile spine: a review of 21 cases treated at a single center. Spine 2012;37:119–126

15. Fisher CG, Keynan O, Boyd MC, Dvorak MF. The surgical management of primary tumors of the spine: initial results of an ongoing prospective cohort study. Spine 2005;30:1899–1908

16. Hsieh PC, Xu R, Sciubba DM, et al. Long-term clinical outcomes following en bloc resections for sacral chordomas and chondrosarcomas: a series of twenty consecutive patients. Spine 2009;34:2233–2239 10.1097/BRS.0b013e3181b61b90

17. Krepler P, Windhager R, Toma CD, Kitz K, Kotz R. Dura resection in combination with en bloc spondylectomy for primary malignant tumors of the spine. Spine 2003;28:E334–E338

18. Gösling T, Pichlmaier MA, Länger F, Krettek C, Hüfner T. Two-stage multilevel en bloc spondylectomy with resection and replacement of the aorta. Eur Spine J 2013;22(Suppl 3):S363–S368 10.1007/s00586-012-2471-0

19. Foweraker KL, Burton KE, Maynard SE, et al. High-dose radiotherapy in the management of chordoma and chondrosarcoma of the skull base and cervical spine: Part 1—clinical outcomes. Clin Oncol (R Coll Radiol) 2007;19:509–516

10

Osteogenic Sarcoma and Ewing's Sarcoma of the Spine

Derek G. Ju, Patricia L. Zadnik, and Daniel M. Sciubba

▩ Introduction

Osteogenic sarcoma and Ewing's sarcoma are malignant tumors that generally arise in the appendicular skeleton, but in rare cases occur as primary tumors of the spinal column. Together with chondrosarcoma, these three sarcomas account for 90% of all primary sarcomas of the bone.[1] Classic osteogenic sarcoma and Ewing's sarcoma are by definition high-grade tumors, and, left untreated, they are associated with aggressive local and metastatic spread. The goals of management are to control localized disease and prevent metastatic spread, which may be accomplished by utilizing a combination of chemotherapy, radiation, and surgery. Surgical control of malignant tumors in the spinal column presents a complex challenge due to anatomic constraints that make it difficult to obtain a wide margin of excision.[2]

Diagnostic and Management Strategies

- Definitive diagnosis is needed in order to start patients on neoadjuvant chemotherapy prior to definitive local control for Ewing's sarcoma and osteosarcoma.
- Fine- or core-needle biopsy are appropriate methods if a specific diagnosis is suspected and a limited amount of tissue is required for diagnosis.[3] If an open biopsy is required, the incision should be permanently marked to facilitate a wide excision at another time if necessary.[3]
- When metastatic disease is present, consultation with a medical oncologist and radiation oncologist is helpful to determine if the patient is a surgical candidate. If there is direct soft tissue extension with bowel involvement, consultation with a general surgeon may further facilitate surgical planning.
- En-bloc procedures are designed to achieve wide margins, and the three main techniques in the spine are spondylectomy, sagittal resection, and resection of the posterior arch.
- Sagittal resections involve a wedge resection of the vertebral body with excision of the posterior elements, and are ideal in situations when tumor is confined to an eccentric portion of the vertebral body, pedicle, or transverse process.[3]
- En-bloc resection of the posterior arch is performed only when the tumor is located in the posterior arch without pedicle involvement.
- Spondylectomy involves the removal of the entire tumor in one piece together with portions of the posterior elements.[4] This is the procedure of choice when the tumor is centrally located and involves no more than one pedicle.[3]
- Previous data from our group has demonstrated success with posterior-only approaches for en-bloc resection of sacral tumors.[5]
- If more than half of the sacroiliac joint is removed for tumor resection, hardware reconstruction with a transiliac bar or femoral allograft is required.
- Lesions not involving the sacroiliac joint can be removed with a low sacral amputation without any hardware reconstruction.

This chapter reviews the epidemiology, clinical presentation, radiographic findings, pathology, and recommended multidisciplinary management options of the most common sarcomas affecting the bone: osteogenic sarcoma and Ewing's sarcoma. Chondrosarcoma of the spine is discussed in Chapter 9.

Osteogenic Sarcoma (Osteosarcoma)

Epidemiology

Osteogenic sarcoma is a primary malignant tumor of connective tissue origin, characterized by bone or osteoid matrix formation within the tumor mass. There are many tumor variants with different morphologies, with the most common type being classic osteoblastic osteogenic sarcoma. It is the most frequent malignant condition of the bone, accounting for 35% of primary bone malignancies.[6] Within the spine, osteogenic sarcoma is the most common sarcoma and makes up 3 to 15% of all primary spinal tumors.[7,8] The peak incidence of osteogenic sarcoma in the spine occurs in the fourth decade of life.[9,10] In contrast, most patients with osteogenic sarcoma in the long bones are under the age of 30.

Primary osteogenic sarcoma rarely arises from the cervical spine and occurs at a proportionally higher frequency in the thoracic spine and sacrum, with the sacrum being the primary site in 68 to 75% of patients.[7,10] According to an analysis of 430 patients with spinal osteogenic sarcoma from the Surveillance, Epidemiology, and End Results (SEER) database maintained by the National Cancer Institute, the incidence is essentially equal between the sexes (1.2 to 1), and spinal tumors are rare in people of Asian, Native American, and African descent.[10]

Other conditions associated with increased risk of developing osteogenic sarcoma include Paget's disease of bone, enchondromatosis, hereditary multiple exostoses, and fibrous dysplasia.[4] Degeneration into a pagetoid osteosarcoma occurs in less than 1% of patients, and of those cases only 6% develop in the vertebrae or sacrum.[11] Nonetheless, these cases have been documented to account for as much as half of the spinal osteogenic sarcoma cases in some tumor databases.[8] Another important risk factor for osteogenic sarcoma is prior radiation exposure, with those subjected to high doses at a younger age having an elevated risk.[12]

Clinical Manifestation

The most frequent presenting symptom is axial or radicular pain.[2,7] Neurologic deficits are the second most frequent presenting symptom and can occur in over 50% of patients.[7,13] Bowel and bladder symptoms are less common, and usually present later as the tumor progresses.[2] In the Cooperative Osteosarcoma Study Group trial, the median delay in diagnosis from the onset of symptoms was 5 months.[7] According to the SEER database, 28% of patients diagnosed with osteogenic sarcoma of the spine presented with gross metastatic disease.[10]

Radiographic Features

The role of computed tomography (CT) and magnetic resonance imaging (MRI) has become increasingly important in the diagnosis and staging of spinal osteogenic sarcoma. Conventional plain radiographs are usually obtained prior to oncological referral, and are useful in determining the aggressiveness of a bone lesion. Plain radiographs typically reveal a dense, solid, and smooth appearance of osteogenic sarcoma.[9] However, the findings may be variable, ranging from a osteosclerotic appearance in 20% of patients to a seemingly normal radiograph.[2,7] For this reason, CT is the recommended modality for diagnostic imaging of osteogenic sarcoma, and scans show significant matrix calcification in 80% of cases.[14]

On MRI, the solid, nonmineralized portions of the tumor are hypointense on T1-weighted sequences and hyperintense on T2-weighted sequences[9] (**Fig. 10.1**). There may be focal regions of hypointensity on all pulse sequences, and fluid–fluid levels are common in the telangiectatic subtype.[15] In contrast, mineralized tumors appear isointense to bone on T1- and T2-weighted sequences[4] (**Fig. 10.1**). Edema in

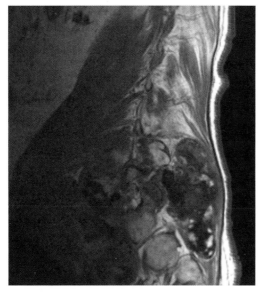

a

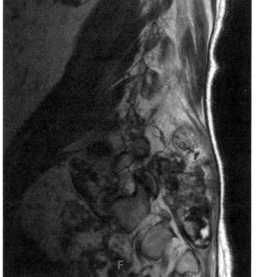

b

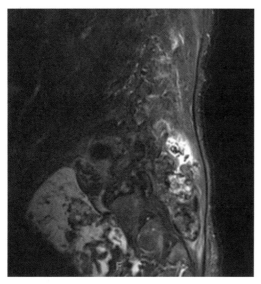

c

Fig. 10.1a–c Sagittal T1 **(a)**, T2 **(b)**, and fat-suppressed **(c)** magnetic resonance imaging (MRI) scans demonstrating large sarcoma of the left hemipelvis extending into the left retroperitoneum, with extension into the left psoas, iliacus, and iliopsoas muscles. The lesion is heterogeneously enhancing secondary to inconsistent mineralization of the tumor.

the surrounding tissues is often seen, but is not specific for osteogenic sarcoma.[9]

The majority of osteogenic sarcoma patients who present with metastatic disease have detectable lung metastases, and a CT of the chest, abdomen, and pelvis can assist with tumor staging.[16] Chest CT is the most sensitive imaging technique in detecting lung metastases, and should be used when available.[16] A technetium-99m methylene diphosphonate (^{99m}Tc) bone scan may be necessary to identify additional bone metastases and skip lesions.

Histopathology

Grossly, osteogenic sarcoma exhibits a red, gritty, granular quality due to osteoid formation.[4] Foci of hemorrhage or necrosis are common histological findings.[4] The majority of osteogenic sarcomas are by definition high grade and have a medullary origin.[17] On a cellular level, osteogenic sarcoma is characterized by spindle cells with nuclear pleomorphism.[18] The histological hallmark of osteogenic sarcoma is the production of bone or osteoid matrix within the tumor, and is the key to diagnosis.[9] Conventional osteogenic sarcoma cells produce different types of extracellular matrix, hence the division into osteoblastic, chondroblastic, and fibroblastic subtypes.[18] However, most tumors do not sort neatly into a subcategory and present with a mixed histology, and there is no significant difference in prognosis or treatment between the subtypes.[17]

Other rare but notable histological types include telangiectatic, small-cell, and epithelioid osteogenic sarcomas. Telangiectatic osteogenic sarcoma shares features with aneurysmal bone cysts, and the lesion is composed of multiple blood-filled sinusoids.[17] With the application of modern-era chemotherapy agents, the prognosis for telangiectatic osteogenic sarcoma has improved and now carries a prognosis similar to that of the conventional type.[18] Small-cell osteogenic sarcoma may be confused with Ewing's sarcoma due to its round, hyperchromatic nuclei and CD99 positivity.[17] Further, translocations mimicking Ewing's sarcoma between chromosomes 11 and 22 have also been observed[17] (see Histopathology, in the Ewing's Sarcoma section of the chapter, below). Finally, epithelioid osteogenic sarcomas are poorly differentiated and may resemble carcinomas.[17]

Management

Currently, there are no standard oncological staging scales used for osteogenic sarcoma. Application of bone tumor staging systems, such as those from the Musculoskeletal Tumor Society and the American Joint Committee on Cancer are limited in efficacy due to the high-grade nature of osteogenic sarcoma and its lack of lymph node involvement.[1] Further, the unique anatomic constraints for patients with osteogenic sarcoma of the spine compared with that of the extremities may limit the application of a generalized grading scheme. Recently, a grading scale for malignant osseous spinal neoplasms, including osteogenic sarcomas, has been proposed in order to enhance risk stratification of treatment candidates.[19] The most important prognostic variables are patient age, metastatic status, and extent of local tumor invasion.[19]

The gold standard of treatment for patients with localized osteogenic sarcoma involves a multidisciplinary approach, consisting of neoadjuvant chemotherapy with wide local surgical excision. The landmark data for multimodal treatment of osteogenic sarcoma of the limbs was provided by Link et al,[20] in which patients undergoing limb resection were randomly assigned to adjuvant chemotherapy or observation only. The relapse-free survival at 2 years was statistically significant between the two cohorts, with 17% of the control group achieving relapse-free survival compared to 66% in the adjuvant chemotherapy group. Gherlinzoni et al[21] performed a retrospective review on 355 patients with osteogenic sarcoma of the limbs, and found that the incidence of local recurrence was related to surgical margin and to tumor necrosis induced by neoadjuvant chemotherapy.

Chemotherapy has also been shown to provide improved local control and survival for patients with osteogenic sarcoma of the spine, although high-quality studies are lacking.[7,13,22] Current neoadjuvant chemotherapy protocols use a combination of methotrexate, cisplatin, doxorubicin, ifosfamide, BCD (bleomycin, cytoxan, dactinomycin), etoposide, and muramyl tripeptide.[6] Shives et al[13] evaluated 27 patients with spinal osteogenic sarcoma and found a longer survival in patients with adjuvant therapy, although no statistical analysis was performed. Reflecting these results, the 2009 consensus recommendation of the Spine Oncology Study Group (SOSG) stated that neoadjuvant chemotherapy offers significant improvements in local control and long-term survival for spinal osteogenic sarcoma.[6]

The only effective surgical treatment of localized spinal osteogenic sarcoma is total spondylectomy or wide local excision with vertebral column reconstruction[4] (**Fig. 10.2**), Although the strongest evidence for aggressive surgery derives from treatment of patients with limb tumors, as evidenced by Link et al[20] and Gherlinzoni et al,[21] there is evidence of spinal osteogenic sarcoma as well. DeLaney et al[23] retrospectively reviewed 41 patients with osteogenic sarcoma, including eight patients who had a spinal tumor. The authors found a higher

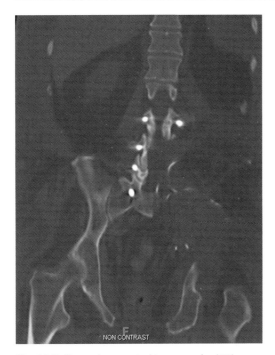

Fig. 10.2 Coronal computed tomography (CT) demonstrating an L4-5 vertebrectomy and hemipelvectomy with hardware reconstruction.

local control rate for patients undergoing gross total resection with negative versus positive margins (78% vs 68%), although the difference was not statistically significant.

Ozaki and colleagues[7] evaluated 22 patients with osteogenic sarcoma of the axial spine. There was a significant survival difference between five patients who underwent wide or marginal surgery and 17 patients who did not, leading the authors to conclude that at least marginal excision is warranted in potentially resectable tumors. Likewise, Sundaresan et al[22] reviewed the results of 24 patients with spinal osteosarcoma who underwent aggressive treatment (aggressive resection, radiation, and chemotherapy) compared with patients who underwent less aggressive treatment (limited resection and radiation). The authors found that patients with a more aggressive treatment had an improved survival, although no statistical analysis was done due to the low sample size.

More recently, Mukherjee and colleagues[24] examined 158 patients in the SEER database with localized spinal osteogenic sarcoma and found a threefold survival (hazard ratio [HR], 0.382; 95% confidence interval [CI], 0.21–0.69) for patients with surgical resection over biopsy alone. The dramatic enhancement in survival was independent of other variables such as tumor location or patient age; however, the extent of resection and surgical margins were not available in the SEER database. The SOSG strongly recommends the use of en-bloc resection of osteogenic sarcoma with wide margins, as it provides improved local control and potentially improved survival.[6] The morbidity and mortality of en-bloc procedures are considerable, and they should be performed only at experienced centers with multidisciplinary teams.

The overall 5-year survival rate in all patients who have spinal osteogenic sarcoma is 18%.[10] The estimated median survival in patients who present with localized disease and receive aggressive treatment is 18 months.[10] An estimated 7% of patients with spinal osteogenic sarcomas present with metastatic disease, and have an approximate median survival of 7 months.[10] Radiation therapy may play a role in palliative care for those with unresectable or metastatic disease; however, osteogenic sarcomas are radioresistant and do not respond well to standard doses.[4] An improvement in survival rates has also been associated with the use of radiation when combined with surgery.[23,24] This may be due to the efficacy of radiation treatment in treating microscopic or minimal residual disease after surgery.

▨ Ewing's Sarcoma

Epidemiology

Ewing's sarcoma represents a family of neoplasms originating from a precursor neural cell, including classic Ewing's sarcoma and primitive neuroectodermal tumor.[4,25] Ewing's sarcoma is the second most common cancer of bone in adolescents and young adults, after osteogenic sarcoma, with an incidence of 2.1 per 1 million children in the United States.[26]

This sarcoma of the spine tends to present at a young age, with a peak incidence in the second decade and an age range spanning the first through third decades.[9] There is a slight male predominance in the spine (1.8 to 1). The condition is exceedingly rare in people of Asian, Native American, or African ancestry.[10] The cause of Ewing's sarcoma is not clear, and is most likely due to spontaneous genetic translocations rather than familial or environmental factors.[25] Further, unlike osteosarcoma, there is no associated risk from prior exposure to radiation.[4]

The spine is an uncommon site, with only 3 to 15% of Ewing's sarcoma occurring in the spine.[2] However, Ewing's sarcoma is the most common malignant vertebral tumor found in children.[27] It can affect any segment of the spine, as well as originate within the paravertebral muscles and invade into the epidural space.[4] Within the axial skeleton, Ewing's sarcoma is most commonly found in the sacrum and lumbar spine, with common involvement of the sacral ala and posterior elements, respectively.[3] Within the sacrum, the tumor may grow to a large size before the onset of pain. Therefore, the insidious malignancy may remain undetected for a prolonged period of time.[4]

Clinical Manifestation

On presentation, the primary symptom of spinal Ewing's sarcoma is localized pain with variable intensity, which occurs in virtually all patients.[2] This pain is often mistaken for normal growing pains or sports-related injuries in the adolescent population.[25] Neurologic deficits are often seen, occurring in 40 to 60% of patients.[2] Bowel and bladder symptoms are rare and tend to occur later in the disease progression.[2] Systemic symptoms such as fever and indicators of a chronic inflammatory state may also occur and lead to a mistaken diagnosis of infection.[4,25] These fairly nonspecific symptoms commonly lead to a delay in the establishment of diagnosis, allowing the malignant tumor to progress. According to the SEER database, 34% of 430 patients with Ewing's sarcoma of the spine present with gross metastatic disease.[10]

Radiographic Features

The most important diagnostic imaging modalities for evaluation of potential Ewing's sarcoma are CT and MRI. Unlike osteogenic sarcoma, plain radiographs are rarely useful in diagnosing Ewing's sarcoma, as this disease process causes a "moth-eaten" destruction of bone rather than complete osteolysis.[2,15] Radiographic images of early disease can range from a seemingly negative radiograph to subtle findings such as osteolysis and haziness of the end plates.[28]

Computed tomography is a useful complementary modality to evaluate the bony elements affected by Ewing's sarcoma. An osteolytic mass is detected in approximately 90% of cases, with rare variants that may present with a mixed lytic/sclerotic or purely sclerotic morphology.[28] The majority of tumors in the mobile spine involve the posterior elements, whereas most tumors in the sacrum involve the sacral ala[28] (**Fig. 10.3**). A CT of the chest, abdomen, and pelvis is recommended for surgical staging. The most common sites for metastatic disease are the lungs, bone, and bone marrow. Further, a ^{99m}Tc bone scan demonstrates intense tracer uptake in Ewing's sarcoma.[9,16]

The recommended modality to evaluate Ewing's sarcoma is MRI with gadolinium enhancement, which enables sufficient evaluation of the soft tissue mass and its surrounding anatomy (**Fig. 10.4**). The tumor bulk is isointense to bone marrow on T1-weighted sequences and isointense to hyperintense to bone marrow on T2-weighted sequences.[9] The cortex of the bone is usually preserved, and patients may present with a pathological fracture if the lesion occurs within the vertebral column.[15]

Histopathology

Grossly, Ewing's sarcoma appears as a gray-white tumor with areas of hemorrhage and necrosis.[3] Evidence of necrosis and atypical histological features have been found to have worse prognostic value in patients with primary Ewing's sarcoma of the extremities.[4] On a microscopic level, Ewing's sarcoma consists of small,

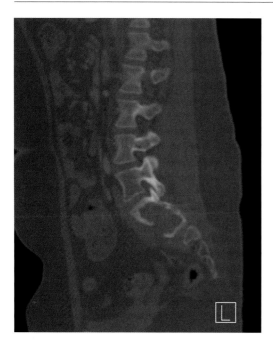

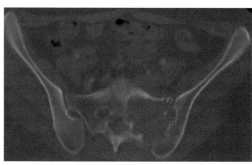

b

a

Fig. 10.3a,b Preoperative axial **(a)** and sagittal **(b)** CT scan demonstrating osteolytic destruction of the left-side sacral ala. T1- and T2-weighted MRI scans (not shown) demonstrated tumor growth and extension.

round cells with oval, uniform nuclei.[9,18] The cellular boundaries are indistinct, and give the appearance of a syncytium with multiple nuclei.[9] Occasionally present are mitotic figures, with apoptotic and karyopyknotic cells.[3] The differential diagnosis for small, round cell tumors includes lymphoma of bone, metastatic neuroblastoma, embryonal rhabdomyosarcoma, small cell osteosarcoma, and osteomyelitis; thus, diagnosis of Ewing's sarcoma is difficult on light microscopy alone.[1,4]

Definitive diagnosis is aided by the use of immunohistochemistry, electron microscopy, and cytogenetic methods. Viable tissue for histopathology, sterile tissue for cytogenetic, and a small sample for electron microscopy should be taken during biopsy for pathological evaluation. On immunohistochemistry, strong expression of the integral membrane glycoprotein CD99 (MIC2) is characteristic of Ewing's sarcoma, but CD99 is not a specific marker for Ewing's sarcoma.[29] Vimentin positivity is another sensitive but not specific marker for Ewing's sarcoma.[29]

Genetically, Ewing's sarcoma, like primitive neuroectodermal tumor, is characterized by a reciprocal translocation between the *EWS* gene on chromosome 22 and a member of the ETS family of transcription factors.[29] Approximately 85% of the tumors contain a t(11;22)(q24;q12) translocation resulting in a EWS-FLI1 fusion protein, and 10% of tumors contain a t(21;22) (q22;q12) translocation resulting in a EWS-ERG transcript.[29] These chimeric transcription factors retain their potent ability to induce transcription of various target genes required for tumor growth. Notably, the type 1 EWS-FLI1 fusion protein is recognized to be an indicator of favorable prognosis due to its less potent transactivation capabilities.[25] Additionally, up to 20% of Ewing's sarcomas exhibit other genetic abnormalities such as mutations of the tumor suppressor genes *p53* and *ink4A,* which are associated with a worse prognosis.[29]

Management

Currently, there are no universally accepted oncological staging systems for Ewing's sarcoma. Staging systems for primary bone tumors are available from the Musculoskeletal Tumor Society and the American Joint Committee on Cancer, but they are not completely applicable and may have limited utility in Ewing's sarcoma.[25] Although the most important prognostic variables—presence of metastatic

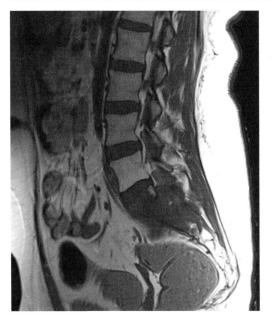
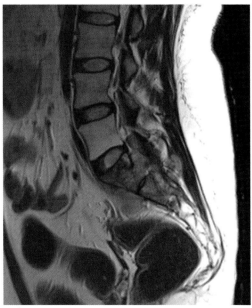

Fig. 10.4a,b **(a)** Gadolinium-enhanced sagittal T1-weighted MRI demonstrating a lesion that is hypointense to the bone marrow occupying S1-S3. There is involvement of the anterior and posterior elements at these levels. **(b)** T2-weighted gadolinium-enhanced sagittal T2-weighted MRI demonstrates a heterogeneously enhancing lesion in S1-S3.

disease and primary tumor size—are included in these staging systems, the nodal status and grade are irrelevant because Ewing's sarcoma rarely has lymph node involvement and is high grade by definition.[25,30] Further, the staging systems do not take into account the location of the primary tumor, which can have significant prognostic value.

For patients with no evidence of metastases at diagnosis, age less than 15 years and tumor less than 8 cm in size were found to be independent predictors of improved survival based on a large cohort of patients with Ewing's sarcoma of the bone from various primary locations.[31] Spinal location is associated with a worse prognosis, due to the anatomic limitations and difficulty in obtaining local control in the axial skeleton. For patients with metastatic disease, those with isolated pulmonary metastasis and skip metastases have a better prognosis than other sites of metastatic spread.[25] The time from diagnosis to recurrence is a significant prognostic factor; recurrence within 2 years of diagnosis is associated with a decreased 5-year survival.[31] As mentioned earlier,

certain histological or genetic characteristics of the patient's tumor may confer some prognostic value.

Regardless of tumor location or extent, systemic chemotherapy is the mainstay of treatment for all patients with Ewing's sarcoma unless contraindicated.[25] The classic chemotherapeutic agents used in Ewing's sarcoma are vincristine, actinomycin D, cyclophosphamide, and doxorubicin (VACD). The development of effective multiagent therapy for Ewing's sarcoma has been a major treatment breakthrough, contributing to an increase in the 5-year survival from 5 to 10% in the 1980s to the current 5-year survival of 65 to 70%.[32–34] The value of chemotherapy was illustrated in 1981 by the first Intergroup Ewing's Sarcoma Group that documented that the addition of doxorubicin to VAC conferred an improved survival over VAC therapy alone.[34] The VACD regimen was further established as standard care of Ewing's sarcoma, as at least eight clinical trials from 1973 to 2001 using VACD demonstrated improved survival.[25,33] Later, second-generation regimens incorporated ifosfamide and etoposide to the standard VACD regimen, which improved event-free survival for patients with localized disease.[33] Throughout these periods the role of chemotherapy has been supported for Ewing's sarcoma in all tumor locations, including the spine.[32,35,36] Due to the potential for chemotherapy-induced cardiac, renal, and hepatic toxicity, evaluation of these organs should be a critical part of the pretreatment assessment.

The treatment of patients with localized Ewing's sarcoma of the spine begins with neoadjuvant chemotherapy, which is designed to facilitate future local interventions by shrinking the soft tissue mass.[25] For patients who present with evidence of spinal cord compression but are neurologically stable, an additional benefit of chemotherapy may be relief of spinal cord compromise.[37] In 2009 the SOSG strongly recommended the use of neoadjuvant chemotherapy for patients with Ewing's sarcoma of the spine due to significant improvements in local control and long-term survival.[6] Following chemotherapy, restaging of the tumor should be performed prior to planning of definitive local control via radiation therapy or surgery. Radiation therapy for local control has historically been the preferred treatment due to the radiosensitivity of Ewing's sarcoma. However, this approach is used less frequently in practice now

due to concern over inducing secondary malignancies, adverse effects on bone growth, and the improvement of advanced surgical techniques for wide resections in the spine and sacrum.[25,37] Radiotherapy should be used in cases of unresectable tumors or after an intralesional or marginal surgical resection. As the majority of Ewing's sarcoma patients are pediatric patients, the field of radiation must carefully outline the vertebral body of interest in order to prevent asymmetric growth.[29]

Surgery for local control of Ewing's sarcoma should be considered in all cases in which the primary tumor can be completely removed in an en-bloc fashion, and subsequent reconstruction with hardware should be performed (**Fig. 10.5**). Bacci et al[38] in 2006 reviewed the outcomes of 512 patients with Ewing's sarcoma over a 20-year span at a single institution, comparing patients who underwent surgery alone or surgery plus radiation with patients treated with radiation alone. A significant improvement in local control (88.8% vs 80.2%, respectively; $p < 0.009$) and 5-year disease-free survival (63.8% vs 47.6%, respectively; $p < 0.0007$) was found in patients treated with surgery, a finding that was especially pronounced in patients who were found to have adequate surgical margins. Generally, aggressive extralesional surgical

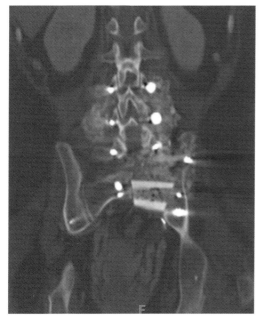

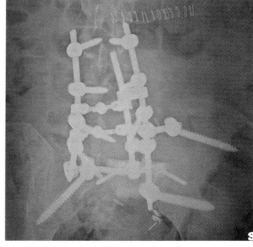

Fig. 10.5a,b **(a)** Coronal CT scan demonstrating femur allograft and hardware reconstruction. **(b)** An anteroposterior (AP) radiograph demonstrating the extent of the surgical reconstruction.

resection provides an improvement in overall survival and local control.[35,38–40] However, it is important to note that statistically significant improvements in these studies were found in patients with tumors in the limbs, not the axial spine, as high-quality studies supporting surgical treatment of Ewing's sarcoma in the spine are lacking. The SOSG issued a weak recommendation in 2006 indicating that en-bloc resection provides improved local control, but not improved overall survival for spinal Ewing's sarcoma.[6] The recommendation also supports the alternative use of radiotherapy for local control alone or to supplement an incomplete resection.

More recently, Mukherjee et al[24] studied 182 patients with spinal Ewing's sarcoma and found a more than twofold survival advantage (HR, 0.494; 95% CI, 0.26–0.96) for patients treated with surgical resection over biopsy alone. Generally, the 5-year event-free survival for patients with localized spinal Ewing's sarcoma is reported to be 50 to 60% with aggressive multimodality treatment.[4] Based on data from the SEER registry, the median survival of patients with localized spinal tumors was 90 months.[10]

Patients with metastatic or recurrent Ewing's sarcoma have a poor prognosis and remain a therapeutic challenge, and the 5-year survival remains approximately 25 to 30% with a median survival of 20 months.[10] The use of high-dose chemotherapy and autologous bone marrow transplantation has not improved survival rates, and is actually associated with an 8% incidence of treatment-related leukemia and myelodysplastic syndromes.[25] Patients with recurrent disease fare even worse, with a 5-year survival of less than 20%.[37] Although the rare solitary lesion may be surgically cured, the majority of patients may only be treated with salvage chemotherapy regimens.

▓ Clinical Considerations

When presented with a patient with suspected Ewing's sarcoma or osteogenic sarcoma, first perform a biopsy and involve medical oncology early in the treatment plan. En-bloc resection offers the best chance for prolonged survival in patients with osteogenic sarcoma and to a lesser extent for Ewing's sarcoma patients; however, there is no definitive cure for either disease. Neoadjuvant chemotherapy can improve local control and survival for Ewing's and osteosarcoma patients, but due to the potential for chemotherapy-induced cardiac, renal, and hepatic toxicity, evaluation of these organs should be a critical part of the pretreatment assessment. Radiation may serve a role for patients who refuse surgery, or in cases of intralesional resection.

Prognosis

- The Spine Oncology Study Group (SOSG) states that neoadjuvant chemotherapy offers significant improvements in local control and long-term survival for spinal osteogenic sarcoma.
- The SOSG strongly recommends the use of en-bloc resection of osteogenic sarcoma with wide margins, as it improves local control and potentially improves survival.
- The overall 5-year survival rate in all patients who have spinal osteogenic sarcoma is 18%. The estimated median survival in patients who present with localized disease and receive aggressive treatment is 18 months.
- The 5-year survival of Ewing's sarcoma has increased from 5 to 10% in the 1980s to the current 5-year survival of 65 to 70%. Based on data from the SEER registry, the median survival of patients with localized spinal tumors is 90 months.
- Patients with metastatic or recurrent Ewing's sarcoma have a poor prognosis; the 5-year survival remains approximately 25 to 30% with a median survival of 20 months.
- The SOSG strongly recommends the use of neoadjuvant chemotherapy for patients with Ewing's sarcoma of the spine due to significant improvements in local control and long-term survival.
- The SOSG issued a weak recommendation promoting en-bloc resection for improved local control, but not improved overall survival for spinal Ewing's sarcoma. The recommendation also supports the use of radiotherapy for local control alone or to supplement an incomplete resection.
- Osteosarcoma is radioresistant; Ewing's sarcoma is radiosensitive, but radiation exposure may increase the risk of secondary malignancies and should be used with extreme care in the pediatric population.

▓ Case Examples

Osteosarcoma

A 76-year-old man presented with pain in his left hip and left lower extremity weakness, with left foot drop. MRI demonstrated a large tumor (**Fig. 10.1**), and a biopsy of the lesion was consistent with chondroblastic osteosarcoma. He was given three cycles of chemotherapy with cisplatin and doxorubicin, but progressed in his disease. A staged surgical approach was offered for en-bloc resection of the mass.

For the first, posterior stage of the operation, L3-S4 was exposed. The tumor was immediately evident posterior to the sacrum on the left side; thus, the musculature was left intact on the left side to maintain a negative margin. The left side paraspinous muscle and fascia was transected at the L3-L4 level. Pedicle screws were placed at L3-S1 on the right side and L3 on the left, with two right-sided iliac screws. Right-sided hemilaminectomies were performed at L4-S3, extending bilaterally at S4. The left side L4-S3 nerve roots were identified, ligated, and cut. Then a midline osteotomy was made from L4 to S4, extending laterally through L4 to generate a hemivertebrectomy at L4 and L5 (**Fig. 10.2**). Due to intraoperative blood loss, the patient required platelets and pressors and remained in the intensive care unit for several days prior to the second stage of his surgery. He developed extensive bilateral deep vein thromboses (DVTs) requiring an inferior vena cava (IVC) filter placement.

For the second stage of the procedure, a radical left hemipelvectomy was completed by the orthopedic surgery team, followed by complex wound closure by the plastic surgery team. The second stage of the procedure was complicated by a left common iliac vein injury with direct repair and ligation of the left internal iliac artery. The plastic surgery team assisted in complex wound closure. The surgery was further complicated by a suspected intraoperative air embolism. The patient's postoperative course was complicated by bilateral subdural hematomas, deep wound infection requiring irrigation and debridement, *Entero-coccus* sepsis, percutaneous endoscopic gastrostomy (PEG) tube placement, and respiratory failure requiring tracheostomy. After a lengthy hospital stay, he was discharged to inpatient rehabilitation. One year after surgery, he is doing well with no evidence of recurrent or metastatic disease and complaints of minimal pain, with strong left and right quadriceps function but loss of left lower extremity function below the knee.

Ewing's Sarcoma

A 26-year-old woman has a history of Ewing's sarcoma in the thoracic spine and sacrum. Her disease remained stable with radiation therapy and multiple cycles of chemotherapy for 2 years; however, in time she developed worsening left lower extremity pain, numbness, and left foot drop. Imaging demonstrated growth of the sacral tumor, but a partial response of her thoracic lesion to medical management (**Fig. 10.4**). Surgery was offered.

A posterior procedure was performed for en-bloc resection of the tumor. A T-shaped incision was made from L2 to the coccyx, extending from the midline to the left posterior iliac crest. Periosteal dissection was performed from L3 to S5. L4-L5 laminectomies and left-sided S1-S5 laminectomies were performed, as well as a left-sided L4-L5 facetectomy. The left-sided L4-S5 nerve roots were identified, ligated, and resected. A high-speed drill was used to create an osteotomy through the midline of the sacrum, extending to the L5-S1 disk space. The L5-S1 disk was excised and the left-side lateral sacroiliac joint was detached from the ilium using a high-speed drill. The left hemisacrum and tumor were retracted dorsally, with careful anterior dissection of the iliac vessels and the rectum away from the tumor mass.

The left side of the pelvis was then reconstructed using a femur shaft, so that an appropriate femur allograft was cut to fill in the defect, extending from the medial aspect of the remaining ilium to the S1 vertebral body, superiorly making contact with the L5 end plate. The femur shaft was secured in place using reconstruction screws through the graft into the S1 vertebral body and the remaining ilium.

Then the pedicle screws were inserted at the L3, L4, and L5 levels bilaterally. Two pelvic screws were inserted on the left side and two on the right side. These screws were then connected to the lumbar screws with several rod attachments and multiple close connectors. The plastic surgery service was called to assist in closure.

The patient's postoperative course was complicated by multiple wound washouts and revisions for her wound closure, as well as a cerebrospinal fluid leak requiring a lumbar drain and, later, a ventriculoperitoneal shunt. She also experienced chronic urinary tract infections and urinary retention requiring a suprapubic tube. Six months after her surgical procedure, she returned to her native country and was lost to follow-up.

■ Chapter Summary

Osteogenic sarcoma and Ewing's sarcoma of the spine are rare. As in most spinal primary tumors, presenting symptoms are often nonspecific and may delay diagnosis and treatment. Currently, patients with osteogenic sarcoma and Ewing's sarcoma are treated with multiple modalities, including surgery, radiation, and chemotherapy. For both tumors, neoadjuvant chemotherapy followed by a wide surgical excision is recommended for patients who have localized disease and resectable tumors. The prognosis for patients presenting with metastatic disease is grim, and current treatments are generally limited to palliative care.

Pearls

♦ Osteogenic sarcoma and Ewing's sarcoma of the spine are high-grade tumors, with the goals of management being to control localized disease and prevent metastatic spread.
♦ Osteogenic sarcoma is the most common sarcoma of the spine and makes up 3 to 15% of all primary spinal tumors, with the majority occurring in the fourth decade of life.
♦ Neoadjuvant chemotherapy is strongly recommended in the management of both osteogenic sarcoma and Ewing's sarcoma due to significant improvements in local control and long-term survival.

Pitfalls

♦ As in other primary spinal tumors, symptoms are often vague and ill-defined, which can lead to a delay in diagnosis, with a significant number of patients presenting with gross metastatic disease.
♦ Ewing's sarcoma is the most common malignant vertebral tumor found in children, with a peak incidence in the second decade.
♦ En-bloc resection offers the best chance for prolonged survival in patients with osteogenic sarcoma and to a lesser extent in patients with Ewing's sarcoma; however, there is no definitive cure for either disease. The morbidity and mortality of en-bloc procedures are considerable, and these procedures should be performed only at experienced centers with multidisciplinary teams.
♦ Avoid the following:
  ○ Intralesional resection or excisional biopsies for tumor resection
  ○ Surgical resection without neoadjuvant chemotherapy
  ○ Forgetting to restage Ewing's sarcoma after neoadjuvant chemotherapy.
  ○ Proceeding with surgical resection without prior staging.

References

Five Must-Read References

1. Gebhardt MC, Springfield D, Neff JR. Sarcomas of bone. In: Abeloff MD, ed. Abeloff's Clinical Oncology. Philadelphia: Churchill Livingstone, 2008:1945–2008
2. Wang VY, Potts M, Chou D. Sarcoma and the spinal column. Neurosurg Clin N Am 2008;19:71–80
3. Kim HJ, McLawhorn AS, Goldstein MJ, Boland PJ. Malignant osseous tumors of the pediatric spine. J Am Acad Orthop Surg 2012;20:646–656
4. Sundaresan N, Rosen G, Boriani S. Primary malignant tumors of the spine. Orthop Clin North Am 2009; 40:21–36, v
5. Clarke MJ, Dasenbrock H, Bydon A, et al. Posterior-only approach for en bloc sacrectomy: clinical outcomes in 36 consecutive patients. Neurosurgery 2012;71:357–364, discussion 364
6. Sciubba DM, Okuno SH, Dekutoski MB, Gokaslan ZL. Ewing and osteogenic sarcoma: evidence for multidisciplinary management. Spine 2009;34(22, Suppl): S58–S68
7. Ozaki T, Flege S, Liljenqvist U, et al. Osteosarcoma of the spine: experience of the Cooperative Osteosarcoma Study Group. Cancer 2002;94:1069–1077

8. Kelley SP, Ashford RU, Rao AS, Dickson RA. Primary bone tumours of the spine: a 42-year survey from the Leeds Regional Bone Tumour Registry. Eur Spine J 2007;16:405–409

9. Ropper AE, Cahill KS, Hanna JW, McCarthy EF, Gokaslan ZL, Chi JH. Primary vertebral tumors: a review of epidemiologic, histological and imaging findings, part II: locally aggressive and malignant tumors. Neurosurgery 2012;70:211–219, discussion 219

10. Mukherjee D, Chaichana KL, Gokaslan ZL, Aaronson O, Cheng JS, McGirt MJ. Survival of patients with malignant primary osseous spinal neoplasms: results from the Surveillance, Epidemiology, and End Results (SEER) database from 1973 to 2003. J Neurosurg Spine 2011;14:143–150

11. Unni KK, Inwards CY. Dahlin's Bone Tumors: General Aspects and Data on 10,165 Cases. Philadelphia: Lippincott Williams & Wilkins, 2009

12. Hayden JB, Hoang BH. Osteosarcoma: basic science and clinical implications. Orthop Clin North Am 2006; 37:1–7

13. Shives TC, Dahlin DC, Sim FH, Pritchard DJ, Earle JD. Osteosarcoma of the spine. J Bone Joint Surg Am 1986;68:660–668

14. Rodallec MH, Feydy A, Larousserie F, et al. Diagnostic imaging of solitary tumors of the spine: what to do and say. Radiographics 2008;28:1019–1041

15. Sciubba DM, Wasserman BA, Gokaslan ZL. Tumors of the spine. In: Khanna AJ, ed. MRI for Orthopaedic Surgeons. New York: Thieme, 2010:316–337

16. Meyer JS, Nadel HR, Marina N, et al. Imaging guidelines for children with Ewing sarcoma and osteosarcoma: a report from the Children's Oncology Group Bone Tumor Committee. Pediatr Blood Cancer 2008; 51:163–170

17. Klein MJ, Siegal GP. Osteosarcoma: anatomic and histologic variants. Am J Clin Pathol 2006;125:555–581

18. Unni KK, Inwards CY. Tumors of the osteoarticular system. In: Fletcher CM, ed. Diagnostic Histopathology of Tumors. New York: Churchill Livingstone, 2007: 1527–1592

19. McGirt MJ, Gokaslan ZL, Chaichana KL. Preoperative grading scale to predict survival in patients undergoing resection of malignant primary osseous spinal neoplasms. Spine J 2011;11:190–196

20. Link MP, Goorin AM, Miser AW, et al. The effect of adjuvant chemotherapy on relapse-free survival in patients with osteosarcoma of the extremity. N Engl J Med 1986;314:1600–1606

21. Gherlinzoni F, Picci P, Bacci G, Campanacci D. Limb sparing versus amputation in osteosarcoma. Correlation between local control, surgical margins and tumor necrosis: Istituto Rizzoli experience. Ann Oncol 1992;3(Suppl 2):S23–S27

22. Sundaresan N, Rosen G, Huvos AG, Krol G. Combined treatment of osteosarcoma of the spine. Neurosurgery 1988;23:714–719

23. DeLaney TF, Liebsch NJ, Pedlow FX, et al. Phase II study of high-dose photon/proton radiotherapy in the management of spine sarcomas. Int J Radiat Oncol Biol Phys 2009;74:732–739

24. Mukherjee D, Chaichana KL, Parker SL, Gokaslan ZL, McGirt MJ. Association of surgical resection and survival in patients with malignant primary osseous spinal neoplasms from the Surveillance, Epidemiology, and End Results (SEER) Database. Eur Spine J 2013;22:1375–1382

25. Ludwig JA. Ewing sarcoma: historical perspectives, current state-of-the-art, and opportunities for targeted therapy in the future. Curr Opin Oncol 2008; 20:412–418

26. Arndt CA, Crist WM. Common musculoskeletal tumors of childhood and adolescence. N Engl J Med 1999;341:342–352

27. Chi JH, Bydon A, Hsieh P, Witham T, Wolinsky JP, Gokaslan ZL. Epidemiology and demographics for primary vertebral tumors. Neurosurg Clin N Am 2008;19:1–4

28. Ilaslan H, Sundaram M, Unni KK, Dekutoski MB. Primary Ewing's sarcoma of the vertebral column. Skeletal Radiol 2004;33:506–513

29. Bernstein M, Kovar H, Paulussen M, et al. Ewing's sarcoma family of tumors: current management. Oncologist 2006;11:503–519

30. Mukherjee D, Chaichana KL, Adogwa O, et al. Association of extent of local tumor invasion and survival in patients with malignant primary osseous spinal neoplasms from the surveillance, epidemiology, and end results (SEER) database. World Neurosurg 2011; 76:580–585

31. Cotterill SJ, Ahrens S, Paulussen M, et al. Prognostic factors in Ewing's tumor of bone: analysis of 975 patients from the European Intergroup Cooperative Ewing's Sarcoma Study Group. J Clin Oncol 2000;18: 3108–3114

32. Evans RG, Nesbit ME, Gehan EA, et al. Multimodal therapy for the management of localized Ewing's sarcoma of pelvic and sacral bones: a report from the second intergroup study. J Clin Oncol 1991;9:1173–1180

33. Grier HE, Krailo MD, Tarbell NJ, et al. Addition of ifosfamide and etoposide to standard chemotherapy for Ewing's sarcoma and primitive neuroectodermal tumor of bone. N Engl J Med 2003;348:694–701

34. Nesbit ME Jr, Gehan EA, Burgert EO Jr, et al. Multimodal therapy for the management of primary, nonmetastatic Ewing's sarcoma of bone: a long-term follow-up of the First Intergroup study. J Clin Oncol 1990;8:1664–1674

35. Sluga M, Windhager R, Lang S, et al. A long-term review of the treatment of patients with Ewing's sarcoma in one institution. Eur J Surg Oncol 2001;27: 569–573

36. Paulino AC, Nguyen TX, Mai WY. An analysis of primary site control and late effects according to local control modality in non-metastatic Ewing sarcoma. Pediatr Blood Cancer 2007;48:423–429

37. Marco RA, Gentry JB, Rhines LD, et al. Ewing's sarcoma of the mobile spine. Spine 2005;30:769–773

38. Bacci G, Longhi A, Briccoli A, Bertoni F, Versari M, Picci P. The role of surgical margins in treatment of Ewing's sarcoma family tumors: experience of a single institution with 512 patients treated with adjuvant and neoadjuvant chemotherapy. Int J Radiat Oncol Biol Phys 2006;65:766–772

39. Talac R, Yaszemski MJ, Currier BL, et al. Relationship between surgical margins and local recurrence in sarcomas of the spine. Clin Orthop Relat Res 2002; 397:127–132

40. Schwab J, Gasbarrini A, Bandiera S, et al. Osteosarcoma of the mobile spine. Spine 2012;37:E381–E386

11

Margins in Spine Tumor Resection: How Much Is Enough? Is Planned Transgression Okay?

Ilya Laufer, Mari L. Groves, and Jean-Paul Wolinsky

▦ Introduction

Cure, or long-term local control, represents the primary goal in the treatment of primary tumors. Various staging systems were developed in order to facilitate prognostication of the probability of cure and survival and to help direct treatment decisions. Physicians most commonly use the Enneking staging system when discussing primary musculoskeletal tumors.[1] Because primary extradural tumors of the spine represent a subset of musculoskeletal tumors, the Enneking system and principles that were initially developed in the context of appendicular tumors have been applied to spinal tumors. Although spinal and appendicular tumors may be histologically identical, the anatomic challenges encountered in the spine distinguish the spinal tumors from their appendicular counterparts.

The Weinstein-Boriani-Biagini (WBB) surgical system and the Tomita surgical classification of vertebral tumors were developed in order to facilitate the application of the Enneking concepts to the spine and to describe the specific vertebral elements that harbor the tumor and the extent of intra- and extraosseous extension.[2,3] Based on the circumferential extent of the tumor and the amount of paraspinal and epidural extension, the systems help predict the margins that may be achieved during surgery. The surrounding structures, tissue planes, and associated neural elements change along the course of the spinal column; therefore, the safety and feasibility of attempting a resection of a clear surrounding margin or en-bloc excision also must be considered in the context of the specific tumor level. Thus, although amputation of a large portion of the sacrum with surrounding musculoskeletal structures and sacral nerve roots may result in minimal structural and neurologic compromise, higher amputation would generally be associated with profound neurologic deficits and require extensive reconstruction.

How much margin should there be, and is a margin necessary, are frequent questions that arise with regard to spinal tumors. To answer this, an understanding of the definition of a margin is critical. Surgical margins in spinal surgery are defined by conventions adopted from the orthopedic extremity literature. But the terms in use are frequently misused, which has contaminated the spinal tumor surgical literature. In addition to understanding what the definition of a margin is, correlating the type of margin that is required with the pathology being treated is critical to delivering the appropriate treatment to a specific patient.

▦ Margin Definition

Margins can be defined as positive, marginal, wide, and radical.[1] A positive margin means that residual tumor remains within the patient. A marginal margin indicates that tumor comes up to the margin of the specimen, but it is contained within the capsule of the tumor. A wide margin indicates that a tumor has been excised and at least 1 cm of healthy tissue has been excised surrounding the tumor. A radical resection means that the tumor is removed and the entire compartment within which the tumor resides is also removed. The margin gives no information on how a surgical resection was undertaken; it only describes the resultant surgical bed.

Often, in spinal oncology, unfortunately, only marginal margins are surgically feasible. Resection of sacral chordomas, even with nerve sacrifice, and resection of soft tissues including skin, fat, and muscle, and planning an osteotomy rostral to the extent of tumor usually still results in a marginal margin. It is rare that sacral chordomas do not have ventral extension of the tumor into the pelvis behind the rectum. In most cases, the tumor capsule is preserved at this margin, but the resection margin is at the mesorectum. Without resection of the rectum, sacral chordoma resections are marginal at the ventral margin or the mesorectum (**Fig. 11.1**).

Patients with mobile spine osseous tumors typically present with epidural extension. In this situation, without dural resection, the best margin will be a marginal margin at the tumor capsule along the dura (**Fig. 11.2**).

Wide margin resections are possible with spinal tumors in rare situations. Some patients may present with small tumors completely contained within the vertebral body (**Fig. 11.3**), and, in these situations, complete resection of the vertebral body with the tumor can result in a wide margin.

Radical resections of the spine are technically possible but are not performed. A radical resection requires resection of the tumor and the entire compartment within which the tumor lies. In an extremity tumor, this would involve resection of the tumor, the bone from which it arises, and the muscles inserting into the bone through their distal insertions. An example would be a tumor arising in the tibia, with a planned resection being an above-the-knee amputation, above the muscular insertions of the muscles surrounding the tumor. In the spine, a conceivable example would be a sacral tumor, contained within the sacrum, with no ventral extension through the sacrum, and no extension

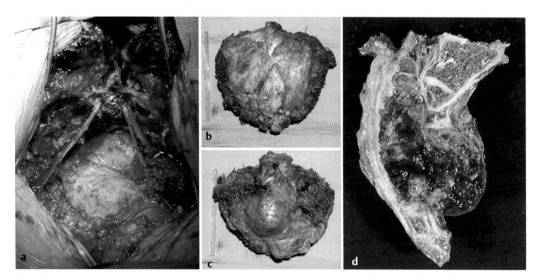

Fig. 11.1a–d A large sacral chordoma with ventral extraosseous extension. **(a)** The postoperative surgical field demonstrates the proximity of the tumor to the intrapelvic organs. **(b)** Posterior view of the specimen demonstrates the wide margin of healthy tissue, which can be obtained. On the other hand, the anterior **(c)** and lateral **(d)** views of the specimen show a marginal margin at the site of ventral extraosseous extension of the tumor. (Courtesy of Jean-Paul Wolinsky, MD.)

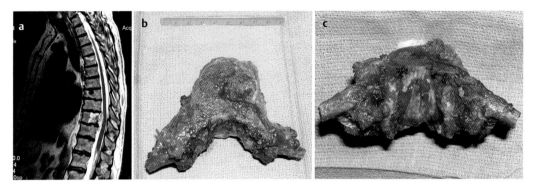

Fig. 11.2a–c **(a)** Sagittal T2-weighted magnetic resonance imaging (MRI) of a T10 chordoma with epidural extension. Superior **(b)** and posterior **(c)** views of the vertebrectomy specimen demonstrate that only a marginal margin was obtained due to the dorsal extension of the tumor into the epidural space, with tumor displacing the posterior longitudinal ligament. (Courtesy of Jean-Paul Wolinsky, MD.)

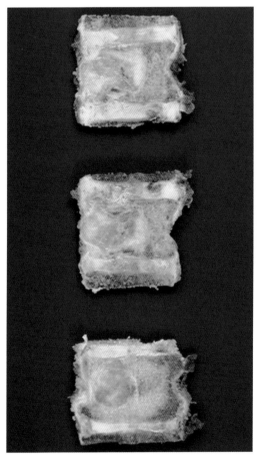

Fig. 11.3 A malignant peripheral nerve sheath tumor entirely confined to the vertebral body without extraosseous extension. This tumor was resected with a wide margin of bone. (Courtesy of Jean-Paul Wolinsky, MD.)

of the tumor to the dura, where a hemicorporectomy is performed. This operation would most likely never be proposed for such tumor architecture, irrespective of the pathology, as the morbidity of the operation would be unacceptable. With extension of the tumor to the dura, a radical resection, even with a hemicorporectomy would not be possible, as resection of the dural "compartment", would require resection of the dura throughout the entire spine and cranium.

The Spine Oncology Study Group evaluated the reliability of the application of the Enneking and WBB staging systems in the spine using a series of primary tumor case examples.[4] Moderate interobserver reliability was demonstrated in the use of the Enneking staging system, an Enneking-recommended surgical margin, the WBB layers, and the WBB-recommended resection. The intraobserver reliability was near-perfect for the Enneking staging system and substantial for the WBB system. The Enneking tumor extent determination proved particularly challenging, with only slight to fair interobserver reliability.

A multicenter cohort study examined the correlation between the ability to achieve an Enneking-recommended margin and the outcome of surgery for primary osseous tumors of the spine.[5] Patients harboring tumors that were amenable to resection with the margin that is recommended by the Enneking staging system had significantly lower local recurrence rates compared with patients in whom an optimal margin could not be achieved. However, we must emphasize that the resectability of the tumor with an appropriate margin is largely an intrinsic characteristic associated with the individual histology, grade, location, and size. This is supported by the observation that in the study cohort, the Enneking-recommended margin could not be achieved in a significant majority of high-grade tumors and tumors located in the cervical and thoracic spine, but could be achieved in a significant majority of benign tumors and tumors located in the sacrum. Furthermore, the risk of blood loss of more than 5,000 mL and the risk of infection were significantly higher in patients who underwent surgery for Enneking-recommended margins.

Surgical Technique Terminology

Further complicating the literature is the misuse of the terms *spondylectomy, en-bloc spondylectomy, total en-bloc spondylectomy (TES), intralesional,* and *en-bloc resection. Spondylectomy* means removing the entire segment of the spine (the vertebral body, pedicles, superior and inferior articulating processes, pars, transverse processes, lamina, and spinous process) (**Fig. 11.4**). It is a surgical technique, but does not specify if the tumor is removed in an en-bloc or intralesional fashion. An entire spinal segment can be removed "piecemeal" and result in a spondylectomy, but this should not be confused with an en-bloc resection.

The terms *en-bloc spondylectomy* and *total en-bloc spondylectomy (TES)* are frequently used in the primary tumor literature,[6] but in the mobile spine they are seldom, if ever, performed. An en-bloc spondylectomy would require resection of the spinal segment without violating any portion of it. Because each spinal segment of the mobile spine contains the spinal cord or the cauda equina, removal of the vertebra without opening of the spinal canal ring would require transection of these neural elements with the specimen. This does occur in the sacrum, when sacral amputations are

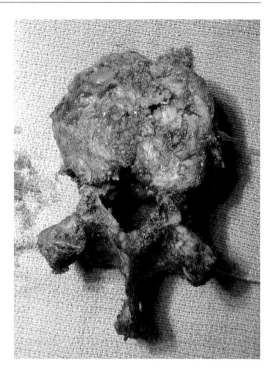

Fig. 11.4 Spondylectomy specimen. (Courtesy of Jean-Paul Wolinsky, MD.)

performed, as the sacrifice of nerves roots in this region is usually undertaken to achieve a meaningful resection.[7]

The term *intralesional resection* should be used anytime the tumor capsule is violated and the tumor is entered. Even if the intent of the tumor resection is to remove the entire specimen in one piece, if the specimen demonstrates that the margin was violated on pathological review, then this is an intralesional resection. If a surgery plan incorporates the need for a planned transgression of the tumor[8] (**Fig. 11.5**) in order to achieve a resection, this is, by definition, an intralesional resection despite complete removal of the tumor.

The term *en bloc* is used if the tumor is removed in one piece without violation of the tumor margin. Certain tumor pathologies require en-bloc resections with negative margins to achieve local tumor control. In certain circumstances, an en-bloc resection might be used to control blood loss in vascular tumors even if the tumor pathology does not require an en-bloc resection for tumor control. Likewise, an

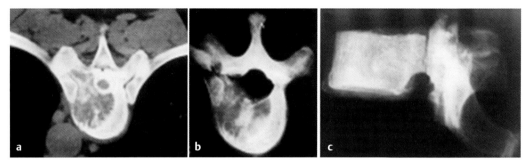

Fig. 11.5a–c (a) A computed tomography (CT) scan of a T10 solitary breast metastasis with invasion of the vertebral body, epidural space, pedicle, and the costovertebral joint. Horizontal **(b)** and lateral **(c)** radiographs of the specimen showing the intralesional resection of the tumor with intentional transgression of the pedicle with tumor invasion.[10] (Reproduced with permission from Lippincott Williams & Wilkins.)

en-bloc resection may be employed to achieve a complete resection if the tumor and surrounding anatomy have become distorted, and the interpretation of tumor margins would be complicated by an intralesional resection.

■ Treatment Options

The type of surgery indicated, en bloc versus intralesional, is determined by the pathology being treated (**Table 11.1**). Thus, prior to doing the resection, it is most important to obtain a definitive diagnosis, which usually requires a biopsy. The margin that is needed to control the tumor is also dictated by the tumor pathology. Many times, the planned surgical margin that is required hinges on the available adjuvant therapies for a given pathology. Furthermore, although en-bloc excision may be the desired method of tumor removal for certain tumors, some evidence suggests that an optimal final margin may be the more meaningful goal and predictor of local control.[9]

Certain tumor pathologies have a very good response to adjuvant therapies such as chemotherapy and radiation therapy, and therefore

Table 11.1 Histology-Specific Recommended Minimal Margin

Pathology (Primary Bone Tumors)	Minimal Margin Needed
Plasmacytoma/multiple myeloma	Biopsy
Eosinophilic granuloma/Langerhans cell histiocytosis	Biopsy
Ewing's sarcoma	Biopsy, en-bloc resection in rare instance of residual tumor after chemotherapy/radiation
Chordoma	En-bloc resection
Osteogenic sarcoma	En-bloc resection
Chondrosarcoma (mobile spine and pelvis)	En-bloc resection
Chondrosarcoma (skull base)	Intralesional resection
Giant cell tumor	En-bloc resection
Aneurysmal bone cyst	Intratumoral chemotherapy vs intralesional resection
Osteoid osteomas	Intralesional resection
Osteoblastoma	En-bloc resection if path unclear
Hemangioma	Intralesional resection

the surgical role may be minor in those instances. Examples of such pathologies include plasmacytoma, multiple myeloma, eosinophilic granuloma (Langerhans histiocytosis), and Ewing's sarcoma. Advances in chemotherapy have changed the approach to Ewing's sarcoma from a surgical lesion to one that is now treated primarily with chemotherapy and radiation therapy. One implication of this new approach occurs in rare situations where there is only a solitary residual focus of tumor; in these situations, a negative margin resection is advocated by some authors to try to eradicate any gross disease in Ewing's sarcoma.[10]

There are certain tumors where an en-bloc resection with a negative margin is critical to achieving long-term control of the disease. The textbook/quintessential representation of such a tumor is a chordoma. It is clear from the surgical literature that piecemeal resection of chordomas has a high propensity for local recurrence.[11] In addition, it is also clear that if an en-bloc resection is planned, but the final pathological margin is contaminated, these patients have a significantly worse prognosis and higher likelihood of recurrence. There are probably two reasons for this finding: (1) chordomas have a high propensity to seed the surrounding tissue if spilled, and (2) adjuvant chemotherapy and radiation therapy have very limited effectiveness in the treatment of chordomas. It is unclear how wide a negative margin needs to be for resection of chordomas, as no studies have suggested an answer.

In our experience in the sacrum, local recurrences never occur at the margin of the rostral or lateral osteotomies. They do not occur at the ventral margin at the rectum, which is frequently the most marginal margin. If there is a local recurrence, it is in the muscle, usually along the piriformis muscle. Of note, this is usually the widest margin that is possible, and it is unclear why the tumor would recur in this area. One possibility is that undetected microscopic tumor exists in these muscles already, and these cells are already beyond the surgical margin. In an attempt to decrease the chance of recurrence in this region, wider margins have been taken by sectioning these muscles at their insertions in the greater trochanter (**Fig. 11.6**).

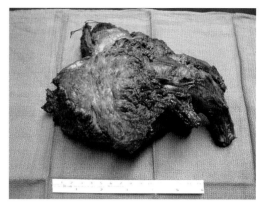

Fig. 11.6 A sacrectomy specimen of a chordoma with resection of piriformis muscles. The muscles are sectioned at the attachment of the piriformis to the greater trochanter. (Courtesy of Jean-Paul Wolinsky, MD.)

Alternatively, some centers are delivering preoperative radiation to these regions in an attempt to reduce the chance of recurrence in this region.[12] But too few patients have undergone this more extended resection or preoperative radiation treatments to know if this approach has a positive impact.

Osteogenic sarcoma is another tumor that tends to behave in a malignant and locally aggressive fashion, but it is unclear if the tumor actually seeds the local environment. It is clear that if the margins for resection are positive, then the overall prognosis for the patient is poor. In general the prognosis for osteogenic sarcoma, even with negative margins, is also poor.[13] En-bloc resection for osteogenic sarcoma may have impact on local control but not on survival. This most likely is not a consequence of the surgical margin, but has more to do with the behavior of the tumor, especially its aggressiveness and its propensity for metastatic spread. Without a good response to chemotherapy, patients with osteogenic sarcoma do poorly.[14] Neoadjuvant chemotherapy is usually employed with the treatment of these tumors, and the percent necrosis of the tumor within a surgical specimen has overall predictive value.[15] An inability to achieve a negative margin may be more a marker that the tumor is very aggressive and that micro-metastatic disease has already occurred.

Chondrosarcoma appears to behave differently in different parts of the body. Histologically, chondrosarcomas of the skull base, spine, and pelvis may appear identical, but they do not behave in the same manner.[16] Skull base chondrosarcomas, given their location, cannot be resected in an en-bloc fashion with negative margins. The morbidity of an en-bloc resection precludes this option in the skull base. These tumors in the skull base are usually resected in a piecemeal, subtotal fashion. Adjuvant radiation therapy in the form of proton beam irradiation can achieve local control rates up to 98% at 10 years.[17] This has not been the experience in the mobile spine and pelvis. In these locations, subtotal resection, even with adjuvant radiation therapy, is associated with very high recurrence rates at 1 year.[18,19] It is not clear, though, if these tumors absolutely need an en-bloc resection or if the tumor margin can be violated as long as ultimately the resection bed is negative. It is our practice to resect these tumors in an en bloc-fashion, if possible. If the tumor architecture precludes doing so, such as a mobile spine chondrosarcoma that circumferentially encases the spinal cord (**Fig. 11.7**), then the plan is to transgress the tumor so as to resect it entirely. The concept of a planned transgression of the tumor is supported by what

has been seen with pelvic chondrosarcomas. Reoperation of chondrosarcomas with residual or locally recurrent tumors can have favorable long-term disease-free survival if complete resection of the tumor with negative margins can be achieved.

Giant cell tumors are thought to be low grade but to have some malignant potential. These tumors have been noted to metastasize to the lung and have demonstrated the potential for malignant transformation.[20] It is unclear if this malignant transformation is a result of adjuvant radiation therapy or is de novo transformation of the tumor. Giant cell tumors presenting in the extremities are usually treated with intralesional resection and postcurettage treatment of the surgical bed with a caustic substance such as phenol.[20] With this treatment, there has been reasonable control with limited recurrences. In the spine, our experience with intralesional resection of giant cell tumors is that it entails a recurrence rate of up to 90%. The reason for this higher recurrence rate for spinal compared with extremity giant cell tumors may lie with the fact that caustic substances such as phenol cannot be used in the surgical bed, especially in the presence of sensitive neural tissue. Tumor recurrences in the spine can be very difficult to treat, and they

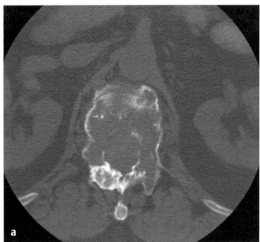 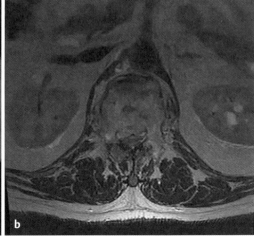

Fig. 11.7a,b A CT scan **(a)** and MRI **(b)** of a clear cell chondrosarcoma with circumferential encasement of the spinal cord. Excision of this tumor requires transgression of the tumor margin in order to preserve the integrity of the spinal cord. (Courtesy of Jean-Paul Wolinsky, MD.)

result in significant morbidity; therefore, we advocate en-bloc resection with a marginal margin of these tumors if the morbidity of the operation is acceptable. As our understanding of these tumors is evolving, this treatment paradigm may change. There has been some evidence that administration of denosumab results in giant cell tumor growth arrest and decrease in size through RANK-L (receptor activator of nuclear factor kappa-B ligand) inhibition and offers a promising medical therapy in the treatment of these tumors.[21]

Aneurysmal bone cysts (ABCs) are vascular low-grade tumors. They can occasionally harbor other tumors within them.[22] Oncologically, these tumors can be treated with an intralesional resection.[23] However, subtotal intralesional resections can result in a recurrence. Given the vascularity of these tumors, preoperative embolization is often employed and en-bloc techniques may be used to decrease operative blood loss. Treatment with intratumoral injection of calcitonin and corticosteroids can result in tumor resolution,[24] and therefore tumors that respond to this treatment may not need surgical resection.

Osteoid osteomas are small tumors without malignant potential. Surgical resection is aimed at gross tumor resection for pain control, but en-bloc resection is not needed.[25] The larger variant of osteoid osteomas, osteoblastomas, are also benign tumors, but given their size, sampling error can be an issue, and care must be taken to distinguish them from osteosarcomas.[26] If differentiation of an osteoblastoma from an osteosarcoma cannot be made preoperatively based on imaging and biopsy, then aggressive management with an en-bloc resection is indicated (**Fig. 11.8**).

Hemangiomas are benign tumors without malignant potential. They tend to be contained within the vertebral body, but in rare cases can grow beyond the anterior column and cause neurologic compromise.[27] Histologically, these atypical hemangiomas are no different from other hemangiomas. Treatment is aimed at neu-

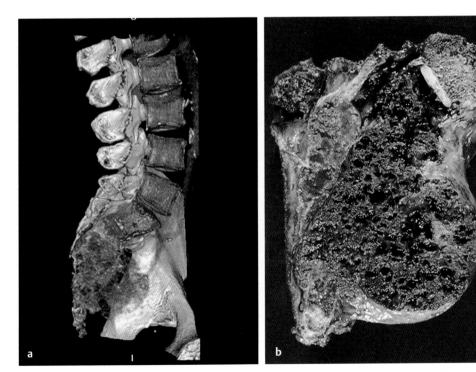

Fig. 11.8a,b **(a)** A three-dimensional CT reconstruction of a giant sacral osteoblastoma. **(b)** A sagittal view of the surgical specimen after en-bloc resection of the tumor. (Courtesy of Jean-Paul Wolinsky, MD.)

rologic protection and tumor control. To prevent recurrences, complete resection should be undertaken. En-bloc resection is not necessary, but, as with ABCs, en-bloc resection may be employed to decrease blood loss during resection.

Chapter Summary

Surgery represents the main treatment modality in the treatment of primary spinal osseous tumors. The histology of the tumor remains the strongest determinant of survival and local control. The surgical margin in the spine ranges from intralesional to wide, with wider margins indicated for more aggressive tumors. The ability to achieve a wide margin in the treatment of spinal tumors is often limited by the contact of the tumor with neural elements, and the goal of wide margin must be balanced with the functional deficit that may result from such surgery. Furthermore, the spinal cord often limits the surgeons' ability to achieve an en-bloc resection, necessitating tumor transgression. Surgical data indicate that failure to achieve the indicated margin in primary tumor resection is associated with increased risk of tumor recurrence. Although surgical technique plays an important role in achievement of the desired margin, tumor biology and stage often act as the ultimate determinant of the ability to carry out an en-bloc resection or the indicated margin. A clear understanding of the desired surgical margin and of the anatomic challenges of the spinal column enables surgeons to devise a surgical plan that minimizes the risk of local recurrence and surgical morbidity.

The behavior of primary spinal tumors ranges from benign to highly malignant. Although asymptomatic benign tumors may be monitored, symptomatic and malignant tumors require treatment with the goal of cure or long-term local control. The spinal column presents unique anatomic challenges, and the oncological surgical principles used in the treatment of appendicular musculoskeletal tumors have been successfully applied to spinal tumors. The propensity of malignant tumors to form satellite and skip lesions outside of the clear radiographic and histological tumor boundaries requires tumor excision with a wide margin of healthy tissue surrounding the tumor and the use of radiation and pharmacological therapy in order to increase the probability of local control. Gross excision of low-grade and benign tumors may provide cure without the use of adjuvant therapy.

The description of the surgical margin must be distinguished from the description of the surgical technique used to remove the tumor. The tumor may be removed in a piecemeal fashion or en-bloc fashion; the latter refers to excision of the whole specimen without violation of the tumor capsule. The description of the margin and the type of tumor excision provide complementary information about the manner in which the tumor was removed. Although the histology of the tumor generally serves as the primary determinant of prognosis, in most instances failure to obtain a histology-appropriate tumor margin has been shown to be an adverse prognostic indicator associated with local recurrence. Therefore, every effort must be made to perform an optimal oncological resection while balancing the morbidity of trying to achieve the indicated margin.

Pearls

- Margins: intralesional, marginal, wide, radical
- Surgical plan: piecemeal, en bloc
- Surgical technique: spondylectomy
- Biopsy: critical for determining the margin requirement, the surgical plan, and the surgical technique

Pitfalls

- Failure to understand the definition of terms for literature descriptors or to understand tumor outcomes
- Failure to identify pathology before formulating the treatment plan

References
Five Must-Read References

1. Enneking WF. A system of staging musculoskeletal neoplasms. Clin Orthop Relat Res 1986;204:9–24
2. Boriani S, Weinstein JN, Biagini R. Primary bone tumors of the spine. Terminology and surgical staging. Spine 1997;22:1036–1044
3. Tomita K, Kawahara N, Baba H, Tsuchiya H, Nagata S, Toribatake Y. Total en bloc spondylectomy for solitary spinal metastases. Int Orthop 1994;18:291–298
4. Chan P, Boriani S, Fourney DR, et al. An assessment of the reliability of the Enneking and Weinstein-Boriani-Biagini classifications for staging of primary spinal tumors by the Spine Oncology Study Group. Spine 2009;34:384–391
5. Fisher CG, Saravanja DD, Dvorak MF, et al. Surgical management of primary bone tumors of the spine: validation of an approach to enhance cure and reduce local recurrence. Spine 2011;36:830–836
6. Tomita K, Kawahara N, Baba H, Tsuchiya H, Fujita T, Toribatake Y. Total en bloc spondylectomy. A new surgical technique for primary malignant vertebral tumors. Spine 1997;22:324–333
7. Fourney DR, Rhines LD, Hentschel SJ, et al. En bloc resection of primary sacral tumors: classification of surgical approaches and outcome. J Neurosurg Spine 2005;3:111–122
8. Tomita K, Kawahara N, Kobayashi T, Yoshida A, Murakami H, Akamaru T. Surgical strategy for spinal metastases. Spine 2001;26:298–306
9. Virkus WW, Marshall D, Enneking WF, Scarborough MT. The effect of contaminated surgical margins revisited. Clin Orthop Relat Res 2002;397:89–94
10. Marco RA, Gentry JB, Rhines LD, et al. Ewing's sarcoma of the mobile spine. Spine 2005;30:769–773
11. Boriani S, Bandiera S, Biagini R, et al. Chordoma of the mobile spine: fifty years of experience. Spine 2006; 31:493–503
12. Wagner TD, Kobayashi W, Dean S, et al. Combination short-course preoperative irradiation, surgical resection, and reduced-field high-dose postoperative irradiation in the treatment of tumors involving the bone. Int J Radiat Oncol Biol Phys 2009;73:259–266
13. Schoenfeld AJ, Hornicek FJ, Pedlow FX, et al. Osteosarcoma of the spine: experience in 26 patients treated at the Massachusetts General Hospital. Spine J 2010;10:708–714
14. Rosen G, Marcove RC, Huvos AG, et al. Primary osteogenic sarcoma: eight-year experience with adjuvant chemotherapy. J Cancer Res Clin Oncol 1983; 106(Suppl):55–67
15. Bacci G, Mercuri M, Longhi A, et al. Grade of chemotherapy-induced necrosis as a predictor of local and systemic control in 881 patients with non-metastatic osteosarcoma of the extremities treated with neoadjuvant chemotherapy in a single institution. Eur J Cancer 2005;41:2079–2085
16. Andreou D, Ruppin S, Fehlberg S, Pink D, Werner M, Tunn PU. Survival and prognostic factors in chondrosarcoma: results in 115 patients with long-term follow-up. Acta Orthop 2011;82:749–755
17. Rosenberg AE, Nielsen GP, Keel SB, et al. Chondrosarcoma of the base of the skull: a clinicopathologic study of 200 cases with emphasis on its distinction from chordoma. Am J Surg Pathol 1999;23:1370–1378
18. Bergh P, Gunterberg B, Meis-Kindblom JM, Kindblom LG. Prognostic factors and outcome of pelvic, sacral, and spinal chondrosarcomas: a center-based study of 69 cases. Cancer 2001;91:1201–1212
19. York JE, Berk RH, Fuller GN, et al. Chondrosarcoma of the spine: 1954 to 1997. J Neurosurg 1999;90(1, Suppl):73–78
20. Errani C, Ruggieri P, Asenzio MA, et al. Giant cell tumor of the extremity: a review of 349 cases from a single institution. Cancer Treat Rev 2010;36:1–7
21. Thomas D, Henshaw R, Skubitz K, et al. Denosumab in patients with giant-cell tumour of bone: an open-label, phase 2 study. Lancet Oncol 2010;11:275–280
22. Fang Z, Chen M. Chondroblastoma associated with aneurysmal cyst of the navicular bone: a case report. World J Surg Oncol 2013;11:50
23. Zenonos G, Jamil O, Governale LS, Jernigan S, Hedequist D, Proctor MR. Surgical treatment for primary spinal aneurysmal bone cysts: experience from Children's Hospital Boston. J Neurosurg Pediatr 2012;9: 305–315
24. Ohashi M, Ito T, Hirano T, Endo N. Percutaneous intralesional injection of calcitonin and methylprednisolone for treatment of an aneurysmal bone cyst at C-2. J Neurosurg Pediatr 2008;2:365–369
25. Gasbarrini A, Cappuccio M, Bandiera S, Amendola L, van Urk P, Boriani S. Osteoid osteoma of the mobile spine: surgical outcomes in 81 patients. Spine 2011; 36:2089–2093
26. Boriani S, Amendola L, Bandiera S, et al. Staging and treatment of osteoblastoma in the mobile spine: a review of 51 cases. Eur Spine J 2012;21:2003–2010
27. Jankowski R, Nowak S, Zukiel R, Szymaś J, Sokół B. Surgical treatment of symptomatic vertebral haemangiomas. Neurol Neurochir Pol 2011;45:577–582

12

Principles Behind Determining the Right Approach

Nicolas Dea and Rowan Schouten

Introduction

Primary tumors of the spine are rare. As a result, clinical expertise has been concentrated in selected quaternary referral centers. In recent years these centers have collaborated and combined the best available evidence with their collective expert opinion to enhance the published literature and further define the essentials of successful surgical care.

Surgery plays a key role in the management of most primary spinal tumors. Historically, inferior results and high recurrence rates were reflective of a poor understanding of the fundamentals integral to the successful operative management of these rare entities, coupled with the technical complexities of their surgical approach. More recently, technological advances and technical descriptions of a number of surgical approaches have demonstrated the feasibility of following evidence-based oncological care principles. Despite this, and because of the potential for severe and unacceptable neurologic deficits and the intrinsic stability function of the spinal column, surgery remains challenging.

This chapter discusses the key principles to consider when selecting a surgical approach and illustrates them with representative cases.

Enneking Classification

Originally described in the 1980s for primary tumors of the appendicular skeleton, the Enneking classification remains the fundamental foundation for approaching primary mesenchymal tumors, including those originating from the spine.[1] This system classifies primary tumors based on three factors: a grade of their biological aggressiveness (G), its local extent (T), and the presence or absence of metastasis (M).

Histological, radiological, and clinical features correlate to identify benign (G0), low-grade malignant (G1), or high-grade malignant (G2) lesions. Benign (G0) lesions are then further subcategorized as being latent (stage 1), active (stage 2), or aggressive (stage 3) based on characteristics of the tumor host margin. Stage 1 benign lesions are slow growing or static, and characterized by mature fibrous tissue or cortical bone encapsulation. Stage 2 benign lesions grow steadily and are bordered by a thin capsule surrounded by an area of reactive tissue. Stage 3 benign tumors extend rapidly, usually preceded by a thick pseudocapsule of reactive tissue with a penetrated or absent capsule.

The location of the tumor is categorized as intracapsular (T0), intracompartmental (T1), or

Table 12.1 Enneking Staging System

Stage	Grade	Local extension	Metastases
Benign			
1	G0	Intracompartmental (T0)	No (M0)
2	G0	Intracompartmental (T0)	No (M0)
3	G0	Intra- or extracompartmental (T1/T2)	No (M0)
Malignant			
1A	Low (G1)	Intracompartmental (T1)	No (M0)
1B	Low (G1)	Extracompartmental (T2)	No (M0)
2A	High (G2)	Intracompartmental (T1)	No (M0)
2B	High (G2)	Extracompartmental (T2)	No (M0)
3	Any	Any	Yes (M1)

Source: Adapted from Enneking WF. A system of staging musculoskeletal neoplasms. Clin Orthop Relat Res 1986;204:9–24.

extracompartmental (T2). Absence of metastases is denoted as M0 and the presence of distant metastasis as M1. These three factors combine to create the Enneking stage (**Table 12.1**). For each stage, a specific resection margin is recommended (**Table 12.2**).

Adhering to and respecting the Enneking principles for tumors of the appendicular skeleton has been shown to result in a lower rate of

Table 12.2 Modified Articulation of Enneking Stages with Surgical Margins

Enneking Stages	Margin for Control
1	No management unless for decompression or stabilization
2	Intralesional excision ± local adjuvants
3	Marginal en-bloc excision
1a	Wide en-bloc excision
1b	Wide en-bloc excision
2a	Wide en-bloc excision + effective adjuvants
2b	Wide en-bloc excision + effective adjuvants
3a	Palliative
3b	Palliative

Source: From Chan P, Boriani S, Fourney DR, et al. An assessment of the reliability of the Enneking and Weinstein-Boriani-Biagini classifications for staging of primary spinal tumors by the Spine Oncology Study Group. Spine 2009;34:385. Reproduced with permission.)

recurrence and in improved survival. During recent decades, advancements in imaging and surgical technology along with spinal oncology subspecialization has permitted the safe application of the Enneking principles for tumors of the spinal column. As has been demonstrated in the appendicular skeleton, this standardized approach has been shown to achieve acceptable morbidity, mortality, and health-related quality of life outcomes for primary spine tumors.[2–4] In a multicenter ambispective cohort analysis of 147 patients with primary spine tumors, Fisher et al[5] demonstrated that the adoption of Enneking principles resulted in a significant reduction in rates of local recurrence and improved life expectancy. Studies assessing the recurrence risk and tumor-free survival following surgical resection of spinal column chordomas[6,7] and chondrosarcomas[8] have also confirmed the importance of adhering to Enneking fundamentals.

For spinal column tumors, the Enneking classification does not take into account the presence of a continuous epidural compartment, the neurologic implications, and the need for restoring spinal stability.[9] Furthermore, the size of the tumor, which has been found to be correlated with adverse prognosis,[6] is not considered. The system was originally based on the natural history of mesenchymal tumors and thus is not applicable to tumors originating from bone marrow, the reticuloendothelial system, or metastatic carcinomas.

■ Weinstein-Boriani-Biagini Classification

The Weinstein-Boriani-Biagini (WBB) classification incorporates the Enneking principles into the staging and surgical approach of primary tumors of the spine by addressing the unique complexity of lesions in this anatomic setting.[10] The pioneering work of these authors significantly assists surgical planning by establishing feasibility criteria and strategies for achieving oncological resection of these tumors while sparing the neurologic elements based on the location of the lesion. In this surgical staging system, vertebral bodies are divided into 12 equal radiating zones in the axial plane (**Fig. 12.1**) numbered clockwise from the left side of the spinous process (1) to the right side of the spinous process (12). The tumor is further divided into five concentric layers centered about the dural sac: A, extraosseous soft tissues; B, intraosseous superficial; C, intraosseous deep; D, (extraosseous extradural; and E, extraosseous intradural. Finally, the longitudinal extent of the tumor is recorded as the number of vertebral segments involved. Based on the WBB stages, Boriani et al[4] proposed indications for surgical procedures based on their experience with 29 patients.

For tumors of the spinal column, moderate interobserver reliability and substantial near-perfect intraobserver reliability for both the Enneking and WBB classification, in terms of staging and guidance for treatment, have been reported.[11]

■ Surgical Margins

Standardized terminology, which has been a source of confusion in the literature, is fundamental for the study of primary spinal column tumors. Curettage or piecemeal resection refers to deliberate intralesionnal resection. En-bloc resection, on the other hand, signifies an attempt to resect a tumor in one piece. En-bloc resection on its own has no clear signification without an appropriate histological description of the resection margins (intralesional, marginal, wide, or radical). An intralesional margin

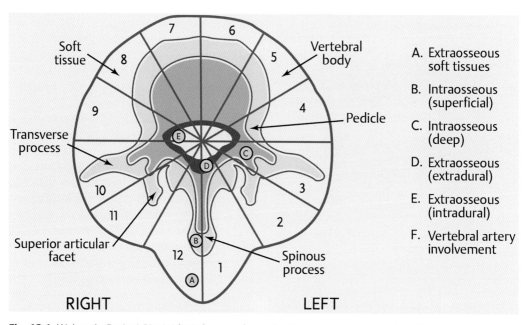

Fig. 12.1 Weinstein-Boriani-Biagini (WBB) surgical staging of spine tumors. (From Boriani S, Biagini R, De Iure F, et al. En bloc resections of bone tumors of the thoracolumbar spine. A preliminary report on 29 patients. Spine 1996;21:1927–1931. Reproduced with permission.)

denotes that the plane of dissection has transgressed into the lesion. A marginal margin refers to dissection within the reactive zone or pseudocapsule surrounding the tumor, whereas a wide resection margin signifies the dissection has occurred beyond the reactive zone through normal tissue. In spine surgery, radical margins, which refer to extracompartmental resection, are rarely feasible, as the epidural space is considered a continuous compartment extending from occiput to the sacrum. The only theoretical scenario is a stage I/IIA tumor totally confined to the vertebra (without epidural disease) where a complete resection including the spinal cord is performed. Achieving wide resection margins in tumors involving the epidural compartment would imply dissection of dural tissue, which would significantly complicate the approach and increase the complication rate. Consequently when there is epidural tumor, marginal resection at the dura is often performed. The cost–benefit ratio of achieving a wide resection at the dura has not been fully evaluated.

When preservation of the uninvolved neural elements cannot be achieved without compromising the surgical margins, the surgeon, conjointly with the patient, has to decide on a compromise. Creating a neurologic deficit can be justified to achieve a potential cure in a patient with a long life expectancy. The alternative is to compromise the Enneking surgical principles and perform a planned tumor transgression to enable delivery of the tumor without neural element sacrifice. Compromising the surgical margins in a planned, predictable fashion has the potential to cause less tumor spillage and a lower rate of local recurrence than a deliberate intralesionnal resection. It cannot be overstated that these decisions must include the patient's personal preferences following a thorough discussion of options. Chapter 11 discusses the issues of surgical margins and planned transgression in detail.

Determining the Diagnosis

The approach to primary spinal tumors begins with determining the appropriate histological diagnosis. Because of the rarity of these tumors, a pathologist experienced with diagnosing these conditions should be consulted. The differential diagnosis includes primary mesenchymal tumors, primary nonmesenchymal tumor (hematological or reticuloendothelial system malignancies), metastatic disease, pyogenic and nonpyogenic spinal infections, inflammatory processes, as well as the more common traumatic and degenerative pathologies. The multitude of primary tumor pathologies and their varying intrinsic biological behaviors make determining an accurate diagnosis of the upmost importance. Ewing's sarcomas, for example, can respond strikingly to neoadjuvant therapies and can thus be considered for medical therapy only.

How tissue is obtained to facilitate a histological diagnosis can have a significant influence on patient outcomes and the surgical strategy subsequently selected. A systematic review addressed this issue.[3] A computed tomography (CT)-guided trocar biopsy appears to be the best oncological way of safely determining a diagnosis, as incisional or open biopsies have been associated with higher recurrence rates and lower disease-free survival. When a primary spinal tumor is suspected, an oncological spine surgeon should be involved early, as the biopsy tract needs to be marked to ensure its inclusion during the definitive resection.

Multidisciplinary Teams

Assembling a multidisciplinary team for preoperative decision making and planning is fundamental to achieving optimal primary spine tumor management. Each case should be discussed in rounds attended by an oncological spine surgeon, radiation oncologist, medical oncologist, pathologist, and radiologist. A group review of the local and systemic workup, histological diagnosis, and staging will enable consensus conclusions to be reached on key issues including the role and feasibility of surgery, and the suitability of neoadjuvant and adjuvant therapies. If a neoadjuvant treatment is deemed necessary, restaging is recommended after completion, before contemplating surgical treatment.

When resection is indicated, various surgical subspecialties can play significant supporting roles to the spine surgeon. When considerable vascular manipulation or reconstruction is necessary, a vascular surgeon is indispensable. Plastic surgeons can assist with the closure of precarious wounds or perform musculocutaneous flap coverage when necessary. When abdominal or pelvic contents and the tumor are closely approximated, a general surgeon can assist in the dissection and create derivation colostomies when required. Complex dissections of the neck can be facilitated by head and neck surgeons, whereas dissection within the chest cavity can be assisted by thoracic surgeons.

▨ Surgical Planning

Because each primary spine tumor has unique characteristics and localizations, surgeons must be flexible about determining the right approach. Each case should be approached individually. The choice of surgical margins according to the Enneking principles is the first step in planning surgical intervention (**Table 12.2**). With advancements in surgical expertise, imaging and technology are important adjuncts in determining the surgical approach to any spinal tumor. We believe there should not be any preset approaches based on localization.

En-bloc resection for tumors of the spinal column was first described in the 1960s. Lièvre et al[12] described a two-stage en-bloc resection of an L4 giant cell tumor. The first stage consisted of resection of the posterior spinal elements, followed by an anterior vertebral body resection 2 weeks later. In the following years, Stener described a similar approach for a giant cell tumor of T11-L1[13] and later reported on his extensive experience (1968–1981) with complete removal of vertebrae for extirpation of tumors in 23 consecutive patients with a minimum of 7-year follow-up.[14] The basic principles used in his case series are still used today.

Stener pioneered the fundamental principle of considering the spinal column to be like a ring through which the neural elements pass. To achieve a resection while adhering to Enneking's principle and preserving neurologic function, a tumor-free window has to be created in that "ring" through which the spinal cord can be delivered during tumor removal. The window can be created by piecemeal resection because it involves nontumoral tissue. A second fundamental principle is to have access to the nerve root at the dural margin via a clear plane of dissection between the tumor and the dura when amputation of a root is necessary. This is often where only a marginal resection can be accomplished, but it is essential for the delivery of the tumor. Another area at risk of oncological contamination is the pedicle.

The localization of the tumor within the "ring" will dictate the feasibility, approach, and method by which the tumor is delivered during en-bloc resection. Boriani et al[10] described three common scenarios for thoracolumbar lesions. First, an en-bloc resection can be performed with an appropriate margin if the tumor is localized in zones 4 to 8 or 5 to 9 of the WBB staging system. In other words, the posterior elements and at least one pedicle have to be free of tumor to be able to achieve oncological resection while safely delivering the spinal cord. This can be achieved via a single posterior or via a staged posteroanterior approach.[15] Second, a sagittal resection can be accomplished when the tumor is confined to zones 3 to 5 or 8 to 10. Again, this can be completed through a single posterior or an anteroposterior approach. Third, when the tumor is confined to the posterior elements only (zones 10 to 3), en-bloc resection can be accomplished using a posterior approach only (**Table 12.3**).

Tumors located in the cervical spine pose a significant challenge because of the many unique anatomic features of this region. The close proximity of the vertebral artery, the peculiar bony architecture, and the functional importance of the cervical roots all make en-bloc resection of a cervical spine tumor demanding. Although the feasibility of en-bloc resection of primary tumors of the cervical spine has been

Table 12.3 Articulation of Weinstein-Boriani-Biagini (WBB) Stages with Surgical Procedures

Radiating Zone	Procedure
4–8 or 5–9	Vertebrectomy (double approach)
2–5 or 7–11	Sagittal resection (double approach)
10–3	Posterior arch resection (posterior approach)

Source: From Chan P, Boriani S, Fourney DR, et al. An assessment of the reliability of the Enneking and Weinstein-Boriani-Biagini classifications for staging of primary spinal tumors by the Spine Oncology Study Group. Spine 2009;34:385. Reproduced with permission.)

demonstrated, because of these anatomic issues significant morbidity and complications are frequent.[16–19] Among others, prolonged intubation, acute respiratory distress syndrome, dehiscence of the posterior pharyngeal wall, prolonged dysphagia, and hardware failure requiring revision have all been reported.[17,19] In the decision-making process these adverse events have to be plotted against the dismal natural history of these tumors and have to be discussed candidly with the patient.

The consequences of unilateral vertebral artery resection are dependent on the variable anatomy of the vertebrobasilar system.[20] An endovascular balloon-occlusion test, cerebral blood-flow studies, and intraoperative temporary occlusion with neuromonitoring are strategies for assessing whether sacrifice can be performed without significant ischemic compromise.

Although the resection of cervical nerve roots frequently carries significant morbidity, in selected cases it can be tolerated. Bailey et al[19] reported no clinically significant consequences following unilateral C2 to C4 nerve root sacrifice despite potential hemidiaphragm paralysis.

Tumors located in the sacrum are associated with a different set of surgical considerations. From a neurologic perspective, sacral roots often need to be sacrificed to achieve a true en-bloc oncological resection, putting bowel, bladder, and sexual function at risk. Todd et al[21] showed that preservation of bowel and bladder continence after major sacral resection occurs in the majority of patients following unilateral sacral root resection or if at least one S3 root is preserved in the case of bilateral sacral resection. Other considerations include the close proximity of major vessels anteriorly and the risk of significant blood loss. The close proximity of the anus and the risk of bowel perforation also increase the risk of surgical-site infection. Derivation colostomies, especially when loss of bowel function is anticipated, have been used to mitigate this occurrence. Wide resection also results in large soft tissue defects. Rotational gluteal or transpelvic vertical rectus abdominis myocutaneous (VRAM) flaps can be used to obliterate this dead space and improve wound healing.[22] Lastly, high sacral resections can interfere with spinopelvic stability, necessitating complex reconstructive techniques (see Chapter 13).

At our institution, preoperative angiography and embolization is routinely attempted. This enhances knowledge of the vascular anatomy and helps with operative planning and the management of intraoperative blood loss. Even though tumoral bleeding should not be a concern if tumor violation is avoided, embolization of involved radicular arteries in the thoracolumbar spine and the vertebral artery in the cervical spine, as well as major tumor feeders, has been effective in reducing blood loss–related complications.

▥ Illustrative Cases

Case 1

History and Examination

A 50-year-old Asian man presented with an 18-month history of progressive right-sided clumsiness, weakness, and numbness, starting initially in his right arm then progressing to involve his right leg. Examination demonstrated bilateral upper extremity altered sensation as well as hyperreflexia and gait disturbance consistent with myelopathy but without objective motor deficit.[19]

Staging

Local staging, with CT and magnetic resonance imaging (MRI), revealed a large C1–3 mass expanding into the surrounding soft tissues and spinal canal, causing marked right-sided spinal cord compression and encasing the right C1, C2, and C3 nerve roots (**Fig. 12.2**). The C2 vertebral body (VB) was primarily involved with extension into the base of the dens. The right vertebral artery (VA) was deviated posterolaterally by the tumor, but remained patent on preoperative angiography. An occlusion test was tolerated without neurologic sequelae. Systemic workup revealed that this was an isolated lesion. A CT-guided core-needle biopsy was performed just lateral to the midline and

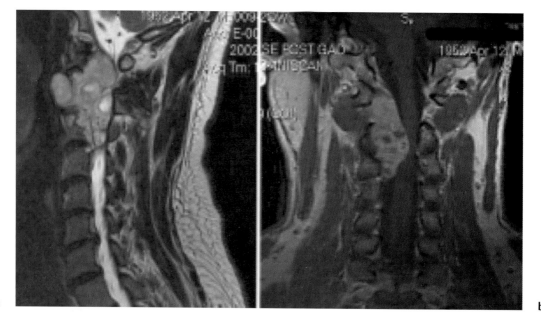

a   b

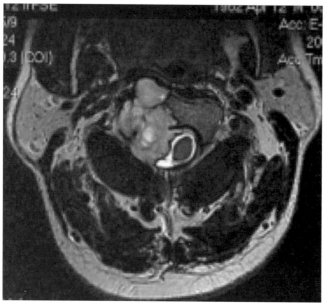

c

Fig. 12.2a–c Case 1: preoperative images. **(a)** Sagittal T2-weighted magnetic resonance imaging (MRI) showing the large tumor centered on C2. **(b)** Coronal postgadolinium image. **(c)** Axial T2-weighted image showing the characteristic features of a chordoma as well as spinal cord displacement by the tumor.

perpendicular to the skin to enable inclusion of the biopsy tract in the subsequent resection. Chordoma was confirmed histologically. The case was subjected to multidisciplinary review.

The first step in surgical planning is to classify the tumor and choose appropriate resection margins. Using the Enneking classification, this is a low-grade malignant tumor with extracompartmental spread (stage 1B), requiring a wide en-bloc resection to achieve cure. Neoadjuvant therapy was not indicated. Surgical staging, using the WBB classification, localized the tumor to areas 1 to 6, A to D. Surgical resection was considered feasible because the two tenets of en-bloc resection were satisfied: first, a window could be created in the spine ring to deliver the tumor from the spinal cord; and second, a plane could be developed from the spinal cord to reach the origin of the roots on the tumor side, allowing them to be divided and taken with the tumor specimen. A detailed preoperative surgical plan was completed. Wide margins were planned, except at the level of the dura, where marginal resection was anticipated.

Surgical Execution (Fig. 12.3)

An ambitious 3-day surgical plan was devised and performed. On the first day, surgical instrumentation from the occiput to C6 was completed. The biopsy tract was incorporated in the resection and the right-sided VA was ligated at the C1-C2 junction proximally and at the C3-C4 level distally. A left-sided C2-C4 laminectomy facilitated visualization of the thecal sac and exiting nerve roots. On the left side, an osteotomy was then performed from above the C2 pedicle to the C3-C4 disk space. The caudal osteotomy through the C3-C4 disk space was then completed from left to right. The right C2-C3-C4 nerve roots were sacrificed at their dural origin.

On the second day, with the patient placed in the right lateral position, the posterior incision was reopened and, with the assistance of a head and neck surgeon, an extended anterolateral approach was undertaken, facilitating visualization of the anterolateral aspects of the VB from the skull base to C4. The left-sided os-

teotomies that were accomplished the day before were then completed anteriorly under direct visualization. The anterior arch of C1 was then resected on the left to facilitate visualization of the odontoid process to complete the osteotomy at that level. Further tumor mobilization was then achieved on the third day to permit the tumor to be rotated and delivered en bloc through the anterior wound. Reconstruction was then completed. Final histological analysis confirmed a chordoma with wide margins throughout the specimen except at the dura, where, as anticipated, marginal resection was noted.

Discussion

This case illustrates the feasibility of a true en-bloc resection of a primary tumor in the cervical spine. Although it is an exhaustive procedure, consuming considerable time and resources, and associated with significant morbidity, this evidence-based approach is well founded to prevent a potentially curable disease from becoming incurable by an intralesional resection.

Case 2

History and Examination

A 30-year-old man presented with an 8-month history of right sacroiliac and leg pain. The right leg symptoms were pluriradicular in nature but predominantly involved the S1 distribution. Physical examination revealed 3/5 weakness in the right L4-L5-S1 myotomes.

Staging

Local staging revealed an extensive lesion, centered on the right sacroiliac joint (**Fig. 12.4**). The tumor extended through the greater sciatic foramen and was immediately adjacent to the anterior aspect of the right sacrum at the S2-S3 level. The patient was systemically cleared of any tumoral activity. Tissue obtained with CT-guided, core-needle biopsy was histopathologically analyzed and a chondrosarcoma was diagnosed. According to the Enneking classification, for curative intent this tumor requires

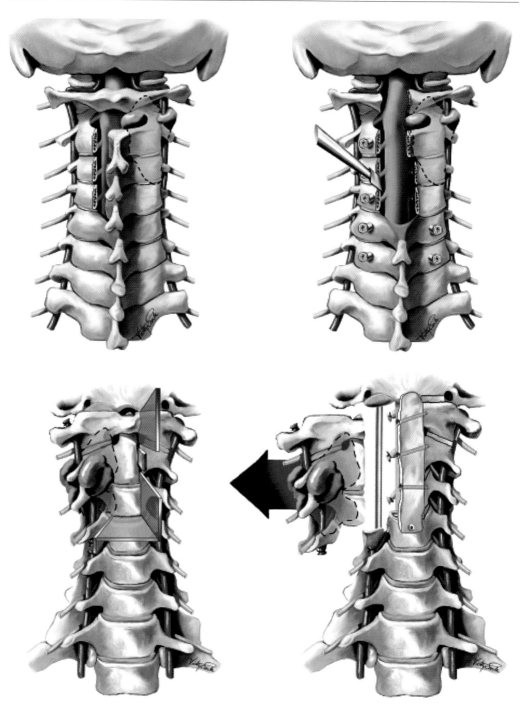

Fig. 12.3 Case 1: artist's illustration of the procedure. (From Bailey CS, Fisher CG, Boyd MC, Dvorak MFS. En bloc marginal excision of a multilevel cervical chordoma. Case report. J Neurosurg Spine 2006;4:409–414. Reproduced with permission.)

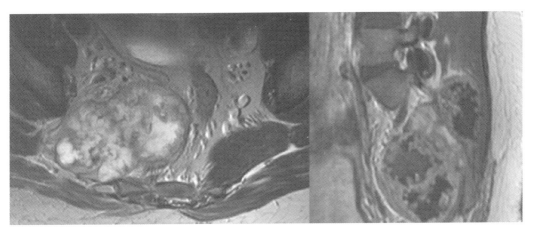

Fig. 12.4a,b Case 2: preoperative images. **(a)** Axial T2-weighted MRI showing the extensive tumor centered on the right sacroiliac joint. **(b)** Sagittal postgadolinium image.

a wide en-bloc resection. However, there are several challenges to achieving this resection, and significant associated morbidity is predicted. The close proximity of the right-sided sacral roots warrant their complete sacrifice along with that of the right sciatic nerve, with the expected associated neurologic deficits discussed above, including the risk of impaired bowel, bladder, and sexual functioning. Given the extent of bony resection necessary to achieve wide margins, reconstruction would also be challenging. However, following application of the oncological principles discussed in this chapter, surgical resection was deemed possible. The diagnosis, proposed surgery, potential complications, and expected deficits were discussed with the patient on multiple preoperative occasions. Because of his age and the chance of a cure, the decision was made to undertake surgical resection.

Surgical Execution

A complex surgical plan was developed by a multidisciplinary surgical team, consisting of a general surgeon, a plastic surgeon, an orthopedic trauma surgeon, and two oncological spine surgeons. The first stage consisted of a posterior approach and posterior release of the tumor. Instrumentation was carried from L3 to the pelvis. The right-sided L5 to S5 nerve root were cut. On the second day, with the pa-

tient placed in the lateral decubitus position, simultaneous anterior and posterior approaches were executed. After a meticulous anterior retroperitoneal release, the osteotomy cuts initiated during the first stage were completed. Once freed the tumor was delivered en bloc posteriorly. Complex reconstruction was then performed utilizing a vascularized fibula graft, and instrumentation bridging L3 to the ischial tuberosity on the right, and L3 to the ileum on the left (**Fig. 12.5**). Surgical margins were all negative.

The patient's postoperative course was complicated by a deep wound infection requiring multiple debridements and closure with a free latissimus dorsi transfer. At 7-year follow-up, he is ambulating, has preserved bowel and bladder function, and no sign of tumor recurrence.

Discussion of Both Cases

These cases illustrate the basic principles leading to definitive surgical management of primary spinal column tumors. When, according to Enneking's evidence-based classification system, an en-bloc resection is indicated and its feasibility is supported by the WBB surgical classification, surgical execution is possible. The expected complications of each specific approach have to be anticipated. Detailed surgical planning is central to the success of these demanding procedures.

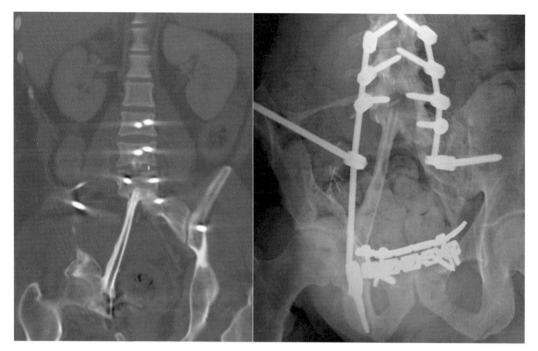

a
b

Fig. 12.5a,b Case 2: postoperative images. **(a)** Computed tomography coronal reconstruction showing solid bony union. **(b)** Anteroposterior X-ray showing the complex reconstruction performed.

Each tumor is unique. Careful consideration has to be given to their individual anatomy and tumor characteristics. When resection is oncologically possible, we now have the surgical expertise, techniques, and reconstruction capability for any approach to achieve this goal in any location of the spine. It is our experience that meticulous preoperative planning using anatomic drawings and the creation of a step-by-step surgical plan helps ensure achievement of evidence-based surgical goals even in extremely challenging scenarios.

Spine surgeons dealing with primary spinal tumors are urged to adopt recognized terminology and classification systems to standardize the treatment and ensure consistent reporting in the published literature, with the ultimate aim of improving patient care.

▪ Chapter Summary

Centers with the necessary surgical experience and subspecialty support are best served to manage primary spine tumors. Careful staging and surgical planning are mandatory for these challenging high-risk procedures. Respecting the resection margins proposed in the Enneking classification has been correlated with lower recurrence rates and increased tumor-free survival. A fundamental concept is to consider the spinal column as a ring through which the neural elements pass. To be able to achieve an en-bloc resection while adhering to Enneking's principles, a tumor-free window has to be created in that "ring" to enable the tumor to be removed while preserving spinal cord integrity. Although these principles determine the feasibility of oncological resection, there are several available surgical dissections, aided by technological advances and subspecialty surgical support, that enable the specific surgical strategy to be individually tailored for each tumor. The morbidity of each approach requires careful consideration. Although inflicting a neurologic deficit is sometimes an acceptable compromise to optimize the chance of a cure, at all times a patient's personal preferences and opinions, guided by an experienced multidisciplinary team, should remain central to this often complex decision-making process.

References

Five Must-Read References

1. Enneking WF. A system of staging musculoskeletal neoplasms. Clin Orthop Relat Res 1986;204:9–24
2. Fisher CG, Keynan O, Boyd MC, Dvorak MF. The surgical management of primary tumors of the spine: initial results of an ongoing prospective cohort study. Spine 2005;30:1899–1908
3. Yamazaki T, McLoughlin GS, Patel S, Rhines LD, Fourney DR. Feasibility and safety of en bloc resection for primary spine tumors: a systematic review by the Spine Oncology Study Group. Spine 2009;34(22, Suppl):S31–S38
4. Boriani S, Biagini R, De Iure F, et al. En bloc resections of bone tumors of the thoracolumbar spine. A preliminary report on 29 patients. Spine 1996;21:1927–1931
5. Fisher CG, Saravanja DD, Dvorak MF, et al. Surgical management of primary bone tumors of the spine: validation of an approach to enhance cure and reduce local recurrence. Spine 2011;36:830–836 10.1097/BRS.0b013e3181e502e5
6. Bergh P, Kindblom LG, Gunterberg B, Remotti F, Ryd W, Meis-Kindblom JM. Prognostic factors in chordoma of the sacrum and mobile spine: a study of 39 patients. Cancer 2000;88:2122–2134
7. Boriani S, Chevalley F, Weinstein JN, et al. Chordoma of the spine above the sacrum. Treatment and outcome in 21 cases. Spine 1996;21:1569–1577
8. Boriani S, Saravanja D, Yamada Y, Varga PP, Biagini R, Fisher CG. Challenges of local recurrence and cure in low grade malignant tumors of the spine. Spine 2009;34(22, Suppl):S48–S57
9. Jawad MU, Scully SP. In brief: classifications in brief: Enneking classification: benign and malignant tumors of the musculoskeletal system. Clin Orthop Relat Res 2010;468:2000–2002
10. Boriani S, Weinstein JN, Biagini R. Primary bone tumors of the spine. Terminology and surgical staging. Spine 1997;22:1036–1044
11. Chan P, Boriani S, Fourney DR, et al. An assessment of the reliability of the Enneking and Weinstein-Boriani-Biagini classifications for staging of primary spinal tumors by the Spine Oncology Study Group. Spine 2009;34:384–391
12. Lièvre JA, Darcy M, Pradat P, et al. [Giant cell tumor of the lumbar spine; total spondylectomy in 2 states]. Rev Rhum Mal Osteoartic 1968;35:125–130
13. Stener B, Johnsen OE. Complete removal of three vertebrae for giant-cell tumour. J Bone Joint Surg Br 1971;53:278–287
14. Stener B. Complete removal of vertebrae for extirpation of tumors. A 20-year experience. Clin Orthop Relat Res 1989;245:72–82
15. Tomita K, Kawahara N, Baba H, Tsuchiya H, Nagata S, Toribatake Y. Total en bloc spondylectomy for solitary spinal metastases. Int Orthop 1994;18:291–298
16. Cohen ZR, Fourney DR, Marco RA, Rhines LD, Gokaslan ZL. Total cervical spondylectomy for primary osteogenic sarcoma. Case report and description of operative technique. J Neurosurg 2002;97(3, Suppl):386–392
17. Rhines LD, Fourney DR, Siadati A, Suk I, Gokaslan ZL. En bloc resection of multilevel cervical chordoma with C-2 involvement. Case report and description of operative technique. J Neurosurg Spine 2005;2:199–205
18. Fujita T, Kawahara N, Matsumoto T, Tomita K. Chordoma in the cervical spine managed with en bloc excision. Spine 1999;24:1848–1851
19. Bailey CS, Fisher CG, Boyd MC, Dvorak MFS. En bloc marginal excision of a multilevel cervical chor-

doma. Case report. J Neurosurg Spine 2006;4:409–414

20. Hoshino Y, Kurokawa T, Nakamura K, et al. A report on the safety of unilateral vertebral artery ligation during cervical spine surgery. Spine 1996;21:1454–1457

21. Todd LT Jr, Yaszemski MJ, Currier BL, Fuchs B, Kim CW, Sim FH. Bowel and bladder function after major sacral resection. Clin Orthop Relat Res 2002;397:36–39

22. Sciubba DM, Chi JH, Rhines LD, Gokaslan ZL. Chordoma of the spinal column. Neurosurg Clin N Am 2008;19:5–15

13

Spinopelvic Reconstruction/Fixation and Fusion

Peter Paul Varga

▩ Introduction

The tumorous pathologies of the lumbosacral junction requiring surgical intervention are very challenging even for the most experienced spine surgeons. Tumors of this region often grow insidiously without specific symptoms, reaching a large size that makes their complete removal a complex feat. Due to the localization, special issues should be considered when investigating all aspects of the local anatomic and biomechanical properties irrespective of the particular oncological approach. Achievement of the optimal oncosurgical resection margins often entails potential functional losses, resulting in psychological issues that should be considered during the planning process. The patient should be prepared accordingly by the surgeon and psychologists for this technically demanding surgery.

In metastatic lesions (which are more common in the sacrum and in the entire spine than are the primary tumors), surgery is always palliative. The main goal of the palliative procedure is functional improvement, although the literature suggests that debulking of the metastatic mass can be oncologically beneficial and can provide longer survival.[1]

Primary malignant spinal tumors are rare conditions, and the sacrum is the most common location.[2,3] The main aim of surgical treatment in these cases is to be curative. En-bloc resection of a primary malignant sacral tumor with wide oncological margins could significantly influence the biomechanics of the spinopelvic complex, which in turn can result in severe deterioration of the ambulatory status, worsening the postoperative morbidity and mortality. The procedures targeting the spinopelvic soft tissue and bony reconstruction after the resection significantly lengthen the surgery and increase the risk for intra- and postoperative complications. Due to multidisciplinary cooperation, and particularly to the development of the intensive care and to anesthesiology advancements, as well as the spinal implant technology, it is possible to perform these extensive surgeries even routinely in comprehensive oncosurgical centers, where the general medical and technical environment fosters a high level of spinal surgical experience.

This chapter discusses the special considerations of spinopelvic stabilization after sacral tumor resection.

▩ Biomechanical Considerations

The body weight from the axial skeleton is transferred to the lower limbs via the sacroiliac (SI) joints. Resection of the sacrum, involving partially or totally the uni- or bilateral SI joints, can affect the biomechanical integrity of the pelvic ring, resulting in disturbances in the physiological movement of the patient particularly in standing and walking.

There is no consensus among sacral tumor experts regarding the need for stabilization and bony reconstruction after resection of a sacral tumor. Some authors reported that spinopelvic stabilization was not necessary after total sacrectomy.[4,5] In their opinion, based on their clinical observations, the remaining muscles and the developing scar tissue at the site of the spinopelvic defect of the body wall can somewhat stabilize the spine as a sling during the postoperative course. Detailed analysis of functional outcomes after long-term follow-up is still unclear. In contrast, biomechanical studies and case series of patients undergoing total sacrectomy show the benefits of bony reconstruction supported by spinopelvic stabilization.[6-16] In cases of total sacrectomy and in certain cases of high sacrectomy, where the cranial resection plain is above the S I/II junction uni- or bilaterally, spinopelvic stability significantly deteriorates.[17-19] In cases of high sacrectomy, if the resection is done above the S1 foramina, the remaining sacral bone is potentially not strong enough to transfer the loading from the spine to the pelvic ring, yielding a higher risk of subsequent fatigue fractures of the sacral remains.[18]

The immediate advantage of stabilization is that it enables starting rehabilitation immediately after the surgery, starting with in-bed exercises and, a few days later, progressing to walking. The early mobilization of these patients helps prevent the postoperative complications related to long-term inactivity, such as thromboembolism, pneumonia, and pressure sores. The psychological effect of the early mobilization is also considerable. Based on these results, and also supported by our own clinical experience, spinopelvic stabilization is strongly advised after destabilizing sacrectomy surgeries.

There are no gold-standard techniques for spinopelvic stabilization. In vitro studies showed the efficacy of different stabilizing (i.e., motion reducing) techniques, but there is no evidence supporting the absolute advantage of the most rigid fixation construct. It is expected that the optimal spinopelvic fixation method should be shock absorbing and a fusion promoting. There is no doubt that the developing bony fusion between the lumbar spine and the pelvic bones will provide definitive, long-term biomechanical stability. Rigid constructs with structured bone grafts seem to be effective, but there are no available studies (or radiological images published) in the literature with long-term follow-up. The total rigidity of the implant construct can absolutely ease the graft–host surface from loading, whereas a nonrigid construction can enable cyclic loading during walking, promoting the incorporation of the bone graft. At this time the optimal rigidity of the different stabilizing constructs and their effect on graft incorporation are open questions.

Sagittal balance has been reported recently to be a global biomechanical factor influencing the degenerative spinal disorders as well as the progression of deformities. In the natural course of sagittal balance and in the development of imbalance, spinopelvic parameters such as pelvic tilt, sacral slope, and pelvic incidence seem to have some predictive value. Total sacrectomy and spinopelvic reconstruction influence the spinopelvic parameters per se,[20] and there can be long-term consequences of the alteration of sagittal alignment, especially if an imbalanced situation is fixed by the spinopelvic instrumentation. Proper sagittal balance is also assumed to play a role in ambulatory ability and in the development of implant failures or nonunion.

■ Spinopelvic Stabilization After Total Sacrectomy

Spinopelvic fixation (SPF) procedures join the lumbar spine to the pelvis (**Fig. 13.1**). The Galveston L-rod technique with pedicle screws and iliac rods system was among the first published techniques in 1984.[21] The original Galveston technique (GT) performed the SPF with the implantation of the L-rods into the iliac crests, but these directly implanted rods commonly loosened. A modified Galveston technique (mGT)

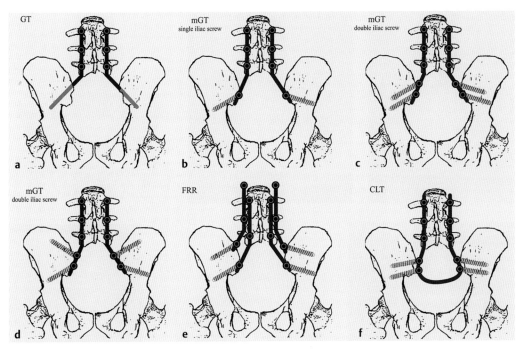

Fig. 13.1a–f Spinopelvic fixation (SPF) methods. **(a)** Galveston technique (GT). **(b–d)** Modified Galveston technique (mGT). **(e)** Four-rod reconstruction (FRR). **(f)** Closed loop technique (CLT).

was introduced in 2000 in which the rods were also fixed to iliac screws in the caudal end of the construct. This procedure has been widely used, and further biomechanical studies showed the positive effect of the use of dual iliac screws, independent of their orientation.[22,23]

The four-rod (FRR) or double-rod double iliac screw system is a further modification of the mGT.[24] In this case, the additional lumbar rods increase the rigidity of the construct but can carry a higher risk of wound healing problems due to the excessive metal implants.[25] The closed loop technique (CLT) for SPF was published in 2009.[15] With this technique, one single U-shaped rod is used to connect all pedicle and iliac screws (bilaterally in the lower double position), providing a better load distribution along the construct (**Fig. 13.2**). This method applies the philosophy of nonrigid fixation to avoid the stress-shielding phenomenon and to promote the bony fusion between the lumbar vertebral body and the pelvis. By this method, safe and strong bony connections develop within the first 24 months after the surgery (**Fig. 13.2g-i**).

Posterior pelvic ring fixation (PPRF) is an additional dimension of spinopelvic stabilization (**Fig. 13.3**). This method uses part of the whole construct to connect the two iliac bones with each other. One published technique is the triangular frame reconstruction (TFR), in which one horizontal rod is used to attach the L5 vertebral body to the two iliac wings and the lower part of the ilia are also connected with another horizontal rod. This technique enables good load distribution across implants, but excessive stress in the iliac bones could entail an increased risk of implant loosening and failure.[13] Another technique was published by authors from Johns Hopkins Hospital (JHH) in 2005.[26] In this technique, an mGT with a transiliac bar inserted through the iliac crests is completed with a horizontal pelvic fixation screw-rod implant and a horizontal femoral allograft placed between the two iliac crests. The different parts of the construct are attached with various connectors.

Anterior spinal column fixation (ASCF) is the third possible dimension of spinopelvic stabilization (**Fig. 13.4**), which consists of adding an

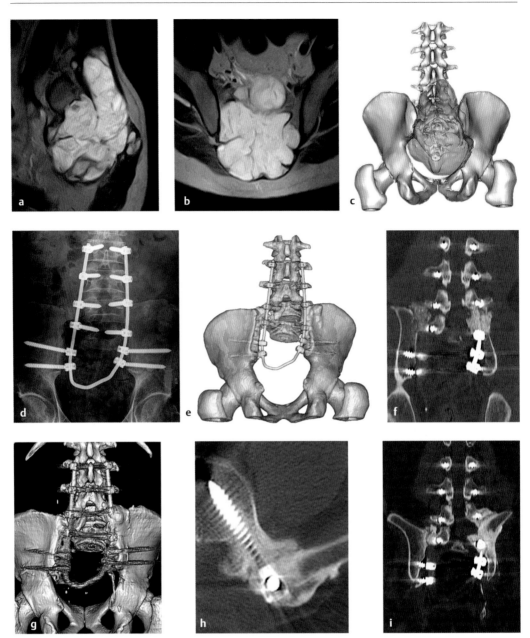

Fig. 13.2a–i A giant sacral chordoma in a 42-year-old man. Sagittal **(a)** and axial **(b)** magnetic resonance imaging (MRI). **(c)** Three-dimensional computed tomography (CT) reconstruction. **(d,e)** After an extended total sacrectomy, the spinopelvic fixation was performed with the closed loop technique. **(f)** Morselized bone graft was placed between the decorticated lumbar laminas and iliac bones. **(g–i)** Two years after the surgery, complete spinopelvic bony fusion can be observed.

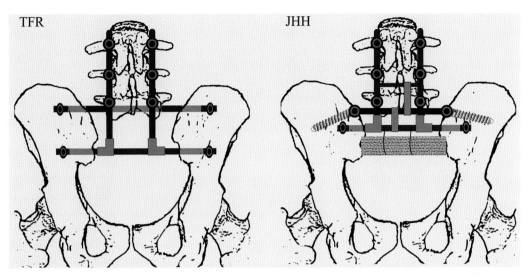

Fig. 13.3 Posterior pelvic ring fixation (PPRF) methods. **(a)** Triangular frame reconstruction (TFR). **(b)** Johns Hopkins Hospital (JHH) method.

anterior support to the lumbar spine. Kawahara et al[9] used a two vertically inserted pedicle screws attached to a sacral rod connecting the two ilia to directly connect the L5 vertebral body to the spinopelvic fixation construct. Their novel technique is a combination of SPF, ASCF, and PPRF techniques using a minimal amount of implants. Dickey et al[7] reported the bilateral fibular graft (BFFR) technique, where two fibular grafts placed between the L5 vertebral body and the bilateral iliopectineal area provide a good anterior support strengthening the ASCF aspect of the construct. It can be combined with any SPF and SPF+PPRF techniques.

There is a wide variety of spinopelvic stabilization methods reported in the literature, but the number of cases and the details of the reported long-term radiological and clinical results are limited or insufficient.

The goals of an optimal spinopelvic stabilization technique after total sacrectomies are not only to restore the spinopelvic stability and to promote the bony fusion, but also to support the different surgical techniques for the soft tissue reconstruction. With the proper stabilization technique, decreasing the size of the large cavity after the removal of the tumorous sacrum can be achieved by pulling caudally the

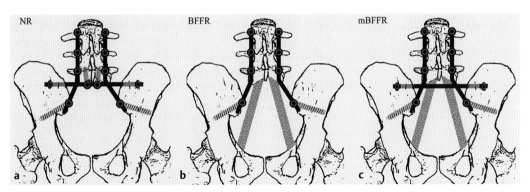

Fig. 13.4a–c Anterior spinal column fixation (ASCF) combined with SPF and PPRF. **(a)** Novel reconstruction (NR). **(b)** Bilateral fibular graft technique (BFFR). **(c)** Modified bilateral fibular graft technique (mBFFR).

remaining part of the lumbar spine and approximating the resection surfaces of the iliac crests. The implant constructions could also provide the possibility of anchoring the soft tissue flaps. The volume of the implant is also a significant factor; the larger the amount of implant, the higher the risk of wound healing problems.[25]

Spinopelvic Fusion

Only a massive and strong bone bridge between the lumbar spine and the pelvis can provide long-term biomechanical stability after total sacrectomy. If true bony fusion is not achieved, the implant will certainly fail, even if it does not cause any symptoms. But the gap between the host surfaces can be very large. Fusion can be expected only 1 to 2 years after the surgery, and delayed fusion or development of pseudarthrosis are common complications. Only a few publications have reported an analysis of the fusion process.

In some constructs the structural graft has an important mechanical role too (see Chapter 14). The BFFR method achieves the ASCF with the implantation of two fibular grafts between the base of the caudal vertebral body and the pelvic bone.[7] The grafts are placed along the force transmission line between the lumbar spine and the hip joints, creating a triangular construct. The proximal and distal docking sites of the graft are under cyclic compression, which can facilitate bone healing. The JHH method represents another solution.[26] In this case, a horizontal structural femur allograft is used to connect the two iliac wings. The allograft is inserted into the host site to bridge the large defect after total sacrectomy and to achieve a bony PPRF.

Nonstructural bone graft is used to bridge the gap between the caudal vertebral body and the iliac wings posteriorly. To create a well-bleeding cancellous host surface, we decorticate the facing bony surfaces with a high-speed drill. The graft is placed into the posterior load transmission lines, which facilitate bony fusion (**Fig. 13.2f**); however, reduction of the gap with the approximation of the bony surfaces is also advised. The amount of disease-free local autograft is limited in such procedures, and cancellous and morselized allograft bone chips as well as synthetic bone grafts are to be used in order to have sufficient graft material. By placing a layer of Gelfoam, we provide a soft but safe anterior and posterior wall around the morselized bony graft mass.

In our clinical experience, the fusion process with routinely used autologous morselized graft from the rest of the posterior iliac crests takes about 12 to 24 months. We did not observe any difference in the timing of fusion comparing the autologous grafts and the synthetic osteoinductive products. By the progression of the fusion process, the new bony mass develops in the line of the load transfer. That part of the bony graft mass, which is out of this line, slowly disappears, and after the second year it is not even detectable on computed tomography (CT) (**Fig. 13.2**).

According to the general biomechanical principles of osteosynthesis, the absolute reduction of motion with spinopelvic fixation is presumably an adverse situation for the development of the bony fusion.[27] A thin, but so far unknown, equilibrium between the rigidity and the micromovement in the construct facilitating the biological process of the bony remodeling would be the optimal solution for spinopelvic fixation, but there are few clinical or experimental reports.

Problems to Avoid

Spinopelvic fixation is a demanding and challenging surgical technique. Numerous studies emphasize the importance of a proper surgical technique in total sacrectomy, but the spinopelvic reconstruction alone also requires high surgical skill and detailed preoperative planning. Otherwise, the oncologically appropriate resection of the sacral tumor cannot provide an optimal surgical and functional outcome because of the deteriorated biomechanics and the subsequent implant failures.

Spinopelvic reconstruction must be planned in detail preoperatively, with consideration given to the margins of the bony resection and to the specific patient's characteristics. Appropriate and thorough planning will result in fewer intra- and postoperative complications. Improvisation should be avoided during the surgery. Because of the complex anatomical, biomechanical, and technical consideration, these surgeries can be safely performed only after a long learning curve. Both the surgeon and the whole team (anesthesiologist, residents, nurses) should be experienced in this procedure. There are few studies available on this procedure, and they lack long-term follow-up of large cohorts, but the biomechanical specifications that these studies discuss must not be underestimated. The fixation construct has to bear very large loading forces; moreover, the construction should absorb some of this load. Otherwise, local shearing stress that is generated around the implants can cause destruction of the vertebral/pelvic bone, particularly in patients with osteoporosis.

Achieving an optimal stress distribution entails some important considerations, such as the length of the implant at the lumbar spine. The number of the lumbar segments involved is highly dependent on the patient's specific measurements and bone quality. For example, we must take into account the long lever arms of a tall person, and we have to extend the stabilization in patients with large body weight. In our experience, the instrumentation of the three lowest segments provides the appropriate stability in most cases, but the patient's specific requirements may entail lengthening the posterior stabilization up to the thoracic spine. For cranial load sharing, the FFR technique can be a good solution. In patients with osteoporosis, the standard methods of augmentation of the transpedicular screws can be performed.

The number of iliac screws required can be underestimated, and their positioning is similarly important. Murakami et al[13] published in vitro data regarding the stress distribution in an mGT construct, demonstrating that the iliac screw is one of the most vulnerable points of the spinopelvic stabilizing construct because maximum stress can be observed around it.[13] The dissipation of the stress is highly recom-

mended by using more iliac screws positioned for better stress distribution. Yu et al[23] compared the biomechanical properties of four different iliac screw-techniques in vitro. They found that bilateral double iliac screws in the lower position optimally manages the local stresses and provides better compressive and torsional stiffness compared with single iliac or double cranially positioned screws.

The postoperative sagittal spinopelvic alignment achieved by the fixation is also an important consideration. Most patients lose some motor activity of the pelvic and lower extremity muscles that are innervated by the nerves resected during the en-bloc sacrectomy. If the plane of the nerve resection is more cranial, the postoperative bony sagittal balance is of greater importance. Due to the important role of the gluteal muscles in hip joint stabilization in the erect position, the loss of bilateral L5 roots presents a great challenge for the patient's rehabilitation. If the bony stabilization fixes the new spinopelvic junction in an unbalanced condition, the patient cannot walk or stand without external support. Patients with good postoperative spinopelvic balance can learn to walk without crutches within 6 months. In our clinical experience only elderly patients need aid in walking or standing; younger patients are stabilized in good (or tolerable) balance and do not need any support (**Fig. 13.5**).

Due to the increasing stresses at the bone–metal interfaces, an unbalanced postoperative spinopelvic alignment increases the risk of early implant failure (i.e., rod or screw breakage). It is often difficult to predict preoperatively the appropriate positioning of the lumbar spine to the pelvis, and it is often difficult during surgery, too. In the future, this aspect of the surgery will be more easily managed using advanced three-dimensional reconstruction computational tools combined with new intraoperative navigational techniques. With the continuing development of technology, spinopelvic reconstruction will be designed and tested in virtual simulation using modern finite element models. These advances will demonstrate the optimal surgical procedure to apply to the specific patient, and will simulate the patient's long-term mechanobiological function-

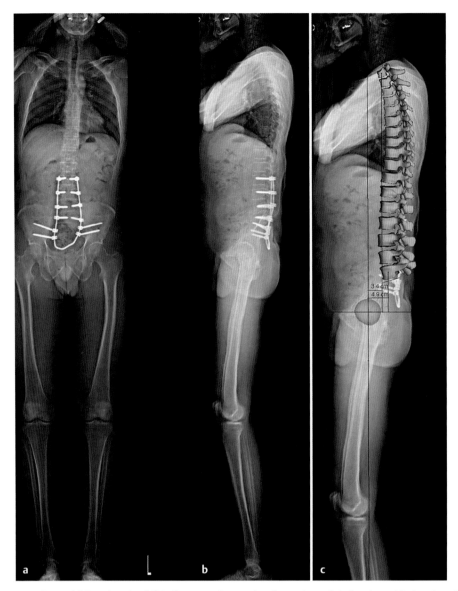

Fig. 13.5a–c Frontal **(a)** and sagittal **(b)** alignment 2 months after spinopelvic fixation with the closed loop technique. **(c)** EOS reconstruction study of the case represented in Fig. 13.2.

ing, highlighting the potential bony fusion or the risk of implant loosening.

One of the key factors in the success of spinopelvic bony reconstruction is the fusion process. Delayed fusion or pseudarthrosis entails the risk of failure. Fatigue fractures can occur in any stage. Because the oncological outcome of these patients is more favorable, they require a stable spinopelvic junction. In our clinical experience the use of morselized autologous bone graft with nonrigid stabilization (closed loop technique) provides an appropriate solution. The bony bridge between the last lumbar vertebral body and the posterior iliac crests develops at the proper site of the load transfer. Between the lumbar segments (to decrease the surgical morbidity), we perform a posterior (interlaminar) or posterolateral (intertransverse) technique instead of the interbody procedures.

Chapter Summary

Fixation and bony reconstruction following sacral tumor resections plays an important role in the early and safe mobilization of the patient after surgery, decreasing the risk of perioperative complications such as thrombo-embolism, pneumonia, and pressure sores.

Strong and safe bony fusion developing between the lumbar spine and the pelvis provides a good base for standing and walking, enabling better functional results and quality of life for this very special group of patients.

Spinopelvic stabilization is a demanding and difficult procedure to perform, requiring surgical experience, proper surgical planning, and appropriate preparation of the patient. Extensive knowledge of spinopelvic biomechanics, surgical anatomy, spinal stabilization, and bone grafting techniques is essential.

There is no gold standard in this field, although there is an increasing number of biomechanical studies and clinical papers published in the literature. The lack of long-term data on fusion rates and functional results encourages researchers to collect and analyze clinical and experimental data from multicenter sources.

With the development of the computerized three-dimensional tools, a better understanding can be achieved of the biomechanical issues of this surgical technique and of the specific patient requirements during the planning process of these challenging surgeries.

Pearls

◆ Spinopelvic bony fusion can provide a good long-term functional outcome after total sacrectomy.
◆ The role of biomechanics and proper sagittal balance cannot be underestimated.

Pitfalls

◆ There is no gold-standard spinopelvic stabilization technique.
◆ This surgery should not be performed without sufficient preoperative planning.

References
Five Must-Read References

1. Ibrahim A, Crockard A, Antonietti P, et al. Does spinal surgery improve the quality of life for those with extradural (spinal) osseous metastases? An international multicenter prospective observational study of 223 patients. Invited submission from the Joint Section Meeting on Disorders of the Spine and Peripheral Nerves, March 2007. J Neurosurg Spine 2008;8:271–278

2. Kelley SP, Ashford RU, Rao AS, Dickson RA. Primary bone tumours of the spine: a 42-year survey from the Leeds Regional Bone Tumour Registry. Eur Spine J 2007;16:405–409

3. Mukherjee D, Chaichana KL, Gokaslan ZL, Aaronson O, Cheng JS, McGirt MJ. Survival of patients with malignant primary osseous spinal neoplasms: results from the Surveillance, Epidemiology, and End Results (SEER) database from 1973 to 2003. J Neurosurg Spine 2011;14:143–150

4. Guo Y, Yadav R. Improving function after total sacrectomy by using a lumbar-sacral corset. Am J Phys Med Rehabil 2002;81:72–76

5. Ruggieri P, Angelini A, Ussia G, Montalti M, Mercuri M. Surgical margins and local control in resection of sacral chordomas. Clin Orthop Relat Res 2010; 468:2939–2947

6. Clarke MJ, Dasenbrock H, Bydon A, et al. Posterior-only approach for en bloc sacrectomy: clinical outcomes in 36 consecutive patients. Neurosurgery 2012;71:357–364, discussion 364

7. Dickey ID, Hugate RR, Fuchs B, Yaszemski MJ, Sim FH. Reconstruction after total sacrectomy. Clin Orthop Relat Res 2005;438:42–50

8. Fourney DR, Rhines LD, Hentschel SJ, et al. En bloc resection of primary sacral tumors: classification of surgical approaches and outcome. J Neurosurg Spine 2005;3:111–122

9. Kawahara N, Murakami H, Yoshida A, Sakamoto J, Oda J, Tomita K. Reconstruction after total sacrectomy using a new instrumentation technique: a biomechanical comparison. Spine 2003;28:1567–1572

10. Kelly BP, Shen FH, Schwab JS, Arlet V, Diangelo DJ. Biomechanical testing of a novel four-rod technique for lumbo-pelvic reconstruction. Spine 2008;33:E400–E406

11. Li G, Fu D, Chen K, et al. Surgical strategy for the management of sacral giant cell tumors: a 32-case series. Spine J 2012;12:484–491

12. Mindea SA, Chinthakunta S, Moldavsky M, Gudipally M, Khalil S. Biomechanical comparison of spi-

nopelvic reconstruction techniques in the setting of total sacrectomy. Spine 2012;37:E1622–E1627

13. Murakami H, Kawahara N, Tomita K, Sakamoto J, Oda J. Biomechanical evaluation of reconstructed lumbosacral spine after total sacrectomy. J Orthop Sci 2002;7:658–664

14. Quraishi NA, Wolinsky JP, Bydon A, Witham T, Gokaslan ZL. Giant destructive myxopapillary ependymomas of the sacrum. J Neurosurg Spine 2010;12:154–159

15. Varga PP, Bors I, Lazary A. Sacral tumors and management. Orthop Clin North Am 2009;40:105–123, vii

16. Zhu R, Cheng LM, Yu Y, Zander T, Chen B, Rohlmann A. Comparison of four reconstruction methods after total sacrectomy: a finite element study. Clin Biomech (Bristol, Avon) 2012;27:771–776

17. Gunterberg B, Romanus B, Stener B. Pelvic strength after major amputation of the sacrum. An experimental study. Acta Orthop Scand 1976;47:635–642

18. Hugate RR Jr, Dickey ID, Phimolsarnti R, Yaszemski MJ, Sim FH. Mechanical effects of partial sacrectomy: when is reconstruction necessary? Clin Orthop Relat Res 2006;450:82–88

19. Yu B, Zheng Z, Zhuang X, et al. Biomechanical effects of transverse partial sacrectomy on the sacroiliac joints: an in vitro human cadaveric investigation of the borderline of sacroiliac joint instability. Spine 2009;34:1370–1375

20. Gottfried ON, Omeis I, Mehta VA, Solakoglu C, Gokaslan ZL, Wolinsky JP. Sacral tumor resection and the impact on pelvic incidence. J Neurosurg Spine 2011;14:78–84

21. Allen BL Jr, Ferguson RL. The Galveston technique of pelvic fixation with L-rod instrumentation of the spine. Spine 1984;9:388–394

22. Yu BS, Zhuang XM, Li ZM, et al. Biomechanical effects of the extent of sacrectomy on the stability of lumbo-iliac reconstruction using iliac screw techniques: What level of sacrectomy requires the bilateral dual iliac screw technique? Clin Biomech (Bristol, Avon) 2010;25:867–872

23. Yu BS, Zhuang XM, Zheng ZM, Li ZM, Wang TP, Lu WW. Biomechanical advantages of dual over single iliac screws in lumbo-iliac fixation construct. Eur Spine J 2010;19:1121–1128

24. Shen FH, Harper M, Foster WC, Marks I, Arlet V. A novel "four-rod technique" for lumbo-pelvic reconstruction: theory and technical considerations. Spine 2006;31:1395–1401

25. Chang DW, Friel MT, Youssef AA. Reconstructive strategies in soft tissue reconstruction after resection of spinal neoplasms. Spine 2007;32:1101–1106

26. Gallia GL, Haque R, Garonzik I, et al. Spinal pelvic reconstruction after total sacrectomy for en bloc resection of a giant sacral chordoma. Technical note. J Neurosurg Spine 2005;3:501–506

27. Rüedi TP, Buckley RE, Moran CG. AO Principles of Fracture Management. New York: Thieme, 2007

14

Structural Graft Selection

Y. Raja Rampersaud

Introduction

Resection of primary spinal or paraspinal tumors with direct spine invasion typically requires complex and at times innovative reconstruction techniques. Furthermore, for primary tumors for which curative intent is typically the main objective, long-term durability is paramount to reconstruction goals. Reconstruction of single or multiple vertebral body en-bloc resections involving more than one third to one half of the vertebra(e) and unilateral or bilateral posterior column resection typically involve extensive instrumentation and structural grafts or grafts to fill the osseous spinal defect(s). Specific to structural graft selection, the goal is to provide durable structural support across the defect(s) and achieve biological integration with the host bone (i.e., fusion). This chapter discusses factors that should be considered for structural graft selection and the options available for reconstructing spinal defects following primary tumor resection.

Due to the rarity of primary spinal tumors, most relatively large case series describing reconstruction and graft selection techniques are surgeon/center specific, using a variety of graft selection and surgical techniques that are often unique to each patient and anatomic defect requiring reconstruction.[1-3] The majority of reports understandably focus on the oncological outcome and technical aspects of each case;

however, very few provide any long-term outcome information specific to the graft selection or reconstruction durability.[1,2] In addition, due to clinical and technological advancements, the reconstruction techniques and graft choices have evolved within different centers that perform a higher volume of these cases.[1-3] Consequently, there is gross variability in graft selection and reconstruction techniques from surgeon to surgeon and from center to center. Also, there are numerous case reports describing innovative and very complex reconstruction for very large tumors that push the limits of resection and reconstruction expertise. Although crucial to the understanding of rare conditions or procedures, these case reports do not provide us with generalizable information regarding structural graft selection and are often limited by relatively short-term follow-up.

Survey of Practitioners

To provide a contemporary and broad representation of decision making in these complex reconstructions, I and my colleagues C.P. DiPaola and C.G. Fisher recently conducted an international Web-based survey to elicit expert opinion regarding decision making about the type of bone grafting choice for reconstruction following resection of primary spinal tumors. Thirty-one (61%) of the 51 members of AO Spine North America–Spine Net Oncology and AO International Oncology Knowledge Forum responded. The respondents were equally divided between orthopedic surgeons and neurosurgeons. The majority of respondents (71%) have been in clinical practice for over 10 years. The average number of primary spine tumor cases performed per year by the respondents in this group was 16, with a range of 2 to 100. Comparatively, the average number of metastatic cases per year for this group was 35, with a range of 7 to 150.

The response for each survey question varied from 28 to 31 / 31 respondents. For primary tumors, the majority (93%) of respondents attempt to generate a fusion, with 63% of them noting that they use bone graft or bone graft substitutes every time and 30% using them almost every time. The preferred choice of bone graft material was equally split between morselized iliac crest (39%) and allograft (39%). The use of local bone alone was the preferred choice of only 16% of respondents. Ceramics (e.g., cal-

cium phosphates) were not preferred by any respondent, and off-label use of bone morphogenetic protein (BMP) was preferred by only two (6.5%) respondents. The majority of respondents typically used combinations of morselized iliac crest, allograft, and local bone.

When anterior structural support was required, structural allograft was preferred by 47% of respondents, followed closely by a prefabricated prosthetic replacement device (i.e., a "cage") preferred by 40%. The use of vascularized fibula or rib was preferred by only three (10%) respondents, and polymethylmethacrylate (PMMA) was preferred by no one (**Table 14.1**). In the event of a 360-degree spondylectomy, the respondents overwhelmingly reported routine anterior column and bilateral posterior column reconstruction, with 42% doing so every time and 42% doing so almost every time. Anterior column reconstruction only and primary spinal shortening (i.e., host bone-on-bone, for a single-level resection) were occasionally/sometimes performed by 30% and 19% of respondents, respectively.

Table 14.1 Structural Graft Selection: Summary of International Survey

Graft Choice*	Preferred by Respondents (%)	Author/Editor Consensus
Structural iliac crest	3.3%	Will consider for 1- to 2-level cervical reconstruction, or 1-level thoracic, particularly with associated radiation. Donor morbidity must be discussed with the patient.
Structural allograft	46.7%	Preferred if available. Provides excellent integration, enables accurate tumor surveillance and lower cost than prefabricated prosthesis, but has limited availability and is susceptible to fracture if unprotected by instrumentation.
Prefabricated prosthetic replacement (i.e., cage)	40%	Preferred. Greater flexibility regarding sizes, shape (can also get custom or modular implants), and availability compared with allograft. Metal cages create imaging artifact, which may delay detection of local recurrence.
Bone cement	0%	Will consider in patients with short life-expectancy (palliative/intralesional procedure) and/or very low likelihood of fusion (e.g., high-dose postoperative radiation will be required).
Vascularized fibula or rib	10%	Will utilize when there is a high risk of nonunion, in a revision case, or to supplement or provide soft tissue reconstruction (i.e., myo-osseous or osteocutaneous flap).

*Survey question: "Considering only primary spine tumor cases, when anterior reconstruction with structural support is necessary, what is your preference for structural support?"

General Factors to Consider in Graft Selection

As noted above, there is often significant case-to-case variability even from the same surgeon or center. This is due to a variety of key factors that need to be considered when deciding on an optimal graft selection. These factors can be broadly categorized into patient, local, tumor, and health system factors. Patient factors include, but are not limited to, age, medical comorbidity, and life expectancy. Local factors can include the anatomic location of the lesion (discussed below), the circumferential and longitudinal degree of the defect, the bone quality, the adequacy of soft tissue coverage, and pre- and postoperative radiation. In addition, when considering autologous grafts such as an iliac crest or a vascularized osseous or composite graft, the morbidity and functional consequences from the donor site also need to be considered and weighed against alternatives to the local reconstruction needs. Tumor factors include histology, perioperative chemotherapy, ability to achieve negative margins, and the need for lifetime local surveillance. Health system factors include, but are not limited to, available multiteam expertise (e.g., for microvascular flaps or resection and reconstruction of associated vascular or visceral involvement), graft availability, and cost.

In our survey we also asked the experts to rank, in order of importance, the factors that influence their decision regarding graft selection. The top five factors ranked as extremely important in graft selection were patient's life expectancy, achieving a clear margin, tumor histology, bone quality, and adequacy of soft tissue coverage (**Table 14.2**). The top three factors ranked as moderately important were graft availability, grafts that enable local tumor surveillance, and pre- or postoperative radiation therapy. A detailed discussion of each factor is beyond the scope of this chapter, but the following discussion provides a brief perspective on the key issues for each of the top factors.

A short life expectancy, not achieving a clear margin, and tumor histology typically relate to a higher likelihood of persistent or recurrent tumor and the probable need for ongoing adjunctive treatment (e.g., postoperative radiation)

Table 14.2 Factors that Influence Bone Graft Selection: Summary of International Survey

Decision Making Factors*	Percent of Respondents
Extremely important:	
Life expectancy	63.3%
Likelihood of achieving a clear margin	51.5%
Tumor histology	43.3%
Bone quality	43.3%
Adequacy of soft tissue coverage	43.3%
Moderately important:	
Graft availability	56.7%
Enable local tumor surveillance	53.3%
Radiation therapy pre- or postoperative	46.7%

*Survey question: "Considering only primary spine tumor cases, rate the importance of each factor that may affect bone graft selection in primary spine tumor reconstructions." Factors included patient age, tumor histology, likelihood of achieving a clear margin, life expectancy, anatomic location, history of preoperative chemotherapy, radiation therapy pre- or postoperative, bone quality, adequacy of soft tissue coverage, enable local tumor surveillance, graft cost, and graft availability.

or future surgery.[4] In these scenarios, a more inert graft such as PMMA that will be resistant to biological effects of local treatment and tumor invasion should be considered. Poor bone quality may necessitate consideration of techniques that utilize PMMA to augment or incorporate adjacent segments into the anterior structural graft and increase the required number of posterior fixation levels.[3] Adequate soft tissue coverage is required to maintain or enable local vascularization and healing as well as reduce the likelihood of wound breakdown and infection. In this scenario a vascular graft would be given high consideration if adequate coverage were not achievable by other means.[2] Graft availability and need for adequate tumor surveillance are self-evident. The negative effects of radiation on soft tissue healing are well known. However, preoperative radiation alone may not significantly adversely affect local bony healing, but it certainly results in local osteopenia.[5] Acute postoperative radiation (planned or due to intraoperative tumor contamination or unexpected positive margin) does have a profound effect on bony healing of anterior interbody strut grafts.[5] In the scenario where the need for acute postoperative radiation is likely or is imposed due to positive margins, the use a vascular graft or PMMA, depending on other factors previously discussed, should be considered.

▪ Specific Considerations Based On Anatomic Site

As noted above, the recommended structural graft choices (**Table 14.1**) in most regions of the spine are typically allograft or prefabricated cages (packed with allo- or autograft bone) that are appropriately sized with respect to diameter (preferably contacting the apophyseal rim of the endplate) and length. Structural bone allograft has the advantage of direct biological fusion (**Fig. 14.1**) where graft union with the host is possible.[6] Allograft also enables unimpeded imaging for assessment of fusion and tumor surveillance. For structural allografts, the options are as follow: for the

cervical spine—radius, fibular, or ulna; for the thoracic spine—tibia or humerus (upper thoracic); and for the lumbar spine—tibia or femur.

Perhaps the greatest current limitation of structural allograft pertains to its relative availability. Due to the possible risk of disease transmission as a result of poor regional procurement and sterilization processes or cultural beliefs, allograft is not available in many countries. Specific to the reconstruction of segmental defects, there is an associated risk of fracture, particularly for irradiated or freeze-dried allograft.[6] However, due to the load sharing and torsional stability that is offered by spinal instrumentation, this is an uncommon occurrence in spinal cases. Comparatively, prefabricated prostheses often referred to as "cages" offer the advantage of greater availability and more size and shape options. Furthermore, for complex defects with transitional anatomy such as at the cervicothoracic junction, contoured or custom options are available.

Most prefabricated prostheses do not directly integrate with the host, and consequently need to be packed with morselized bone (auto- or allograft) to enable fusion. For primary tumor reconstruction, metallic cages have the distinct disadvantage of metal artifact on magnetic resonance imaging (MRI) and to a lesser extent on computed tomography (CT), which may delay the detection of local disease recurrence on tumor surveillance (the clinical sequelae of which can be debated). Furthermore, the cost of cages, particularly contoured or custom devices, may be prohibitive in certain health care systems. Reconstruction of complete uni- or bilateral posterior column defects is also variable from case to case, but appropriately sized load-sharing strut graft(s), typically allo- or autograft, are preferable. At our center, we have had excellent success with using rib grafts for this purpose.[7] In cases where there is a high risk of failure (revisions or postoperative radiation), a vascularized rib can be considered.

Junctional regions of the spine typically present with further unique anatomic and mechanical challenges that warrant discussion. Due to the frequent need for massive resections, reconstruction of lumbar-pelvic defects typically represents the most variable and dif-

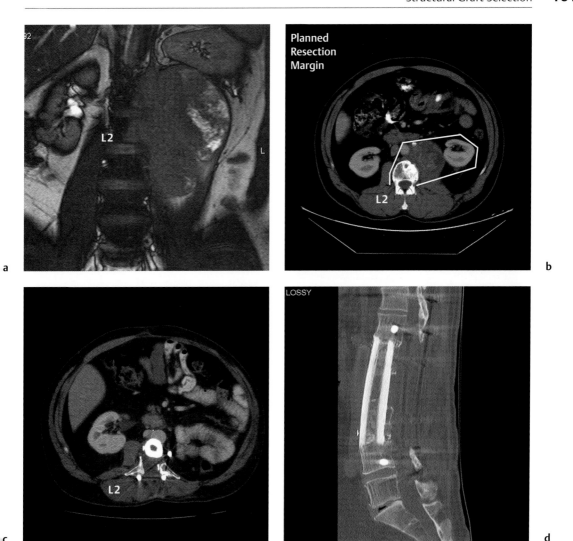

Fig. 14.1a–d Coronal magnetic resonance imaging (MRI) **(a)** and axial computed tomography (CT) of a large retroperitoneal primitive neuroectodermal tumor (PNET) in a 46-year-old man. **(b)** The planned resection is demonstrated on the axial CT. The patient is 6 years postresection, working on his farm, and is disease free at last assessment. **(c)** A 5-year axial CT demonstrating the allograft femur and aortic stent anteriorly and the posterolateral bony elements that were retained to provide vas0 cularized bone in the posterior column. **(d)** Sagittal CT at 5 years demonstrating excellent incorporation at the host–allograft junctions.

ficult reconstructions, with the greatest risk of complication. This topic is discussed in Chapter 13. Due to the straight alignment, structural graft selection at the thoracolumbar junction does not present any additional specific issues beyond those already discussed. On the other hand, the transitional anatomy (rapid change in size and contour) of the cervicothoracic junction (CTJ) often requires the use of contoured cages or unique allograft step-cuts, particularly for multilevel resection that cross the CTJ. The occipitocervical junction (OCJ) is associated with unique access and reconstruction challenges for marginal or wide en-bloc resections.[8] This is particularly so for resections that require high anterior access and the possible resection of the posterior pharyngeal wall, wherein adequate soft tissue coverage is critical to avoid infection and enable osseous healing. In the latter scenario, a myo-osseous vascularized fibular strut graft (i.e., with attached muscle and fascia) is recommended to provide structural support (clivus to cervical spine) and posterior pharyn-geal wall reconstruction (**Fig. 14.2**). Alternatively, if the posterior pharyngeal wall is intact, then posterior reconstruction with cages or autograph struts from the occipital condyles to the cervical lateral masses can be utilized due to the sagittal vertebral axis being posterior in the upper cervical spine.[9] The terminal

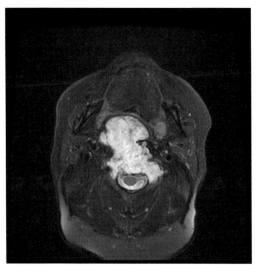

a

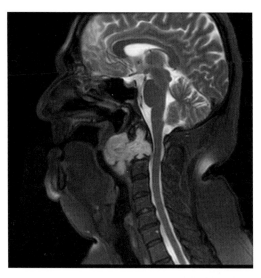

b

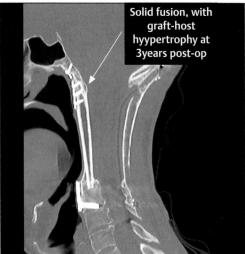

c

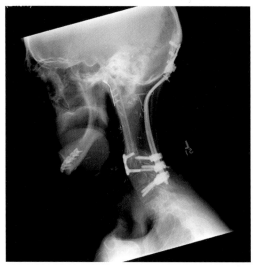

d

Fig. 14.2a–d Axial (**a**) and sagittal (**b**) MRI scans of a C1-C4 chordoma in a 59-year-old mam. The chordoma entailed bilateral vertebral artery involvement at C2. Management involved a multistage en-bloc R0 resection that included the posterior pharyngeal wall, unilateral vertebral artery bypass, myo-osseous vascularized fibular strut graft, posterior central rib graft, and circumferential instrumentation. Patient is disease free at 4 years with persistent dysphonia and dysphagia. (**c**) Post-operative sagittal CT scan at 3 years demonstrating solid integration of both grafts, with hypertrophy at the terminal ends of the vascularized fibular graft. (**d**) Lateral radiograph at 3 years demonstrating the reconstruction.

ends of the cages can be compressed into the condyle and cervical lateral mass to provide immediate stability of the graft.

Reconstruction Results

Despite the extremely high-risk environment for osseous healing, nonunion following en-bloc resection is less common than one would expect. In the largest published series of en-bloc resections (n = 134, including n = 90 for primary tumors), at a median follow-up of 47 months Boriani et al[1] reported 7% instrumentation failure using a posterior pedicle screw fixation connected with a modular anterior carbon fiber system packed with autogenous graft or bone substitutes. They attributed the failure to short segment posterior fixation. In a much smaller clinical series, Matsumoto et al[10] reported on late instrumentation (anterior mesh cage and pedicle screw fixation) failures following en-bloc resections in 15 patients; seven of the resections were for primary tumors. At a mean follow-up of 41.5 months, an 40% overall instrumentation failure rate (rod or cage fracture) was reported, with most failures occurring after 2 years. In the seven primary tumor total en-bloc spondylectomies (TESs), two failures (29%) occurred. Cage subsidence ($\geq$ 5mm), preoperative radiation, and the number of levels of posterior instrumentation ($\leq$ 4 levels) were reported to be significantly associated with late instrumentation failure.

The pitfall of short-segment posterior fixation is supported by the biomechanical study from Disch et al.[11] Using a one-level TES model, the authors demonstrated that it is the number of levels of posterior fixation that predominantly determines stability even with anterior fixation. Anterior-alone or short-segment (one level above and below) circumferential fixation is not recommended following TES. For a one-level TES, posterior pedicle screw fixation two adjacent segments or more above and below with anterior column structural support is recommended.

In another intermediate-term (mean follow-up of 41.5 months) prospective case series of 26 en-bloc resections for primary tumors, Fisher et al[2] reported a revision rate of 10%, with two of 20 surviving patients requiring revision instrumentation for nonunion (one each in the thoracic and the lumbar spines). The authors used multilevel posterior fixation in all cases with a variety of anterior structural graft choices.

In a series of highly complex en-bloc resections for cervical chordoma, Hsieh et al[8] reported late nonunion and instrumentation failure in three of the five cases reconstructed with instrumented anterior cages and post rod-screw fixation. The mean clinical follow-up was 4.5 years. Unfortunately, the authors did not comment on the specific mode(s) of failure in these cases. In my personal series of two such cases, one requiring C1-C3 en-bloc resection following an incomplete intralesion resection performed at another center, and the other a C1-C4 en-bloc resection, a vascularized myo-osseous fibular graft has successfully incorporated in both cases (**Fig. 14.2**).

These reports demonstrate the critical importance of structural graft selection and reconstruction techniques that incorporate sound biomechanical principles and long-term goals to achieve fusion. Revision surgeries in these cases with already significantly compromised host tissue can be daunting, and the best strategy is optimization of the index procedure. Sound knowledge of what has been tried and resulted in failure or success is paramount to sound decision making for structural graft selection and reconstruction following en-bloc resection for primary tumors.

Chapter Summary

Although the literature on spinal instrumentation and fusion techniques is extensive, the literature pertaining to reconstruction of structural defects following en-bloc primary tumor resection of the spine is relatively limited. Due to the rarity of primary spinal tumors, case series describing reconstruction and graft selection techniques are surgeon/center and patient specific, and they focus on the oncological and technical aspects of the cases. Very few reports provide long-term data on the durability of the graft selection and reconstruction. Furthermore, there are numerous case reports that describe very specific and complex reconstructions typically for very large multilevel resections. Consequently, no case-specific (i.e., significant heterogeneity will always exist between cases) evidence-based best practices can be clearly stated on this topic. The ultimate goal of spinal fusion following en-bloc resection of a primary tumor represents a significant challenge due to a variety of potentially unfavorable factors that negatively affect osseous healing; these include gross instability of the spine, poor vascularity due to wide dissection of the surrounding soft tissues, and a hostile local environment secondary to radiation or chemotherapy.

tion (directly or indirectly) with the host bone (i.e., fusion).
◆ General key factors in structural graft selection fall into four broad categories: patient, local, tumor, and health system.
◆ To successfully achieve access, soft tissue coverage, biomechanically sound fixation and long-term structural graft integration, unique technical requirements based on the anatomic location of the defect, particularly at junctional segments, need to be carefully considered and planned for each case.

Pitfalls

◆ Thinking of only the short-term rather than the long-term goals will almost always be a regrettable decision in these cases.
◆ Not all centers have the necessary multidisciplinary expertise and equipment required to achieve the end goals of reconstruction in these cases. Ensure that all goals will be met and contingency plans are identified and executable before proceeding with the index procedure.
◆ Regardless of appropriate graft selection, inadequate fixation will lead to a poor outcome. Avoid anterior-alone or anterior and short-segment posterior (i.e., one level above and below) fixation in these types of cases.

Pearls

◆ The overall goal of structural graft selection should be to provide durable structural support across the spinal defect(s) and enable biological integra-

References
Five Must-Read References

1. Boriani S, Bandiera S, Donthineni R, et al. Morbidity of en bloc resections in the spine. Eur Spine J 2010; 19:231–241
2. Fisher CG, Keynan O, Boyd MC, Dvorak MF. The surgical management of primary tumors of the spine: initial results of an ongoing prospective cohort study. Spine 2005;30:1899–1908
3. Fourney DR, Abi-Said D, Rhines LD, et al. Simultaneous anterior-posterior approach to the thoracic and lumbar spine for the radical resection of tumors followed by reconstruction and stabilization. J Neurosurg 2001;94(2, Suppl):232–244
4. Fisher CG, Saravanja DD, Dvorak MF, et al. Surgical management of primary bone tumors of the spine: validation of an approach to enhance cure and reduce local recurrence. Spine 2011;36:830–836
5. Emery SE, Brazinski MS, Koka A, Bensusan JS, Stevenson S. The biological and biomechanical effects of irradiation on anterior spinal bone grafts in a canine model. J Bone Joint Surg Am 1994;76:540–548
6. Delloye C, Cornu O, Druez V, Barbier O. Bone allografts: What they can offer and what they cannot. J Bone Joint Surg Br 2007;89:574–579 Review
7. Lewis SJ, Kulkarni AG, Rampersaud YR, et al. Posterior column reconstruction with autologous rib graft after en bloc tumor excision. Spine 2012;37:346–350
8. Hsieh PC, Gallia GL, Sciubba DM, et al. En bloc excisions of chordomas in the cervical spine: review of five consecutive cases with more than 4-year follow-up. Spine 2011;36:E1581–E1587
9. Scheer JK, Tang J, Eguizabal J, et al. Optimal reconstruction technique after C-2 corpectomy and spondylectomy: a biomechanical analysis. J Neurosurg Spine 2010;12:517–524
10. Matsumoto M, Watanabe K, Tsuji T, et al. Late instrumentation failure after total en bloc spondylectomy. J Neurosurg Spine 2011;15:320–327
11. Disch AC, Schaser KD, Melcher I, Luzzati A, Feraboli F, Schmoelz W. En bloc spondylectomy reconstructions in a biomechanical in-vitro study. Eur Spine J 2008; 17:715–725

15

Wound Closure Techniques

Justin M. Sacks and Justin M. Broyles

▨ Introduction

Radical oncological resection is warranted for aggressive benign tumors and for low-grade and high-grade malignant tumors of the spine. Advances in neurosurgical technique, instrumentation for spinal stabilization, and adjuvant therapy allow for a greater number of surgical candidates than ever before.[1] However, surgical wounds that contain hardware and vital neural structures can have devastating consequences for patients if the wounds become exposed or infected.

Complex, composite wounds of the spine are managed with immediate soft tissue reconstruction using muscle or fascial flaps.[2] This is particularly indicated for those patients identified as being at high risk for wound-healing complications, such as those with prior operations, infections, potential for planned placement of spinal instrumentation, or medical comorbidities that predispose to complications.[3] The oncological spine surgeon should work in tandem with the plastic and reconstructive surgeon to optimize both the ablative and the reconstructive surgical procedure.

Reconstructive options range from primary closure to local muscle flaps to more complex methods of reconstruction such as microvascular free tissue transfer. Defects in regions that have been exposed to prior irradiation or sur-

gery, or have a paucity of local tissue require more complex types of reconstructive interventions. Using a combination of these techniques, the goal of the reconstructive surgeon, in tandem with the neurosurgical team, is to obliterate dead space and provide coverage of vascularized soft tissue over critical areas in an effort to prevent infection and restore function to these patients.

▨ Preoperative Evaluation

The physiological status of the patient must be considered and balanced with the overall reconstructive plan. The overall prognosis of the patient must also be taken into account as well. Reconstruction to improve a patient's quality of life is often considered even in a palliative scenario.[4]

Medical Comorbidities

The patient's medical history should be thoroughly reviewed to stratify the relative risk of infection. Evidence of malnutrition, smoking, diabetes mellitus, and peripheral vascular disease should be evaluated, as these conditions can have deleterious effects on wound healing as well as flap survival.[5]

Radiation Therapy

Radiation therapy induces tissue injury through changes in the microcirculation of the defect and its surrounding areas, leading to decreased perfusion and impaired wound healing. Indeed, spinal surgery patients who undergo adjuvant radiation have up to three times the rate of wound healing complications as compared with their nonradiated counterparts.[6] For this reason, the reconstructive surgeon should be cognizant of the timing, dosage, and location of any prior or planned radiation. Additionally, the plastic and reconstructive surgeon should utilize tissue outside the field of radiation for flap reconstruction. This will take the form of a pedicled or free tissue transfer. A variable amount of skin, adipose, fascia, muscle, and bone can be rotated or transplanted on a vascular pedicle composed of a specific artery and vein.

Timing of Reconstruction

The timing of spinal soft and hard tissue reconstruction is most often dictated by the status of the tumor and the surgical margins. Certain patient factors such as advanced age, multiple comorbidities, or the need for locoregional control with adjuvant radiotherapy must also be considered in the timing. Primary reconstruction carries a significantly decreased rate of wound healing complications and is preferred to delayed reconstruction.[7] Delayed reconstruction, although not optimal, is occasionally unavoidable for defects with extensive soft tissue deficits or in cases of patient instability. If a patient requires delayed reconstruction, a negative pressure closure device is the preferred temporizing measure until definitive reconstruction can be performed at a later date. Negative pressure closure devices over exposed neural structures in the region of the spinal cord can create both cerebrospinal fluid leaks and pain.

Imaging

Preoperative imaging with computed tomography (CT) and/or magnetic resonance imaging (MRI) should be performed to evaluate the integrity of the surrounding soft tissue, vascular anatomy, and any previously placed hardware. Often, local tissue, such as the paraspinal musculature, will be sought to obliterate surgical defects; however, if this tissue is not available, the reconstructive surgeon will have to plan in advance to utilize regional or distant tissue outside of the zone of injury to reconstruct the defect. Knowledge of the associated vasculature helps with preoperative planning and with the eventual intraoperative decisions.

▓ Reconstructive Surgical Tenets

The core principle underlying reconstructive algorithms used by plastic surgeons is to progress from simple to more complex reconstructions on the basis of the specific wound requirements. The underlying goal for the reconstruction is to close a wound primarily with local tissue that will be tension-free and obliterate dead space. When primary closure is not feasible, local tissue flaps of tissue can be used.

Local tissue flaps enable surgeons to reconstruct soft tissue defects with similar tissue from an adjacent location. "Random" local flaps comprise adjacent skin and subcutaneous tissue and are based on a subdermal plexus vascular supply. By definition, a random flap does not have a distinct, specific blood supply. In contrast, axial-pattern flaps are based on specific blood vessels. Axial flaps can be fasciocutaneous (deep muscle fascia with overlying skin), myocutaneous (muscle with skin), or osteocutaneous (bone with overlying skin); these flaps enable reconstructive surgeons to repair defects with tissue that is similar to the resected tissue.

Microvascular free tissue transfer involves harvesting a tissue construct and its named blood supply from a distant region of the body and placing it into a defect. Vascular anastomosis between the flap's donor vessels and the patient's recipient vessels is performed under magnification provided by a surgical microscope. The decision to use a particular flap is based on the requirements for replacing missing skin, adipose tissue, fascia, muscle, or bone.

The primary advantage of microvascular free tissue transfer is that tissue of a quality similar to that of the resected tissue can be moved from a remote part of the body, thereby enabling optimal aesthetic and functional outcomes. This also enables irradiated or infected tissue to be removed and replaced with soft, pliable, and vascularized tissue. The drawbacks of free tissue transfer are related to donor-site morbidity and the potential for longer operative times. However, with careful coordination, harvests of vascularized osteocutaneous flaps (e.g., free fibula flap) can be performed simultaneously or in concert with oncological resections.

Anatomic Location and Axial Pattern Flap Availability

Spinal soft tissue defects can be classified according to a scheme suggested by Casas and Lewis[8] in which wounds are divided into the upper third, middle third, and lower third. The upper third of the spine includes all cervical vertebrae up to T7. The middle third of the spine includes T1 to T12. The lower third of the spine includes vertebrae L1 to S5.[8]

Upper Third

Defects of the upper third of the spine, defined by the spinous processes of C3 through C7, are among the most commonly encountered by the plastic surgeon and are amendable to a multitude of axial pattern flaps. The majority of these defects can be reconstructed using bilateral paraspinal flaps. Additionally, a unilateral trapezius muscle flap can be used when the paraspinal muscles have been compromised. A latissimus dorsi muscle with or without a skin paddle can be harvested for larger, more extensive defects.[8]

Middle Third

The middle third of the spine is delineated by the spinous processes of C7 to L1. Reconstruc-

tion of this area is similar to that of the upper third, where bilateral paraspinous muscle flaps are able to provide coverage for a majority of defects. If these muscle flaps are unavailable due to trauma, irradiation, or defect size, the latissimus dorsi muscle can provide durable coverage either as a standard, axial pattern flap or by utilizing reverse latissimus muscle flap.[9]

Lower Third

The boundaries of the lower third of the spine are dictated by the spinous processes of L1 to S5. Due to the proximity of this region to the gluteal and posterior thigh regions, there is a multitude of potential flap donor sites available for flap reconstruction. Within this region, the paraspinous muscles are robust and readily available for coverage of most defects. If they are unavailable, other regional flap options are the latissimus dorsi turnover muscle flap, gluteus muscle flap, and pedicled vertical rectus abdominis myocutaneous flap (VRAM) based on the deep inferior epigastric vessels. When utilized in the lower third, the pedicled VRAM is routinely used to obliterate the actual space created by a subtotal or total sacrectomy. In these clinical situations, the bowel can herniate posteriorly and become entangled in spinal hardware or develop a bowel obstruction. In the setting of a total sacrectomy, the free fibula bone can be anastomosed to the superior blood supply of a pedicled VRAM or through a vein graft to the intercostal vessels.[10]

Adjuncts to Flap Surgery

Negative Pressure Wound Therapy

Negative pressure-assisted closure can provide for temporary coverage in soft tissue spinal defects when definitive reconstruction is delayed. When utilized appropriately, this device can promote neovascularization, decrease edema, and increase local granulation tissue, as well as provide contractile force at wound edges.[11] Although this modality can be used to prepare the wound bed for definitive reconstruction with soft tissue flaps in a delayed fashion, it can also be used to promote healing by secondary intention in partial-thickness defects.

Internal Tissue Expansion

Tissue expansion is a process in which an inflatable prosthetic implant with a silicone shell is used to expand local and regional tissues so that they can eventually be advanced into the wound in a delayed fashion. The inflatable implant is inserted at the time of tumor extirpation or during a second procedure. At subsequent office visits, saline is injected through an integrated or remote port to gradually expand the implant. Once the tissue has been sufficiently expanded, it can be advanced into the defect. Because tissue expansion takes time, the method is not feasible for spinal reconstruction that requires immediate coverage of spinal instrumentation or neurovascular structures. Risks of tissue expansion include infection, extrusion, and rupture of the implant.[12]

External Tissue Expansion

A recently adapted alternative to internal tissue expansion is external tissue expansion. This technique relies on the application of a constant, external force to the underlying skin, fascia, and muscle. There are several adapted means of expansion using different tensioning devices that are often secured to the periphery of the wound. As the external forces are applied to the overlying skin and fascia, several cytoskeletal and extracellular changes occur to produce a biochemical response that results in an overall increase of tissue mass and size.[13,14]

Examples of external expander systems include Jacob's ladder, retention sutures, and commercially available external expansion systems. Each of these techniques applies external force and tension to the edge of the defect to produce a gradual closure using autologous tissue. The disadvantages of this technique include the lengthy time required for closure as well as pain and discomfort during the expansion process. These are not primary or secondary options in spinal soft tissue reconstruction but must be considered in the clinical setting of the patient.

Biological Tissue Matrices

Commercially available biological tissue matrices (BTMs) currently come from five different sources: human dermis, porcine dermis, porcine small intestinal submucosa, bovine dermis, and bovine pericardium.[15] These BTMs can be used to reconstruct soft tissue defects where there is a paucity of available donor tissue. Although each BTM is inherently different due to its proprietary processing technique, the central tenet that all BTMs should be based on is the provision of strength and early revascularization capacity in an effort to provide soft tissue coverage and resist infection. Within spinal and sacral reconstruction, BTMs can be used in a multitude of capacities including the provision of durable coverage over implanted hardware as well as the creation of pelvic diaphragms to prevent visceral herniation into low sacral defects.[16] These defects, as mentioned previously, arise from subtotal or total sacrectomy defects.

■ Characterization of Axial Pattern Flaps

Paraspinous Muscle

The paraspinous muscles are a multilayered group of muscles that line each side of the spinal column and have the potential to provide excellent coverage of moderately sized defects at almost any level of the spinal column. Although composed of nine paired muscle groups, the collective flap is referred to as the paraspinous muscle flap and is transposed based on either the medial or lateral perforating intercostal vessels. The superficial layer is composed of the splenius capitis and the splenius cervicis muscles, both of which are found in the cervical spine, or upper third. The intermediate layer of the spinal column is composed of the iliocostalis, the longissimus, and the spinalis muscles, and these span the entire length of the spinal column. Finally, the deepest layer includes the transversospinal, semispinalis, multifidus, and rotatores muscles.

These paired midline muscles are dissected superficially to reveal the extent of the lateral border. Then the dissection proceeds along the medial undersurface of the muscle groups, and the paraspinous muscles are elevated off of the ribs, with care taken to preserve the lateral intercostal perforators. After elevation, the paraspinous muscles are manually advanced toward the midline and sutured together.[17] The advantages of the paraspinous muscle flaps include convenience as well as a relative ease of dissection. Additionally, there is often no donor-site defect, as many times the flap is within the wound bed. However, because of this proximity to the wound, the flap is often compromised secondary to resection and is not available for reconstruction (**Fig. 15.1**).

Trapezius Muscle

The trapezius flap can be harvested as a myocutaneous or muscle-only flap and was first described in 1979.[18] The flap is based off of the descending branch of the transverse cervical artery and vein. In addition to the dominant blood supply from the transverse cervical system, it also receives minor contributions from the dorsal scapular artery and perforating posterior intercostal vessels. This flap is useful for the coverage of defects in the upper third, or cervical region of the spinal column.

The advantages of this flap include a relatively flat and thin cutaneous portion that can be useful in shallow defects. The disadvantages include a relatively limited arc of rotation and significant donor-site morbidity of upper extremity weakness. Additionally, due to the proximity of the muscle to the operative field, the muscle may be damaged or irradiated, leading to inability to use the flap (**Fig. 15.2**).

Latissimus Dorsi Muscle

The latissimus dorsi muscle flap is a versatile flap and can be harvested either as a muscle only or as a myocutaneous flap. This flap can be used to reconstruct upper, middle, and lower areas of the spinal column and has a remarkable arc of rotation.[19] The latissimus dorsi muscle has a dual blood supply. The dominant vascular pedicle is derived from the thoracodorsal artery, and the flap also receives a significant supply from the segmental intercostal vessels that enter the muscle at the midline.

The traditional latissimus dorsi flap can be raised as an axial pattern flap off of the thoracodorsal artery and vein. Conversely, when the latissimus dorsi is detached at its insertion into the humerus, its vascular supply becomes based on the secondary intercostal vessels, and

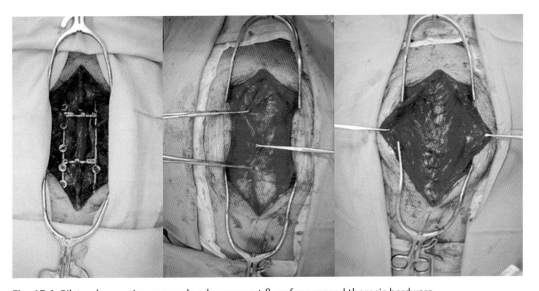

Fig. 15.1 Bilateral paraspinous muscle advancement flaps for exposed thoracic hardware.

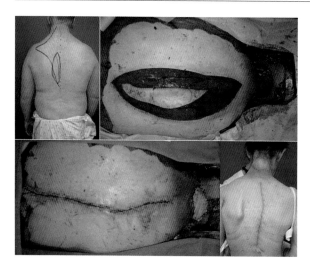

Fig. 15.2 Pedicled myocutaneous trapezius flap for cervical soft tissue defect.

the resulting flap is referred to as the reverse latissimus dorsi flap.[9] The advantages of the flap include a very large area of coverage with a wide arc or rotation. Additionally, this flap is frequently out of the zone of injury, so it provides robust coverage of spinal wounds without the potential for radiation damage. Potential limitations are the donor-site morbidity of harvesting a large skin paddle and the need for skin graft coverage of the back. Additionally, flap harvest can limit upper extremity motion in some patients. Also, the resultant donor-site defect is prone to hematoma and seroma for-

mation. Large-caliber self-suction drains are routinely placed and removed when the output is less than 20 mL of serous fluid for 3 successive days (**Fig. 15.3**).

Gluteus Maximus Muscle

The gluteus maximus muscle is typically harvested as a muscle-only flap, but can be harvested as a myocutaneous flap if needed. The flap is based off of the superior gluteal artery and has a short axis for rotation, rendering it useful only for defects of the lower third of the

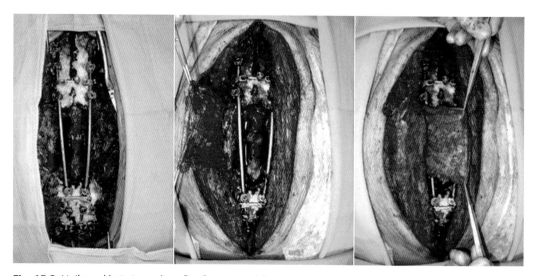

Fig. 15.3 Unilateral latissimus dorsi flap for exposed thoracic hardware.

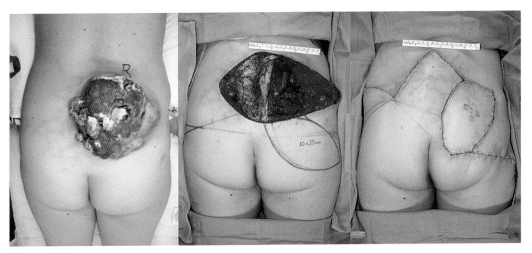

Fig. 15.4 Unilateral pedicled superior gluteal artery perforator flap and rhomboid fasciocutaneous flap for large sacral defect after oncological resection.

spine. The superior half of the muscle is able to provide coverage for the contralateral sacrum, and the inferior half of the muscle is able to provide coverage for the ipsilateral ischium.

The gluteus maximus flap provides a robust, relatively large amount of vascularized muscle and fascia and is able to obliterate the largest of sacral defects.[20] The donor site of the flap can be closed with relative ease using a V to Y advancement closure. Because the flap has such a large muscle, the gluteus maximus is prone to denervation atrophy. Additionally, its proximity to the sciatic nerve represents a potential source of morbidity during dissection (**Fig. 15.4**).

Rectus Abdominis Muscle

The pedicled VRAM flap is a versatile flap based on the inferior epigastric system. It can be harvested as either a muscle-only or a myocutaneous flap and is most useful for defects of the lower third of the spine and the pelvic region. The flap has a robust vascularity and abundant soft tissue bulk, especially in corpulent patients. The flap is most useful for reconstructing and obliterating the dead space that ensues after sacrectomy or pelvic exenteration.[21]

The advantage of this flap is its ability to provide robust, vascularized tissue into the defect that is outside of the field of radiation. In the setting of a subtotal or total sacrectomy this flap is of particular interest as it both obliterates dead space in the base of the pelvis and obturates any small or large bowel segment that may herniate to the posterior aspect and become lodged in spinal hardware or develop into a bowel obstruction. The disadvantage of this flap is that it necessitates performing the surgery from an anterior approach, which can lead to herniation, bulge formation, and wound healing complications or injury to the surrounding viscera (**Fig. 15.5**).

Fibular Bone

The free fibular flap is the ideal choice for treatment of sacrectomy defects that contain vast amounts of dead space and no autologous bone for structural support, as it is a well-vascularized source of both bone and soft tissue. The flap is based off of the perforating arteries from the peroneal artery. If additional soft tissue is needed, it can be used as a chimeric flap with the soleus muscle. This flap can only be harvested and used as a free flap, and therefore can be utilized in any region of the spine for osseous reconstruction; however, its main utility is in pelvic reconstruction and chronic osseous nonunions, as the fibular bone provides a stable buttress to support surrounding hardware.[22]

The rich vascularity of this flap has been shown to promote improved healing and an

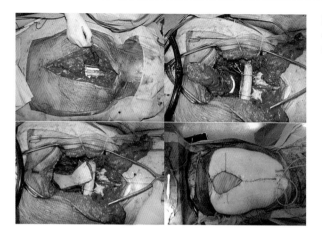

Fig. 15.5 Pedicled vertical rectus abdominis flap for subtotal sacral defect with nonvascularized bone graft.

ability to overcome osteomyelitis. The soft tissue portion of the flap obliterates any residual dead space. Additionally, it can be harvested simultaneously while performing sacral debridement, effectively minimizing operative times. The disadvantage of this flap is that it entails a steep learning curve for dissection and flap harvest (**Fig. 15.6**).

▨ Postoperative Care

Ambulation

In an effort to mitigate the thrombotic effects of surgery as well as potentially offload pres-

sure on the wound closure and flap, ambulation is recommended on the first postoperative day if there has been no dural violation. But if a dural violation has occurred, then bed rest is recommended for 3 days, during which time the patient should be turned every 2 hours to decease the incidence of ischemic ulcer creation as well as to offload incisional pressure. Using this strategy, prolonged pressure on the incision is avoided and the potential for subsequent flap necrosis is mitigated.

Drain Management

When closing wounds over an area of tumor extirpation or hardware implantation, a vast

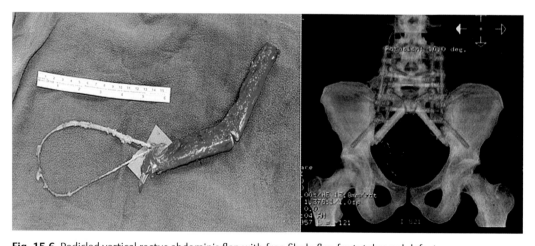

Fig. 15.6 Pedicled vertical rectus abdominis flap with free fibula flap for total sacral defect.

amount of dead space is invariably created. It is critical for the reconstructive surgeon to mitigate this dead space with a combination of vascularized soft tissue and self-suction drains. Closed-suction drains assist in the elimination of seroma and hematoma formation and should be left in place until each respective drain produces less than 20 mL of exudate per day over a span of 3 consecutive days.

Complications

Complications in patients requiring soft tissue coverage of implanted hardware are devastating to the patient and the surgical team.[2] The most commonly encountered complications include seroma, hematoma, wound infection, and flap failure. In patients in whom soft tissue fluid collections are suspected, imaging studies such as CT or MRI are indicated to evaluate the location and extent of the suspected collection as well as the potential for hardware involvement. If there is any indication of infection, culture-directed, broad-spectrum antibiotics should be started, and sharp debridement of all necrotic tissue should be performed. Flap failure, either partial or complete, can occur for a myriad of reasons and should generate an operative evaluation of the flap to interrogate the potential for reversible problems. If flap failure persists, the patient will likely require further operative management to correct the resultant defect.

Chapter Summary

The goal of reconstructive surgery for cancer patients who have undergone extirpative spinal surgery is to restore form and function. The central tenet underlying the reconstructive algorithm is to progress from simple too more complex reconstructions on the basis of the specific wound requirements. Defects in regions that have been exposed to prior irradiation or surgery, or have a paucity of local tissue, require more complex types of reconstructive interventions. Using a combination of these techniques, the reconstructive surgeon aims to obliterate dead space and provide coverage over critical areas in an effort to prevent infection and restore form and function to these patients.

Pearls

♦ Communication between the plastic and neurosurgical teams is of the upmost importance when planning surgery. Adequate communication enables the surgical team to provide full disclosure to the patient with regard to potential donor-site morbidity. Additionally, it enables determining the appropriate preoperative imaging and evaluation of potential flap donor sites.

♦ When closing wounds over the spinal column, it is critical to identify structures that must be covered with vascularized tissue. Local muscle flaps based on axial pattern blood supplies are optimal to obliterate dead space and cover structural grafts and hardware in the upper, middle, and lower third of the spine.

♦ Obliterate all associated dead space in the spinal wound with both vascularized tissue and closed-suction drains. Preventing hematoma and seroma formation is an important component of successful wound closure over the spinal column.

♦ When reconstructing soft tissue defects over the spine, it is critical to maintain a vascularized wound bed free of devitalized tissue. Scar tissue, devitalized adipose, and muscle potentially act as a nidus for infection.

Pitfalls

♦ When closing wounds over the spinal column, it is critical to use closed-suction drains in order to eliminate seroma and hematoma. Early removal of drains leads to seroma formation and potential infection.

♦ Failure to off-load pressure on the midline spinal wound results in pressure necrosis at the wound site. This can subsequently lead to dehiscence and infection of the spinal wound.

♦ Attempting closure of a spinal wound in a primary fashion without muscle flaps leads to higher rates of wound dehiscence and infection. The obliteration of dead space with muscle flaps decreases the formation of fluid collections.

References
Five Must–Read References

1. Ciol MA, Deyo RA, Howell E, Kreif S. An assessment of surgery for spinal stenosis: time trends, geographic variations, complications, and reoperations. J Am Geriatr Soc 1996;44:285–290

2. Stahl RS, Burstein FD, Lieponis JV, Murphy MJ, Piepmeier JM. Extensive wounds of the spine: a comprehensive approach to debridement and reconstruction. Plast Reconstr Surg 1990;85:747–753

3. Few JW, Marcus JR, Lee MJ, Ondra S, Dumanian GA. Treatment of hostile midline back wounds: an extreme approach. Plast Reconstr Surg 2000;105:2448–2451

4. Weigel B, Maghsudi M, Neumann C, Kretschmer R, Müller FJ, Nerlich M. Surgical management of symptomatic spinal metastases. Postoperative outcome and quality of life. Spine 1999;24:2240–2246

5. Thalgott JS, Cotler HB, Sasso RC, LaRocca H, Gardner V. Postoperative infections in spinal implants. Classification and analysis—a multicenter study. Spine 1991;16:981–984

6. Ghogawala Z, Mansfield FL, Borges LF. Spinal radiation before surgical decompression adversely affects outcomes of surgery for symptomatic metastatic spinal cord compression. Spine 2001;26:818–824

7. Chang DW, Friel MT, Youssef AA. Reconstructive strategies in soft tissue reconstruction after resection of spinal neoplasms. Spine 2007;32:1101–1106

8. Casas LA, Lewis VL Jr. A reliable approach to the closure of large acquired midline defects of the back. Plast Reconstr Surg 1989;84:632–641

9. Stevenson TR, Rohrich RJ, Pollock RA, Dingman RO, Bostwick J III. More experience with the "reverse" latissimus dorsi musculocutaneous flap: precise location of blood supply. Plast Reconstr Surg 1984;74:237–243

10. Garvey PB, Clemens MW, Rhines LD, Sacks JM. Vertical rectus abdominis musculocutaneous flow-through flap to a free fibula flap for total sacrectomy reconstruction. Microsurgery 2013;33:32–38

11. Morykwas MJ, Argenta LC, Shelton-Brown EI, McGuirt W. Vacuum-assisted closure: a new method for wound control and treatment: animal studies and basic foundation. Ann Plast Surg 1997;38:553–562

12. Cunha MS, Nakamoto HA, Herson MR, Faes JC, Gemperli R, Ferreira MC. Tissue expander complications in plastic surgery: a 10-year experience. Rev Hosp Clin Fac Med Sao Paulo 2002;57:93–97

13. Lasheen AE, Saad K, Raslan M. External tissue expansion in head and neck reconstruction. J Plast Reconstr Aesthet Surg 2009;62:e251–e254

14. Baird R, Gholoum S, Laberge JM, Puligandla P. Management of a giant omphalocele with an external skin closure system. J Pediatr Surg 2010;45:E17–E20

15. Broyles JM, Abt NB, Sacks JM, Butler CE. Bioprosthetic tissue matrices in complex abdominal wall reconstruction. Plastic and Reconstructive Surgery–Global Open. 2013;1:e91

16. Korn JM, Connolly MM, Walton RL. Single-stage sacral coccygectomy and repair using human acellular dermal matrix (AlloDerm) with bilateral gluteus maximus flaps for hernia prophylaxis. Hernia 2009;13:329–332

17. Hultman CS, Jones GE, Losken A, et al. Salvage of infected spinal hardware with paraspinous muscle flaps: anatomic considerations with clinical correlation. Ann Plast Surg 2006;57:521–528

18. Demergasso F, Piazza MV. Trapezius myocutaneous flap in reconstructive surgery for head and neck cancer: an original technique. Am J Surg 1979;138:533–536

19. Giesswein P, Constance CG, Mackay DR, Manders EK. Supercharged latissimus dorsi muscle flap for coverage of the problem wound in the lower back. Plast Reconstr Surg 1994;94:1060–1063

20. Furukawa H, Yamamoto Y, Igawa HH, Sugihara T. Gluteus maximus adipomuscular turnover or sliding flap in the surgical treatment of extensive sacral chordomas. Plast Reconstr Surg 2000;105:1013–1016

21. Glatt BS, Disa JJ, Mehrara BJ, Pusic AL, Boland P, Cordeiro PG. Reconstruction of extensive partial or total sacrectomy defects with a transabdominal vertical rectus abdominis myocutaneous flap. Ann Plast Surg 2006;56:526–530, discussion 530–531

22. Choudry UH, Moran SL, Karacor Z. Functional reconstruction of the pelvic ring with simultaneous bilateral free fibular flaps following total sacral resection. Ann Plast Surg 2006;57:673–676

16

Complications and Their Avoidance: How to Plan Primary Tumor Resection to Minimize Complications and Maximize Outcome

Michael C. Oh, Vedat Deviren, and Christopher P. Ames

▦ Introduction

Although primary tumors of the spine are rare, their treatment requires some of the most demanding and complex surgical approaches and can result in significant morbidity and mortality.[1] The best chance of cure or minimization of recurrence often requires total en-bloc resection for malignant tumors, whereas some benign tumors may be amenable to intralesional piecemeal removal. Due to technical challenges required for wide-margin en-bloc resection with complex reconstruction, complication rates remain high. These complications include construct failure, alignment failure, pseudarthrosis, infection with or without skin dehiscence, spinal cord or nerve root injury, cerebrospinal fluid leak with pseudomeningocele, excessive bleeding requiring transfusions, large-vessel injury, and intraoperative contamination of malignant tumors. Large tumors may involve nearby nerve roots or dura, with planned and unplanned risk of neurologic deficits; wide-margin en-bloc resection for malignant primary tumors may require sacrifice of neural elements to achieve the best chance of recurrence-free cure.

Depending on the location of the tumor, different vital anatomic structures may be in-volved, including vertebral arteries, the trachea, esophagus, aorta, vena cava, iliac vessels, ureters, and parts of the distal gastrointestinal tract. Other common postoperative complications, such as deep venous thrombosis, pulmonary embolism, urinary tract infection, pneumonia, dysphagia, ileus, and myocardial infarction may be caused by prolonged immobility and extensive surgical resections with long operative times.

Because of the complexity involved in resecting primary spine tumors, careful preoperative planning is mandatory, which includes imaging, biopsy, and, perhaps most importantly, detailed patient counseling and shared decision making. Patients should be well informed of all potential complications, and discussions regarding the risks and benefits of the potential sacrifice of neural elements for the best chance of cure should be part of every preoperative counseling.

This chapter reviews the literature related to complications in surgical resection of primary spine tumors and discusses how best to plan primary spine tumor resection to minimize complications while maximizing outcome. We present several cases from our own experience with primary spine tumors to illustrate some of the more common complications as well as the importance of judicious preoperative planning.

Preoperative Planning and Imaging

Planning of primary spine tumor resection starts with a thorough imaging evaluation. Standing scoliosis X-rays should be utilized to assess the regional and global alignment. This is especially important for lumbar tumors, where the postoperative pelvic incidence (PI) should measure within 11 degrees of lumbar lordosis. The location of the individualized thoracic apex should be noted to ensure that thoracic instrumentation extends beyond the apex when planning thoracic resections. Cervicothoracic kyphosis should be noted when planning cervical resections as well. Because primary tumor patients treated with en-bloc resections often have long survival, conforming to deformity principles is important to optimize functionality and patient-reported satisfaction, and to prevent construct failure.

Computed tomography (CT) is used to evaluate the extent of bony invasions, but is also critical in evaluating the bone qualities of adjacent vertebral bodies for potential instrumentation. The number of involved vertebral levels should be carefully noted. Whether the tumor is confined to the vertebral body or extends into pedicles or laminas should be evaluated and graded by the Weinstein-Boriani-Biagini (WBB) surgical staging system.[2] For example, whether one or both pedicles are involved can change surgical planning, as the sequence and location of osteotomies for total en-bloc spondylectomy differ depending on the extent of tumor invasion into pedicles and posterior bony structures.[2,3] The delivery corridor for the specimen should be decided based on the size and location of the bulk of the mass and its adherence to surrounding structures such as viscera and major vessels.

Magnetic resonance imaging (MRI), specifically T1-weighted scans with gadolinium or T2-weighted scans, can provide additional in-formation regarding the extent of tumor invasion. Involvement of non-bony structures, such as the epidural space, neuroforamina, or paravertebral tissues, should be carefully evaluated.

Although routine preoperative angiograms are not necessary in most cases, selective arterial embolization may provide good outcomes in patients with aneurysmal bone cysts,[4] especially given the finding that surgery can result in 15 to 30% complication rates.[5] Preoperative angiograms in patients with large cervical tumors may be helpful in evaluating the patency of vertebral arteries (VAs).[6] Occlusion tests can also be performed to determine if it is safe to sacrifice the artery, and if sacrificing the VA will assist in tumor resection with wide margins. Coils should be placed distal and proximal to sites of intended VA ligation to prevent inadvertent coil removal and back bleeding at surgery. An example of such case is depicted in (**Fig. 16.1**). In this patient with giant cervical chordoma spanning four levels from C3 to C6, an angiogram was first performed to coil and sacrifice the right VA, which was encased by the tumor. This was followed by intraoperative ligation of the right VA during the first portion of the procedure via a posterior approach. Following posterior osteotomies and ligation of nerve roots, a Silastic sheet was placed between the dura and the posterior longitudinal ligament to provide an easier plane of dissection for the en-bloc removal of tumor from consequent anterior approach.

Preoperative Diagnosis and Biopsy

Proper surgical planning requires biopsy for pathological diagnosis. Although small asymptomatic benign tumors may be observed, symptomatic benign tumors may require surgery for decompression or stabilization.[2] For malignant tumors, a biopsy sheath should be used with the tract carefully noted and marked, as en-bloc resection requires resection of the biopsy tract for the best outcome. The study by Fourney and colleagues[7] suggested that surgery that was performed at the same center where the

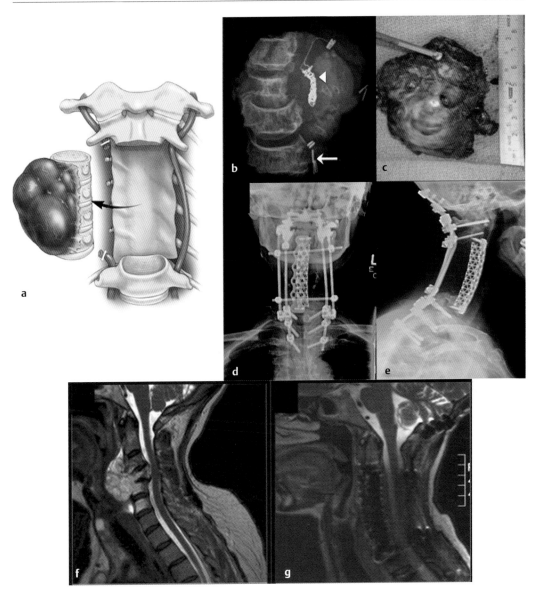

Fig. 16.1a–g A four-level en-bloc resection of a cervical chordoma in a 60-year-old woman who presented with severe neck pain. She was found to have a giant chordoma centered at C4 and expanding the anterior aspects of C3 thru C6, as shown by sagittal T2-weighted magnetic resonance imaging (MRI) **(f).** She underwent a four-level en-bloc resection by a two-stage approach, where the first approach consisted of posterior osteotomies, ligation of right vertebral artery, and placement of a Silastic sheet **(a)**. **(a–c)** This was followed by anterior en-bloc tumor resection. The patient also underwent preoperative coil embolization of the right vertebral artery (**b,** *arrowhead*) and intraoperative surgical clipping (**b,** *arrow*). The right C4 and C5 nerve roots were sacrificed. Stabilization consisted of occiput to T3 posterior spinal fusion and instrumentation with a C3-C6 anterior cage and plate **(d,e). (g)** Postoperative T2-weighted MRI showed good decompression of the spinal cord.

initial biopsy was done had better outcomes. Although not statistically significant, patients who received biopsy and surgery at the same referral center were 78% disease free at the final follow-up, whereas those whose biopsy was done at one center and who were then referred elsewhere for surgery were 55% disease free at final follow-up.[7] Consistent with these results, patients treated for sacral chordomas by biopsy and surgery at the same referral center had a 75% disease-free rate, whereas those initially treated elsewhere had a 42% disease-free rate. Although this finding was also not statistically significant, experts generally agree that biopsy and surgery should be performed at the same institution, preferably one with extensive experience.[1,7]

Following complete imaging and biopsy studies, a systematic surgical staging should be done to formulate consistent surgical planning. We recommend the use of the WBB surgical staging system[2] to help guide more consistent surgical planning and for systematic reporting of surgeries and the extent of tumor invasion.

▧ Surgical Nuances

Extent of Resection

Malignant primary spine tumors, such as chordomas, chondrosarcomas, osteosarcomas, and Ewing's sarcomas, require wide en-bloc resection with adherence to oncological principles for best outcomes.[1,2,8–10] For example, en-bloc resection with wide margins provides good long-term local control for 92.3% of giant cell tumors,[11] 78% of chordomas,[8] and 82% of chondrosarcomas.[9] By comparison, intralesional resection provides local control for 72.2% of giant cell tumors,[11] 22% of chordomas,[8] and 0% of chondrosarcomas.[9] Although it is clear that the best outcomes are provided by en-bloc resection, morbidity remains high, with an overall complication rate of 35.1% with 2.2% overall mortality.[1]

Certain benign tumors, namely giant cell tumors (GCTs) with Enneking stage III[2,11] or posteriorly located aneurysmal bone cysts,[4] also have been shown to have the best outcome

with en-bloc resection. One such patient in our experience was a 29-year-old man who was previously treated in a different country for a T12 GCT with laminectomy, partial anterior corpectomy, and anterior and posterior spinal instrumentation (**Fig. 16.2**). A recurrence of this tumor, just lateral to the anterior cage, was noted on follow-up MRI. We performed en-bloc spondylectomy via thoracotomy, which included the recurrent tumor as well as the anterior cage from the previous surgery as one piece.

Although complete spondylectomy for resection of primary spine tumors was initially described by Roy-Camille's group[12] and by Stener,[13] total en-bloc spondylectomy using a thread-wire saw was first developed by Tomita.[3,14] This technique has also been extended for treatment of metastatic tumors for selected patients. Development of these new surgical techniques and devices has enabled performing en-bloc spondylectomies in the spine. Furthermore, the use of a thread-wire saw has been shown to minimize tumor contamination during en-bloc resections.[14] Future development of new devices, such as the thread-wire saw guide and spinal cord protector device, may help reduce neurologic deficits and other major intraoperative complications involved with technically challenging total en-bloc spondylectomies.

Some total en-bloc spondylectomies require multidisciplinary approaches with multistaged operations (**Fig. 16.3**). In a 38-year-old woman with a giant chordoma spanning from T5 through T8, we performed a three-stage en-bloc resection with assistance from thoracic surgeons to dissect and mobilize the aorta and esophagus. The patient was first treated preoperatively with stereotactic radiosurgery with Cyberknife (2,500 cGy), followed by posterior decompression and osteotomies to release the posterior components. The second stage consisted of a left thoracotomy for dissection of the aorta off the tumor mass with anterior spinal osteotomies at T5 and T8-9. The final stage consisted of dissection and mobilization of the esophagus with en-bloc spondylectomy of T5-T8 and delivery of the tumor. The patient is currently recurrence-free 18 months after surgery and lives a very active life.

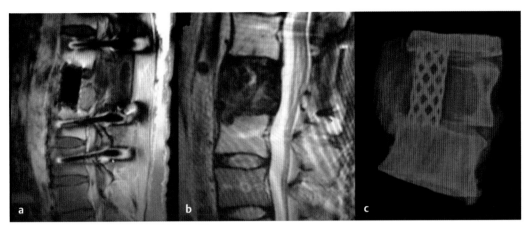

Fig. 16.2a–c En-bloc resection of a recurrent giant cell tumor with previous instrumentation in a 29-year-old man who was previously diagnosed with a T12 tumor and treated at another hospital with a laminectomy, partial anterior corpectomy, and anterior and posterior spinal fusion and instrumentation. Biopsy at the time confirmed giant cell tumor. **(a)** Preoperative MRI. **(b)** On follow-up MRI, recurrence was evident lateral to the anterior cage.

(c) Thus, we performed an en-bloc spondylectomy via a posterior osteotomy and then a thoracotomy with T10 rib resection, followed by T12 anterior spinal osteotomy, L2-L3 diskectomy, and en-bloc corpectomy of T12-L2. Careful planning allowed salvage of this patient with negative surgical margins. Finally, the spine was stabilized with cage reconstruction from T12 to L3 and anterior spinal fusion and instrumentation from T11 to L3.

Tumor Location

Decision making regarding the use of different approaches and multidisciplinary teams, which may include head and neck surgery, thoracic surgery, general surgery, and plastic surgery, are also determined by tumor location. Although the evaluation of tumor extension into surrounding structures is a critical step in preoperative planning, the tumor location (cervical, thoracic, lumbar, or sacral) presents inherent risks to different anatomic structures. Primary tumors of the cervical spine present risks to the VAs, esophagus, trachea, cervical nerve roots, and spinal cord. The aorta, esophagus, and vena cava are at risk in the thoracic spine during surgery. Late aortic dissection causing paraplegia and death has been reported following thoracic tumor surgery.[1] Lastly, surgery in the lumbar and sacral regions presents risks to the cauda equina, aorta, iliac vessels, ureters, and distal gastrointestinal tracts.

In one institutional series by Zileli and colleagues,[6] 66 surgeries were performed in 35 patients with primary tumors of the cervical spine. There were eight complications, both early and late, including graft extrusion, graft donor-site infection, instrument failure and revision, respiratory complication, diabetes insipidus of unknown etiology, postoperative epidural hematoma, seventh nerve palsy, and one postoperative death. Of note, there was one VA bleeding during tumor resection, which was repaired without complications.

Cloyd and colleagues[10] performed a systematic review of the literature to identify patients who underwent en-bloc resection for primary cervical spine tumors. Eight patients had complications. The most common complication was dysphagia. Other complications included pneumonia, respiratory distress, seizure, thrombotic event, and wound dehiscence. Of note, mean operative time, estimated blood loss, and length of stay were 18.6 hours (range, 4.3–56 hours), 2.9 L (range, 0.6–8.7 L), and 34.6 days (range, 16–54 days), respectively. From this study, one can conclude that en-bloc resection of cervical spinal tumors carries a high morbidity rate, and thus, patients should be carefully selected and should be well informed about the risks and

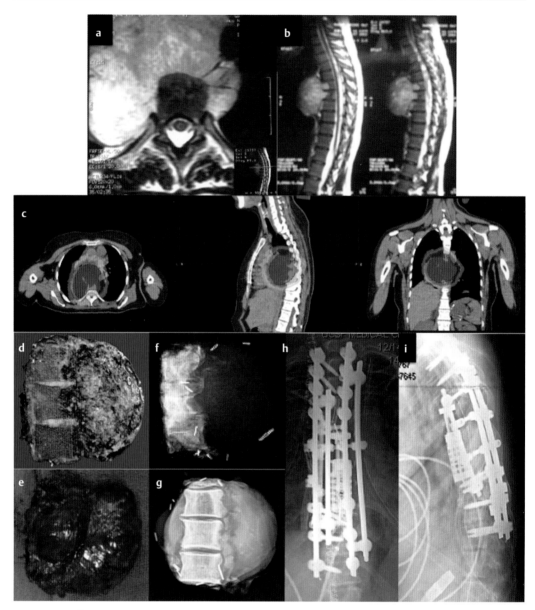

Fig 16.3a–i Three-stage en-bloc resection of giant thoracic chordoma with dissection and mobilization of the aorta and esophagus in a 38-year-old woman who presented with back pain. **(a,b)** She was found to have a giant chordoma spanning T5 to T8 as shown on T2-weighted MRIs. **(c)** She underwent stereotactic radiosurgery with Cyberknife (2,500 cGy), followed by a three-stage en-bloc resection. The first stage consisted of a posterior laminectomy of T5-T9, transpedicular osteotomies of T6-T8, rhizotomies of T6-T8, and rib resection at T6-T9. The second stage consisted of a left thoracotomy for dissection of the aorta off of the tumor mass, with anterior spinal osteotomies at T5 and T8-T9. **(d–i)** The final stage consisted of dissection of the esophagus off of the tumor with en-bloc spondylectomy of T5-T8 with delivery of tumor, cage reconstruction of T5-T9, and anterior spinal instrumentation of T5-T9. The patient tolerated the procedures without major complications and is fully ambulatory at last follow-up.

benefits of surgery. Moreover, due to vital anatomic structures in the cervical spine, wide en-bloc spondylectomies, although achievable, are often difficult in the cervical spine[6,10] (**Fig. 16.1**).

Another location that presents special challenges for the surgeon is the sacrum. Tumors in this region can often grow to very large proportions before becoming symptomatic. High sacrectomy leads to bowel and bladder incontinence, raising risks of infection, motor deficits (loss of plantar flexion), and sensory abnormalities. These complications were found to be dependent on the extent of spinal nerve resection and the level of the sacrectomy.[7,15–17] For example, preserving the S3 nerve root was the best indicator for preserving bowel and bladder function, as unilateral and bilateral S3 nerve root resection resulted in a 37.5% and 75% bowel and bladder incontinence rate, respectively.[16] However, for large tumors that extend above the S3 nerve root, intentional sacrifice of multiple nerve roots may be warranted, with high sacrectomies offering the best chance of recurrence-free cure. Bowel injury during surgery is also a potential major complication,[15] as is postoperative ileus. A diverting colostomy may be of benefit in reducing infection risk due to fecal contamination in total sacrectomy patients.

▨ Complications

Hardware Construct and Alignment Failure

In cases where the spinal column is destabilized, complex circumferential reconstruction with instrumentation is required to restore the three columns of the spine (anterior, middle, and posterior). Once thought to be best achieved by connecting anterior and posterior implants, advances in modern implants often do not require this connection. Autogenous bone grafts or bone substitutes should be used to help form solid fusions. Rib grafts may be placed adjacent to cages to facilitate primary fusion, and multiple rod constructs may also

help prevent rod fracture related to delayed union. Proper stabilization is crucial for early mobilization and timely recovery of muscle function, with the ability to bear weight and thus decrease pressure on the extensive wounds.

For primary sacral tumors, special reconstruction techniques are required following en-bloc sacrectomies to restore the continuity of the pelvic ring and to establish bilateral unions between the lumbar spine and iliac bones,[18] which are key steps in achieving mechanical support for early mobilization. Further studies are needed, however, to evaluate the biomechanics of the pelvic structures in more detail following sacrectomy. In one patient, we performed an en-bloc tumor resection for a giant sacral chordoma involving the lower sacrum below the inferior S2 segment (**Fig. 16.4**). This 65-year-old man underwent a high sacrectomy below S1 without instrumentation. On follow-up pelvic X-ray and CT scans, he was found to have a midsacral fracture and pelvic open-book fracture with destruction of the anterior rami of the bilateral pelvis. Although previous studies have indicated that sacrectomies below the S1 nerve root do not require instrumented reconstruction for early mobilization,[19] this case exemplifies the need for further evaluation of pelvic biomechanics following sacrectomy.

Construct failure, whether early or late, can entail pseudarthrosis, rod fracture, or malposition or migration of the construct. **Fig. 16.5** illustrates a case of construct failure due to pseudoarthrosis and rod fractures following recurrent thoracic chondrosarcoma resection 5 years after en-bloc index surgery. Following en-bloc resection of a T3-T4 chondrosarcoma, the patient developed pseudarthrosis and rod fractures, resulting in severe kyphosis with dorsal migration of the cage into the spinal canal. This required reoperation to reposition the cage, with extension of the previous fusion across the cervicothoracic junction.

In one study by Boriani's group,[1] among 134 patients who underwent en-bloc resection of primary spine tumors, 11 patients had hardware failure or loosening, three with deformity, and one with a malpositioned anterior

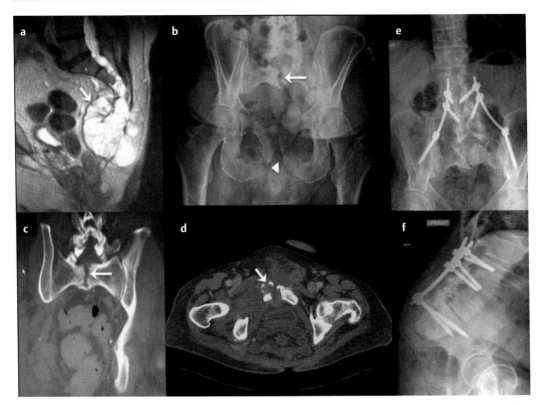

Fig 16.4a–f Sacral and pelvic open-book fractures following a high, but not complete, sacrectomy in a 65-year-old man who presented with sacral and leg pain. **(a)** He was found to have a giant sacral chordoma (*arrow*) involving the lower sacrum up to the inferior S2 segment. Patient underwent high sacrectomy for en-bloc tumor resection. Although S1 was left intact, a follow-up pelvic X-ray **(b)** and CT scans **(c)** revealed a midsacral fracture (*arrow*) and a pelvic open-book fracture (**d**, *arrow*) with pelvis destruction of the bilateral anterior rami. **(e,f)** This patient was later instrumented at another hospital.

cage during surgery that required reoperation. Although reoperation was mostly due to tumor recurrence, hardware failures also contributed significantly to the number of reoperations. In another report, there were eight reported complications from 66 operations for cervical primary spine tumors.[6] Two of the eight complications (25%) were hardware-related (graft extrusion, and instrument failure and revision). Although malposition of the construct during surgery is rare, continued follow-up with X-rays is crucial because, over time, some patients develop pseudarthrosis, hardware failure or loosening, migration of hardware, or deformity.

Because large tumor resection from the spine inevitably destabilizes the spine, it is important to restore both sagittal and coronal balance when reconstructing the spine following resection. The same principles used in deformity surgery apply here. We recommend pre- and postoperative standing scoliosis X-rays to evaluate the patient's global spinal balance. Global alignment can fail following primary spine tumor resection due to infection, pseudarthrosis, and hardware failure, and may require revision with extension of fusion to additional levels (**Fig. 16.6**). One patient who underwent en-bloc resection of an L3-L4 chondrosarcoma did well initially, but then started developing severe low back pain with sagittal and coronal imbalance and a forward tilt. A CT scan was suspicious for deep infection centered at the L4-L5 disk space, with pseudarthrosis and lucency around the allograft. The

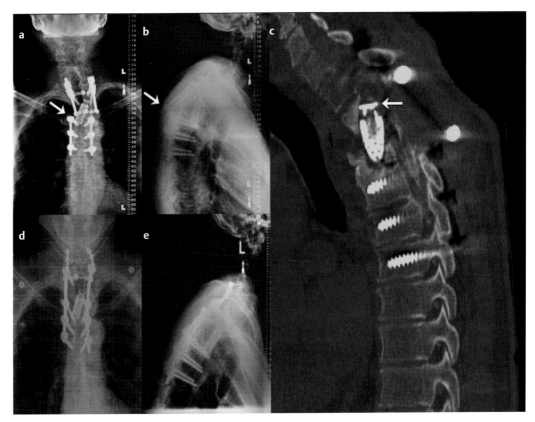

Fig 16.5a–e Construct failure due to pseudarthrosis and rod fractures following recurrent thoracic chondrosarcoma resection 5 years after *en-bloc* index surgery. This is a 57-year-old man with a history of a T3-T4 chondrosarcoma previously resected via a transpedicular T3-T4 corpectomy with anterior cage reconstruction and a T1-T7 posterior spinal fusion and instrumentation. Although this patient did well initially, he later presented with increasing bilateral leg pain and weakness. Workup with X-ray **(a,b)** and CT **(c)** showed pseudarthrosis at T2-T3 **(a,b,** *arrows*) and rod fractures **(c,** *arrow*). This resulted in severe kyphosis with dorsal migration of the cage into the spinal canal. The patient was returned to the operating room for a transpedicular corpectomy of T2 with repositioning of the cage. **(d,e)** Posterior spinal instrumentation was extended up to C5. At the final follow-up, his symptoms improved with a stable construct.

patient was reoperated with extension of the posterior spinal fusion and instrumentation down to the pelvis with restoration of coronal and sagittal balance. Cultures later turned positive for *Pseudomonas aeruginosa*. Revisions near the cervicothoracic and thoracolumbar junctions may require fusion across these segments, when alignment fails due to complications (**Fig. 16.5**). We have also found that four-rod posterior reconstruction following total spondylectomy provides a more solid construct with less potential for failure (**Figs. 16.3** and **16.7**).

Wound Infection

Because of long operative times with complex reconstruction involved, infection rates remain high, often requiring reoperation for wound washout or revision of instrumentation (**Fig. 16.6**). Dead space closure with muscle flaps or via paraspinal mobilization is critical in preventing seroma formation, which presents a high risk of delayed infection. Nonresorbable sutures should be used for fascial closures in high-risk wounds, at the cervicothoracic junction, and in previously radiated areas. One such

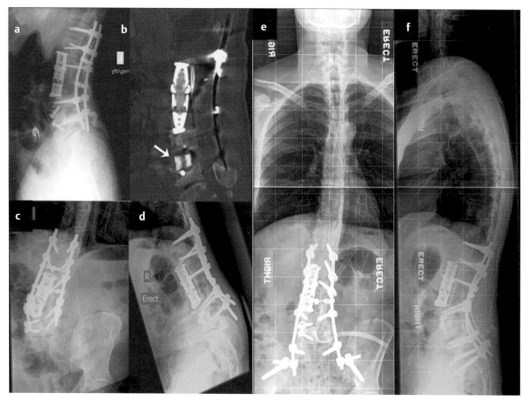

Fig. 16.6a–f Alignment failure with sagittal imbalance following en-bloc resection of an L3-L4 chondrosarcoma in a 48-year-old man. **(a,b)** Anterior cage reconstruction and L1-L5 posterior spinal fusion and instrumentation. **(c,d)** He did well initially but then started developing severe low back pain with sagittal and coronal imbalance and a forward tilt. CT scan was suspicious for deep infection centered at the L4 (**b**, *arrow*) to L5 disk space with pseudarthrosis and lucency around the allograft. **(e,f)** Patient was reoperated with extension of the posterior spinal fusion and instrumentation down to the pelvis with restoration of coronal and sagittal balance via Smith-Peterson osteotomies at L4-L5 and L5-S1. The infected L4-L5 disk space was curetted and then packed with autograft from the iliac crest. Cultures later returned positive for *Pseudomonas aeruginosa*.

case is a 76-year-old man who underwent an en-bloc tumor resection and reconstruction for a C2 chordoma performed from a transmandibular-transglossal approach (**Fig. 16.8**). Following surgery, the patient underwent proton beam therapy. Two months later, he presented with purulent, open drainage from his pharyngeal wound with an exposed anterior cage through the pharyngeal wound. This patient eventually required reoperation with a fat graft with free flap closure and long-term antibiotic therapy. When attempting to prevent postoperative pharyngeal erosion or wound infections after proton beam therapy, a retropha-

ryngeal approach, autograft rather than metal implants, and soft tissue flaps have all be employed. Despite these measures, high anterior cervical reconstructions have high complication rates.

In one seminal study by Boriani's group[1] looking at morbidity associated with en-bloc resections of primary spine tumors, the deep infection rate was found to be 5.4%, and surgical debridement and long-term multiple antibiotics were required. The rate of deep infection was higher (9.8%) in patients previously treated with radiation therapy. Overall, primary bone tumors of the spine carry a higher incidence

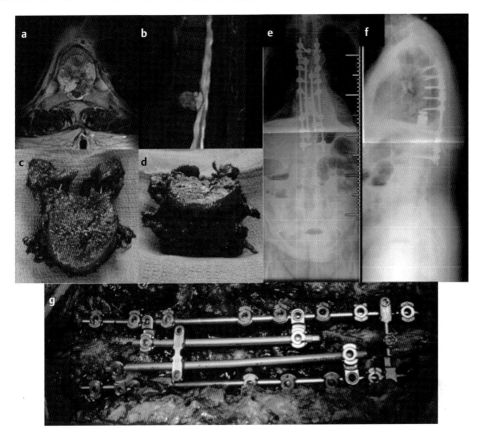

Fig 16.7a–g Supplementation of posterior spinal instrumentation with a four-rod system for increased stabilization in a 78-year-old woman who presented with severe back pain. **(a,b)** She was found to have a hyperintense lesion at T10 on T2-weighted MRI, consistent with chordoma. She underwent a total en-bloc spondylectomy of T10 **(c,d)**, followed by anterior cage reconstruction and a four-rod posterior spinal fusion construct **(e–g)**. She tolerated the procedure without significant complications and remained neurologically intact.

of surgical-site infection compared with other spine tumor surgeries. The infection rate for primary bony spinal tumors was reported to be 13.7%, whereas primary non-bony and metastatic spinal tumors carried an incidence of surgical-site infection of 8.9% and 9.5%, respectively.[20] *Staphylococcus aureus* was the most common organism, found in a third of all surgical-site infections. Major risk factors for infection following spinal tumor surgery were previous spinal surgeries, complex plastic closures, increasing number of comorbidities, presence of a hospital-acquired infection at the time of a previous surgery, previous radiation therapy, and longer hospital stay.[20] In general, combined anterior/posterior approaches, which are commonly required for primary spinal tumor surgeries, age greater than 60 years, smoking, diabetes, previous surgical infection, increased body mass index, and alcohol abuse are all predisposing risk factors for infection following spine surgery.

Postsurgical infection and wound dehiscence following sacrectomy warrant a special review because wound infection rates are especially high given the vicinity close to the large bowel, with increased incidence of bowel incontinence following sacrectomy. One such case was a 52-year-old woman who underwent en-bloc sacrectomy with reconstruction for sacral chondrosarcoma (**Fig. 16.9**). She presented 4 months later with a 3 cm × 1 cm wound dehiscence and

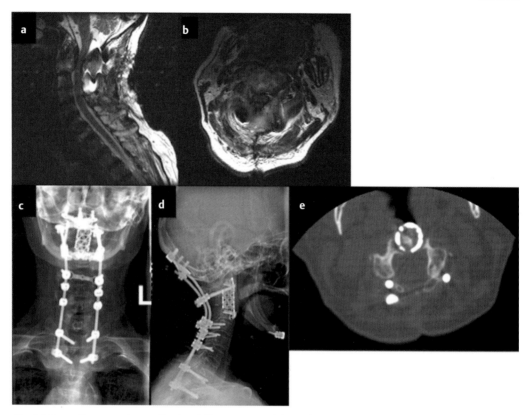

Fig. 16.8a–e Pharyngeal complication following en-bloc tumor resection and reconstruction for C2 chordoma performed from a transmandibular-transglossal approach in a 76-year-old man who presented with severe neck pain, and who underwent a posterior laminectomy and instrumentation with a biopsy confirming a chordoma at another hospital. Patient then started developing leg paresthesia 10 days after his initial surgery. **(a,b)** MRI showed collapse of the C2 vertebral body with retropulsion into spinal canal. Once he was transferred to our hospital, he underwent posterior removal of hardware, exposure and mobilization of bilateral vertebral arteries at C2, osteotomy of C2 pedicles, and occiput to T2 posterior spinal fusion and instrumentation, followed by a pharyngeal en-bloc C2 tumor resection with anterior cage reconstruction via a transmandibular-transglossal approach **(c,d)**. Following surgery, patient underwent proton beam therapy. **(e)** Two months later, he presented with purulent open drainage from his pharyngeal wound. There was an open wound with exposure of the anterior cage in the back of the throat, which required reoperation with fat graft and free flap closure.

Fig. 16.9a–k (*opposite*) Wound infection following en bloc sacrectomy for chondrosarcoma. **(a–e)** This is a 52-year-old woman who underwent en bloc sacrectomy with reconstruction for sacral chondrosarcoma, who presented 4 months following surgery with 3x1cm wound dehiscence and purulent drainage. **(a, b)** Preoperative T2-weighted MRI shows tumor infiltration throughout the sacrum as well as **(c)** paravertebral soft tissue dorsally and off midline. **(d,e)** She underwent instrumentation following sacrectomy. **(f, g)** T1-weighted MRI with gadolinium shows enhancing fluid collection, **(f, g** *arrows***)**, which was also noted on CT **(h** *arrow***)**. She required wound washout with removal of hardware, rotational flap closure, and long-term antibiotic therapy. Culture was positive for vancomycin-resistant enterococcus. **(h, i)** CT scans prior to hardware removal and **(j, k)** after hardware removal are shown. Despite removal of hardware, patient was able to walk 10 weeks following her initial surgery after prolonged recumbancy.

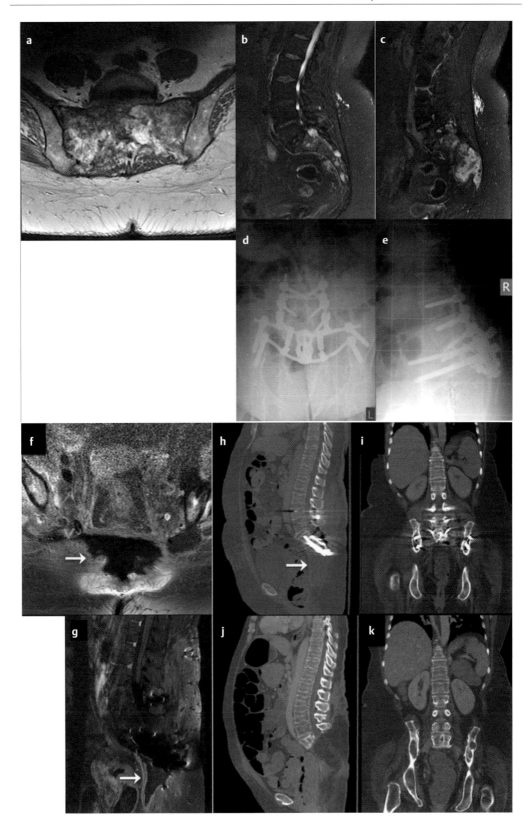

purulent drainage, which required a wound washout with removal of hardware, rotational flap closure, and long-term antibiotic therapy. Culture was positive for vancomycin-resistant enterococcus. Despite removal of all hardware, the patient was fully ambulatory at 8 months following her initial surgery.

Infection rates as high as 25 to 44% following sacrectomies have been reported.[15,17] Infection risks are increased with bowel incontinence,[16] greater extent of resection (i.e., high sacrectomies),[16,17] and long surgery time.[17] The most frequent organisms were *Enterococcus* (23%), *Escherichia coli* (20%), and *Pseudomonas aeruginosa* (18%), and approximately three out of four patients had multimicrobial infections.[17] Although infections can be treated with surgical debridements and long-term antibiotic therapy, almost half of patients require multiple surgical debridements: 52.2% of patients were treated with one surgical debridement, whereas 34.8% and 13.0% of patients required two and three surgical debridements, respectively.[17] Moreover, infections can lengthen the hospital stay, delay healing, and cause pseudarthrosis with hardware failure (**Fig. 16.6**). Long-term wound follow-up is recommended, given that 30% of wound infections occur 4 weeks to 6 months after the sacrectomy[17]; the remaining 70% of infections occurred within 4 weeks of surgery. The prolonged use of negative pressure drains and especially intrawound vancomycin powder, which has shown significant benefit in other areas of spinal surgery, should be strongly considered.

◼ Chapter Summary

Careful preoperative surgical planning and prudent patient selection are absolute requirements for minimizing complications and maximizing outcomes of primary spine tumor surgery. This planning starts with a thorough imaging evaluation followed by a biopsy for pathological diagnosis of the tumor. Although malignant tumors may require en-bloc resection with wide margins for the best outcome, benign tumors may be amenable to intralesional piecemeal removal. However, the morbidity of en-bloc resection should always be weighed against potential neurologic deficits and other major complications involved with extensive wide margin resection. Some surgeries may require multidisciplinary approaches with surgeries at large referral centers with extensive experience for the best outcome.

Pearls

- ◆ Understand the difference between wide-margin en-bloc resection and intralesional piecemeal resection and when each should be utilized.
- ◆ Utilize different imaging techniques (i.e., standing scoliosis X-rays, CT, and MRI) for thorough preoperative evaluation.
- ◆ Proper surgical planning requires biopsy for pathological diagnosis.
- ◆ Understand the different potential complications related to tumor location.
- ◆ Understand the different instrumentation techniques to prevent hardware failure, alignment failure, and pseudarthrosis.

Pitfalls

- ◆ Wide-margin en-bloc resection requires the same principles of deformity surgery to provide solid stabilization with preservation or restoration of global and local spinal balances.
- ◆ Complications such as hardware failure, wound infection with dehiscence, and tumor recurrence may be delayed, requiring long-term follow-up with serial imaging.

References
Five Must-Read References

1. Boriani S, Bandiera S, Donthineni R, et al. Morbidity of en bloc resections in the spine. Eur Spine J 2010;19:231–241

2. Boriani S, Weinstein JN, Biagini R. Primary bone tumors of the spine. Terminology and surgical staging. Spine 1997;22:1036–1044

3. Tomita K, Kawahara N, Baba H, Tsuchiya H, Fujita T, Toribatake Y. Total en bloc spondylectomy. A new surgical technique for primary malignant vertebral tumors. Spine 1997;22:324–333

4. Boriani S, De Iure F, Campanacci L, et al. Aneurysmal bone cyst of the mobile spine: report on 41 cases. Spine 2001;26:27–35

5. Papagelopoulos PJ, Currier BL, Shaughnessy WJ, et al. Aneurysmal bone cyst of the spine. Management and outcome. Spine 1998;23:621–628

6. Zileli M, Kilinçer C, Ersahin Y, Cagli S. Primary tumors of the cervical spine: a retrospective review of 35 surgically managed cases. Spine J 2007;7:165–173

7. Fourney DR, Rhines LD, Hentschel SJ, et al. En bloc resection of primary sacral tumors: classification of surgical approaches and outcome. J Neurosurg Spine 2005;3:111–122

8. Boriani S, Bandiera S, Biagini R, et al. Chordoma of the mobile spine: fifty years of experience. Spine 2006; 31:493–503

9. Boriani S, De Iure F, Bandiera S, et al. Chondrosarcoma of the mobile spine: report on 22 cases. Spine 2000;25:804–812

10. Cloyd JM, Chou D, Deviren V, Ames CP. En bloc resection of primary tumors of the cervical spine: report of two cases and systematic review of the literature. Spine J 2009;9:928–935

11. Boriani S, Bandiera S, Casadei R, et al. Giant cell tumor of the mobile spine: a review of 49 cases. Spine 2012;37:E37–E45

12. Roy-Camille R, Saillant G, Bisserié M, Judet T, Hautefort E, Mamoudy P. [Total excision of thoracic verte-brae (author's transl)]. Rev Chir Orthop Repar Appar Mot 1981;67:421–430

13. Stener B. Total spondylectomy in chondrosarcoma arising from the seventh thoracic vertebra. J Bone Joint Surg Br 1971;53:288–295

14. Tomita K, Kawahara N, Baba H, Tsuchiya H, Nagata S, Toribatake Y. Total en bloc spondylectomy for solitary spinal metastases. Int Orthop 1994;18:291–298

15. Clarke MJ, Dasenbrock H, Bydon A, et al. Posterior-only approach for en bloc sacrectomy: clinical outcomes in 36 consecutive patients. Neurosurgery 2012; 71:357–364, discussion 364

16. Guo Y, Palmer JL, Shen L, et al. Bowel and bladder continence, wound healing, and functional outcomes in patients who underwent sacrectomy. J Neurosurg Spine 2005;3:106–110

17. Ruggieri P, Angelini A, Pala E, Mercuri M. Infections in surgery of primary tumors of the sacrum. Spine 2012;37:420–428

18. Jackson RJ, Gokaslan ZL. Spinal-pelvic fixation in patients with lumbosacral neoplasms. J Neurosurg 2000;92(1, Suppl):61–70

19. Hugate RR Jr, Dickey ID, Phimolsarnti R, Yaszemski MJ, Sim FH. Mechanical effects of partial sacrectomy: when is reconstruction necessary? Clin Orthop Relat Res 2006;450:82–88

20. Omeis IA, Dhir M, Sciubba DM, et al. Postoperative surgical site infections in patients undergoing spinal tumor surgery: incidence and risk factors. Spine 2011; 36):1410–1419

Index

Page numbers followed by *f* or *t* indicate figures and tables, respectively.